BREAST LUMPS: Find o...
lighting a cigarette can help...
by the breast lumps and cys...
cycles. For more tips, turn to p. 149

ADULT ACNE: Have you discovered the hard way that acne isn't just for teenagers? If so, turn to page 24 to learn the simple things you can do to minimize outbreaks—and find out why having acne in your twenties and thirties may mean your skin isn't aging as quickly as you are.

TENSION HEADACHES: An extremely common ailment, tension headaches can make sufferers feel miserable. Turn to page 389 to find out which herbal remedies can help ease the pain by increasing circulation and boosting serotonin levels in the brain.

HEART DISEASE: Onions, oranges, and a few lifestyle changes can simply and effectively protect your heart for years to come. Check out some of these life-saving remedies on p. 411

VISION: Cataracts catch up with everyone as they age. But you can lower your risk fivefold by adding something delicious to your diet—and discovering what popular prescription medication is most likely to rob you of a clear view in the future. Turn to page 175.

GALLSTONES: Believe it or not, you can help stop painful bladder disease with a side order of . . . tuna salad! To learn more about the main course of an antigallstone program, turn to page 348.

HIGH BLOOD PRESSURE: One out of four Americans suffers from high blood pressure, tripling the risk of heart disease and stroke. Yes, diet is important and the right supplements are essential—but becoming aware of something that may be going on while you sleep might literally save your life. Turn to page 445.

THE DOCTORS BOOK
OF
HOME
REMEDIES
FOR Preventing Disease

2,000 Ways to Help Fight Disease and
Prevent Illness . . . with Treatments that
Can Be Found Right in Your Own Home

Edited by Hugh O'Neill

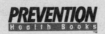

BANTAM BOOKS
New York   Toronto   London   Sydney   Auckland

This edition contains the complete text
of the original hardcover edition.
NOT ONE WORD HAS BEEN OMITTED.

THE DOCTORS BOOK OF HOME REMEDIES FOR
PREVENTING DISEASE

A Bantam Book / published by arrangement with Rodale Press, Inc.

PUBLISHING HISTORY

Rodale Press edition published 1998
Bantam paperback edition / July 2000

Prevention Health Books is a trademark; *Prevention* and *The Doctors Book*
and *The Doctors Book of Home Remedies* are registered trademarks of Rodale
Press, Inc.

Directions for putting on a condom on page 42 were adapted and reprinted
from *A Physician Guide to HIV Prevention*, American Medical Association,
June 1996. Copyright © 1996 by the American Medical Association.
Reprinted with permission.

ISBN: 0-553-58233-X

Published simultaneously in the United States and Canada

Bantam Books are published by Bantam Books, a division of Random
House, Inc. Its trademark, consisting of the words "Bantam Books"
and the portrayal of a rooster, is Registered in U.S. Patent and
Trademark Office and in other countries. Marca Registrada. Bantam
Books, 1540 Broadway, New York, New York 10036.

PRINTED IN THE UNITED STATES OF AMERICA

OPM   10   9   8   7   6   5   4   3   2

ABOUT *PREVENTION* HEALTH BOOKS

The editors of *Prevention* Health Books are dedicated to providing you with authoritative, trustworthy, and innovative advice for a healthy active lifestyle. In all our books, our goal is to keep you thoroughly informed about the latest breakthroughs in natural healing, medical research, alternative health, herbs, nutrition, fitness, and weight loss. We cut through the confusion of today's conflicting health reports to deliver clear, concise, and definitive health information that you can trust. And we explain in practical terms what each new breakthrough means to you, so you can take immediate, practical steps to improve your health and well-being.

Every recommendation in *Prevention* Health Books is based upon interviews with highly qualified health authorities, including medical doctors and practitioners of alternative medicine. In addition, we consult with the *Prevention* Health Books Board of Advisors to assure that all the health information is safe, practical, and up-to-date. *Prevention* Health Books are thoroughly fact-checked for accuracy, and we make every effort to verify recommendations, dosages, and cautions.

The advice in this book will help keep you well-informed about your personal choices in health care—to help you lead a happier, healthier, and longer life.

NOTICE

This book is intended as a reference volume only, not as a medical manual. The information given here is designed to help you make informed decisions about your health. It is not intended as a substitute for any treatment that may have been prescribed by your doctor. If you suspect that you have a medical problem, we urge you to seek competent medical help.

THE DOCTORS BOOK OF HOME REMEDIES FOR PREVENTING DISEASE

EDITORIAL STAFF

SENIOR MANAGING EDITOR: Edward Claflin

SENIOR EDITOR: Hugh O'Neill

RECIPE EDITOR: David Joachim

CONTRIBUTING EDITOR: Sheree Crute

WRITERS: Bill Gottlieb, with Doug Dollemore, Julie A. Evans, Kelly Garrett, Sid Kirchheimer, Gale Maleskey, Bonnie Trachtenberg, Margo Trott

CONTRIBUTING WRITERS: Pamela Boyer, Mary Nagle, Steve Schwade, Therese Walsh, Yun Lee Wolfe

ASSISTANT RESEARCH MANAGER: Jane Unger Hahn

LEAD RESEARCHER: Kathryn Piff

EDITORIAL RESEARCHERS: Jennifer Abel, Elizabeth Brown, Leah B. Flickinger, Grete Haentjens, Lois Guarino Hazel, Mary Kittel, Mary S. Mesaros, Paula Rasich, Staci Sander, Lorna S. Sapp, Lucille Uhlman, Nancy Zelko, Shea Zukowski

SENIOR COPY EDITORS: Amy K. Kovalski, Karen Neely

ART DIRECTOR: Darlene Schneck

COVER AND INTERIOR DESIGNER: Richard Kershner

LAYOUT DESIGNER: Faith Hague

MANUFACTURING COORDINATORS: Brenda Miller, Jodi
  Schaffer, Patrick T. Smith
OFFICE MANAGER: Roberta Mulliner
OFFICE STAFF: Julie Kehs, Suzanne Lynch, Mary Lou
  Stephen

pharmacy and chairman of the department of clinical pharmacy at West Virginia University in Morgantown

WILLIAM J. KELLER, PH.D., Professor and chairman of the department of pharmaceutical sciences in the School of Pharmacy at Samford University in Birmingham, Alabama

ROBERT D. KERNS, PH.D., Associate professor of psychiatry, neurology, and psychology at Yale University and chief of the psychology service and director of the comprehensive pain management center at the Veterans Administration Connecticut Health Care System in West Haven

CHARLES P. KIMMELMAN, M.D., Professor of otolaryngology at Cornell Medical School and attending physician at Manhattan Eye, Ear, and Throat Hospital, both in New York City

JEFFREY R. LISSE, M.D., Professor of medicine and director of the division of rheumatology at the University of Texas Medical Branch at Galveston

SUSAN OLSON, PH.D., Clinical psychologist, transition therapist, and weight-management consultant in private practice in Seattle

DAVID P. ROSE, M.D., D.SC., PH.D., Chief of the division of nutrition and endocrinology at Naylor Dana Institute, part of the American Health Foundation in Valhalla, New York, and an expert on nutrition and cancer for the National Cancer Institute and the American Cancer Society

MARIA A. FIATARONE SINGH, M.D., Associate professor at Tufts University School of Nutrition and Science Policy in Medford, Massachusetts, professor of exercise and sports science and medicine at the School of Health Sciences at the University of Sydney in Australia, and a scientist in the nutrition, exercise physiology, and sarcopenia laboratory at the Jean Mayer

USDA Human Nutrition Research Center on Aging at Tufts University in Boston

YVONNE S. THORNTON, M.D., Associate clinical professor of obstetrics and gynecology at Columbia University College of Physicians and Surgeons in New York City and director of the Perinatal Diagnostic Testing Center at Morristown Memorial Hospital in New Jersey

LILA AMDURSKA WALLIS, M.D., M.A.C.P., Clinical professor of medicine at Cornell University Medical College in New York City, past president of the American Medical Women's Association, founding president of the National Council on Women's Health, director of continuing medical education programs for physicians, and Master and Laureate of the American College of Physicians

ANDREW T. WEIL, M.D., Clinical professor of internal medicine at the University of Arizona in Tucson and director of the program in integrative medicine of the College of Medicine

DOUGLAS WHITEHEAD, M.D., Associate clinical professor of urology at Albert Einstein College of Medicine, associate attending physician in urology at Beth Israel Medical Center in New York City, and co-founder and director of the Association for Male Sexual Dysfunction in New York City

RICHARD J. WOOD, PH.D., Associate professor at Tufts University School of Nutrition and Science Policy in Medford, Massachusetts, and laboratory chief of the mineral bioavailability laboratory at the Jean Mayer USDA Human Nutrition Research Center on Aging at Tufts University in Boston

SUSAN ZELITCH YANOVSKI, M.D., Director of the obesity and eating disorders program in the division of digestive diseases and nutrition at the National Institute of Diabetes and Digestive and Kidney Diseases in Bethesda, Maryland

CONTENTS

INTRODUCTION
Your Health's Best Friend Is You

"What a piece of work is man," said Hamlet.

That line from Shakespeare says it all. When everything's working right, a human being is indeed an impressive creature, a dynamic balance of breathing, bones, and brain waves, of hormones and heartbeats. And this book is meant to help you keep that impressive piece of work in the best possible working order.

Some years ago, *Prevention* Health Books published the original *Doctors Book of Home Remedies*, which went on to sell over 13 million copies in 20 languages. Why was that book so popular? Many reasons. It brought advice from hundreds of leading medical experts into our kitchens and living rooms. And all of the tips were simple things that you could try at home. No prescriptions required. No high-tech tests. No surgical interventions. The advice was plain as day, suggestions you may give your mom if she had a stomachache or your brother if he couldn't sleep. *The Doctors Book of Home Remedies* harvested the experience of our best medical people, translated their advice into regular talk, and empowered people to heal themselves.

Today, that empowerment has grown into a dramatic trend in health care. We are taking responsibility for our health, trying to eat right, exercise, and do everything we can to be strong and stay well. *The Doctors Book of Home Remedies for Preventing Disease* is the next step, a complete book of easy strategies to help you thrive.

As we did for *The Doctors Book of Home Remedies,* the writers and editors of *Prevention* Health Books have gone to the best sources of information to uncover top-level, practical health advice. Our sources include hundreds of doctors, researchers, and leading experts. But this time, instead of asking for cures and remedies, we tried a more probing question: How can we prevent health problems from happening in the first place?

All the answers are here. How black tea can cut the risk of stroke. How bananas minimize muscle cramps. How tuna can inhibit the growth of gallstones. You will learn about stretches that can deter bursitis and how vacuuming can short-circuit postnasal drip. Deep-breathing techniques that can prevent high blood pressure, tai chi moves that can help prevent psoriasis, and yoga positions that discourage sciatica. Or how about an herb that can prevent dry mouth, a spice that prevents motion sickness, or a shampoo that will prevent oily hair? These are just a few of the secrets that doctors and experts gave us—just because we asked. In the pages that follow, you will find hundreds more, along with entire recipes that were tested in the *Prevention* kitchen to help stop problems before they start.

With these invigorating actions to better your health, you don't need to wait for unwanted health problems to suddenly ambush you. You will discover the myriad benefits of small but important actions. The lesson is simple: If we give our bodies at least as much tender loving care as we give our cars and homes, we will get better mileage through life and better shelter from the storms.

To be sure, illness isn't fair. It can strike despite heroic health regimens. But the advice in this book will keep the surprise attacks to a minimum. If you take advantage of our doctors' wisdom, you will have less of the bad stuff—aches and pains, fatigue, infections, hospital bills, and dark nights. And you will get far more of the good stuff—energy, vitality, and years to enjoy with the people you love. Good health itself is an ample reward—and if you take this book to heart, you have a good chance of enjoying the best of your own good health for many years to come.

Hugh O'Neill
Senior Editor
Prevention Health Books

ACCIDENTS
They Will Happen, But Don't Have To

Playground equipment. Golf carts. Baby walkers. Bicycles. Those are just a few of the sly instruments of destruction that can injure and maim. And the list goes on. The tools in the shed. The utensils in the drawer. Even the houseplant hanging in the corner. Truly, almost anything can cause an injury.

In the wrong hands, the innocent item can become dangerous with shocking speed, and often, those wrong hands are children's.

Accidents result in 70,000 deaths and 147 million documented injuries every year in the United States. According to the National Safety Council, unintentional injury deaths are exceeded only by heart disease, cancer, stroke, and chronic obstructive pulmonary disease. In fact, among people under the age of 45, unintentional injuries are the leading cause of death. To read the statistics, you would think that we were just tripping over ourselves to fall into trouble.

The good news is that the National Safety Council says that accidents are nearly always preventable. In fact, accidents are so preventable that many injury prevention specialists don't even think that they should be called accidents. Instead, they prefer to refer to accidents as unintentional injuries.

"We try not to use the word *accident*," says Sharon Thorson, injury prevention specialist and coordinator of the Brain Injury Prevention Program for the Colorado Department of Public Health and Environment in Denver. "That lets people off the hook." What people call accidents are often preventable, she points out. "If a child falls down the stairs, that's not an accident. Somebody should have put something across the stairs that would have prevented the child from falling down."

But despite many precautions, accidents do happen to children, causing as many as 10,500 fatalities and 693,075 injuries to children each year in the United States.

Riding in the Right Style

Parents often hear how important it is for children to use car safety seats, and some hospitals don't even let you leave the premises unless the baby is properly buckled up. A government survey found that placing your child in a safety seat reduces the likelihood of injury by an estimated 69 percent for infants and 47 percent for toddlers. Too often, however, safety seats and booster seats aren't installed correctly, and that puts kids at risk. Here is some advice from car safety experts.

PLEASE BE SEATED . . . PROPERLY. According to the U.S. Department of Transportation, it is essential to use a rear-facing car safety seat for infants up to about 20 pounds and up to one year old. Children over 20 pounds and at least one year old should ride in a car seat that faces the front of the car, van, or truck. Older kids over 40 pounds should ride in a booster seat until the car's lap and shoulder belts fit properly.

And it is essential to make sure that the car seat is installed properly, says Thorson. "In a national study, 85 percent of the car seats that were checked were not correctly attached—that's a lot of potential tragedies."

The problem? "Manufacturers provide good instructions, but some people buy used car seats or get hand-me-downs and don't know how to put the seat in the car," Thorson says. She suggests visiting trained emergency medical technicians or paramedics to check if your seat is properly installed.

BACK AND CENTER. "The child goes in the backseat, never in the front," says Thorson. "The front seat is just too dangerous because of the airbag." In back, the safest position is in the center, adds Janice Yuwiler, director of the California Center for Childhood Injury Prevention at San Diego State University. "There is more cushioning and more car around the child." If you are using a booster seat that requires a lap-shoulder belt, however, and you drive an older model car that doesn't have one, your child may be safer in the front, she says.

According to the U.S. Department of Transportation, only children that are over 12 years of age should be permitted to sit in the front seat.

LOCK 'EM UP. When you install the seat, make sure that you use the special locking clip when it is required for your car, cautions Yuwiler. In some cars, the movement of the belt is unrestricted, so the belt moves freely through the latch. That is why children's safety seats come with a locking clip and instructions for using it. "The locking clip stops the belt from moving," says Yuwiler.

TIGHTEN THE CINCH AND SPARE THE CHILD. The

harness that goes over the child's shoulders should be snug. "There should be no more than two fingers' width of space between the child's chest and the harness," says Yuwiler.

BOOST THEM WHEN THEY ARE OLDER. When children pass the 40-pound mark, they should be moved into a booster seat in the backseat of the vehicle that has been installed following the manufacturer's instructions, says Heather Paul, Ph.D., executive director of the National SAFE KIDS Campaign in Washington, D.C. In fact, this precaution is just as essential as a safety seat for toddlers. In terms of risk, "not using a booster seat puts a five-year-old at a bigger risk than leaving that child on the street corner at night by himself," she says.

Keep using the booster seat until the child weighs about 80 pounds, she advises. "A booster seat allows a child to be better positioned in the belt system; it 'boosts' a child's ability to be restrained," Dr. Paul says. For a small child, the adult harness-belt system doesn't do much good. "If you stick a child of 45 to 50 pounds in the big lap-shoulder belt, he typically takes the shoulder belt off because it hits him in the neck and chin. The shoulder and lap belt need to fit snugly and securely, and for that you need a booster seat," she says.

Watching the Water

According to the National SAFE KIDS Campaign, drowning is the second leading cause of accidental death in children in the United States, and most of those drownings happen not when a child is swimming, but when a child falls into a pool or is left alone in the tub, says Dr. Paul.

If someone is watching the child indoors, all it takes is some small distraction, and the child may slip away. "If the caregiver is distracted for five minutes or so, answering the phone or the front door, the child could get out through a sliding glass door or open window and into the pool or pond or hot tub in the backyard," says Yuwiler.

Like other accidents, these are often preventable.

RAISE THE STAKES. "Put a fence between the house and the pool," says Yuwiler. She also recommends that the gate is one that you *pull* open rather than push open. "This is because young children typically push things in but can't pull things out."

The fence should be four-sided, at least five feet high, and the gate should be self-closing and self-latching, adds Dr. Paul.

In addition, it is a good idea to look for gates that are also self-locking, adds Yuwiler.

DESIGNATE A WATCHER. When you have a group of people over, agree that one person is going to watch the pool, suggests Yuwiler. "What happens is that you have seven kids running in different directions, and everybody else thought somebody else was watching." If one person has the responsibility of watching the pool, your chances of spotting danger will be more effective, she adds.

LIFEGUARD THE TUB, TOO. Even when there are just a few inches of water in a bathtub, a young child can be at risk. "Never leave a child alone or with a sibling in a tub," says Dr. Paul, not even to answer the phone or get a towel.

A related risk—and another reason to watch kids when they are in the tub—is the danger of being burned by scalding water. Set the temperature of your hot water heater no higher than 120°F, says Dr. Paul. (Clothes and dishes will get clean at this temperature, she says.)

BAIL OUT THE BUCKETS. Buckets used for household chores, especially the industrial five-gallon kind, can be very hazardous to small children, says Dr. Paul. She recommends that you empty any liquid out of containers after you are finished using them.

Do's and Must-Do's of Childproofing Your House

Whether you are a parent, grandparent, kindly aunt, or doting uncle, you should look at your house with a critical eye. Where could a child trip, fall, or otherwise stumble into trouble? For childproofing your house, here are some of the basic safety tips from experts.

INSTALL SAFETY GATES. "There are a number of different kinds of safety gates," says Craig Kaminer, founder of Childproofers, a Saint Louis–based company that has installed child safety devices in thousands of homes, and a former paramedic with emergency medical services in New York City. Some gates can be permanently installed so that children can't push or pull the gate out of place. For this reason, permanent gates are safer than temporary gates, he says. According to Kaminer, temporary gates are fine for keeping kids in one area as long as there is adult supervision.

BE WARY OF WALKERS. Baby walkers cause about 27,000 injuries a year in the United States to children under 15 months old.

SAFETY-PROOF THE CRIB. If you have borrowed or inherited a crib, double-check to make sure that none of the screws are loose.

CHECK THE SPACING. Slats in the side of a crib should be no wider than 2⅜ inches apart, says Kaminer.

CHECK THE KID'S CRIB STUFF. If you use bumper pads, they should be firmly anchored so that a child can't dig underneath and get stuck. If there's a mobile over the crib, make sure it's well-secured.

PASS ON POSTS. For optimal safety, the corners of a crib should be the same height as the end panels so clothing won't get caught on a post.

GET A SNUG MATTRESS. You should not be able to place

more than two adult fingers between the mattress and the crib side.

FORGO THE PORTABLE CRIB. Make sure that it is *not* the V-form type with collapsible hinges. The crib could collapse on the child.

GET THE LOWDOWN ON HIGH CHAIRS. When you are putting a child in a high chair, always fasten the belt and crotch strap.

STAND BY YOUR CHILD. A child should never be left alone on the table. "If you need to reach for a diaper, keep one hand on the child to prevent a fall," says Kaminer.

CLEAR THE AREA. The changing-table necessities need to be kept beyond reach of the child, cautions Kaminer.

SOFTEN THE HEARTH. Many children get hurt near the fireplace, where sharp edges can inflict long-lasting wounds. Kaminer recommends a custom-made padded product called Hearth-Guard that fits over the sharp corner edges of your fireplace. It is sold by fireplace specialty stores.

KEEP CORDS OUT OF REACH. "Always try to bundle up loose cords and keep them hidden," cautions Kaminer.

LOCK UP THE POISONS. There are more than one million poison exposures every year in children under age six— and about 50 of those children die. Parents could prevent almost all of those poisonings with a few, simple measures, says Rose Ann Soloway, R.N., administrator of the American Association of Poison Control Centers in Washington, D.C. "Medicine and cleaning products should be stored in their original containers with child-resistant caps," she says. "Potentially dangerous household items and medicine need to be locked out of sight and reach of children."

GUARD THE SECOND STORY. A window guard is a safety device designed to keep children from falling out of windows. "Install window guards above the first floor," says

Janice Yuwiler, director of the California Center for Childhood Injury Prevention at San Diego State University. "Screens are not strong enough to keep your child from falling out the window." You can purchase window guards from major baby specialty retailers.

WATCH OUT FOR OLD PLAYGROUNDS. Playground standards have changed, and the newer ones are more likely to be safe. "In the past five years, considerable effort has been made to create standards that ensure the

Keeping Your Kitchen Safe

Your child may scamper around the kitchen like she owns the place, but Julia Child she is not—and this much-used room in the house can be a dangerous place for kids.

"A kitchen is a dangerous place for small children," says Dr. Paul, and she has numerous examples. Parents have unintentionally knocked scalding food or boiling water on wandering tots. And children have pulled pots of hot food, searing oil, or boiling water down on themselves. Even the act of eating can turn into an all-out emergency if a child gulps down overheated food or starts to choke.

Here are some ways to nip trouble in the bud when you have kitchen duty.

SWIVEL THE HANDLES. Turn all pot handles toward the back of the stove, says Dr. Paul. That way, small hands can't reach up and grab them.

WAVE OFF. Don't use microwaves to heat baby food or formulas, advises Dr. Paul. Microwaves heat unevenly; food that is lukewarm or cool on the outside can have a scalding-hot pocket in the center. That searing-hot surprise can burn your child's mouth.

HOLD THE KID OR THE POT, NOT BOTH. If you are holding something hot—in or out of the kitchen—don't

protection of children from all types of injuries and
potential fatalities," says Arthur Mittelstaedt, Ed.D.,
executive director of the Recreation Safety Institute
in Ronkonkoma, New York. "If the playground is old,
parents should conduct their own visual inspection of
the equipment." In fact, parents should get to know any
area where their children play, Dr. Mittelstaedt advises,
and that includes playing fields, skating areas, and
sledding areas.

hold your child, too, suggests Dr. Paul. If the child needs attention just as the soup comes to a boil, set the soup aside
and then pay attention to the child. If you ever fell holding
both, you and your child could be injured.

MONITOR FOOD. Cut food into slivers so that your
child can't choke on it, Yuwiler recommends. "Think about
a hot dog," she says. "If you cut it crosswise, it is the perfect
circumference of a child's esophagus." Like a cork getting
stuck in a pipe, that round hot dog can get jammed in the
child's throat on the way down. And there are some foods
that you should never give a child who is under the age of
three, says Yuwiler. Popcorn, nuts, and hard candy should be
off-limits to these toddlers.

Be a Road Worrier

Every parent is concerned about children and traffic, and
the old adage, "Look both ways," applies for adults as well
as kids. "Pedestrian injuries are a big cause of injury with
kids," says Yuwiler. But looking both ways is not enough,
she cautions. Here are some other things that guardians and
babysitters should keep in mind.

KEEP UP THE HAND-HOLDING. A child may have
memorized the rules about crossing the street, but that

doesn't necessarily mean that he can see that car racing around a curve. "I think the most important thing that a parent should know is that the child's auditory and visual systems are immature," says Yuwiler. "They don't have the ability to make the judgment about how fast the car is coming, so they shouldn't be walking without any kind of restraint until they are six or seven." And always take a child's hand when crossing the street, she says.

CHECK THE CORNERS. When you are teaching a child how to cross the street, remind him about cars turning corners, says Yuwiler. For instance, a five-year-old might stop at the curb, look both ways, but forget to look for a car that is coming around the corner. So "both ways" is not enough: Show the child how to watch cars that are approaching the intersection or exiting a driveway.

CIRCLE THE CAR. If a small child is behind the car, he is completely invisible to the driver. If you are in any neighborhood that has children, "you should walk around the back of the car before you get in so that you can be certain there is no child in the way," says Yuwiler. "Obviously, children shouldn't play in the driveway," she adds, but even if you have told them that, you always need to check before backing out.

Starting Out with a Sitter

Your babysitters are important allies, and they need to get some basic training if they are going to help prevent the many mishaps of childhood. "Explain everything to the babysitter," says Cheri Stanley, a former public education specialist in Arvada, Colorado, who created a "Babysitting Checklist" for concerned parents. "With first-time babysitters, parents should bring them in for an interview and spend 20 to 30 minutes going over all the items in the house." And if you are a grandparent who is babysitting for

---

Looking Out for Number Two

Don't let your guard down with your second child. "The majority of accidents that we are seeing is to second children, not first," says Kaminer.

"The first child in a family is usually overprotected," he observes. But that doesn't mean the second one should get the short end of the safety measures. "By the time parents have the second child, there are broken latches on drawers and other failed safety devices because the older child is out of the danger zone." Also, more experienced parents may be overconfident, notes Kaminer. "They think, 'Johnny was okay, so why do we need this extra safety stuff?' As soon as you let your guard down, that is when accidents happen."

---

the first time, make sure that you are informed about these items before the parents go out, she advises. Here is what Stanley includes on her checklist for parents to do.

EXPLAIN THE BACKUP. "The babysitter needs to know where you are going and how you can be reached by phone," says Stanley. In addition to leaving your own number, you should also leave the number of a backup person like grandparents or a close neighbor.

GET OUT THE EMERGENCY NUMBERS. "Make sure that the sitter knows where the emergency phone numbers are," says Stanley. "We encourage sitters to keep the list in their pockets because if there is a fire and they have to get out of the house, they have the numbers right there," she says. Put a list near the phone and make sure that the sitter knows where it is.

RUN THROUGH A FIRE DRILL. Activate a smoke detector while the sitter is there so that she knows what it sounds like, says Stanley. "And if there is a fire extinguisher, you need to show the babysitter where it is and how to use it."

Stanley also advises parents to take the babysitter on a tour of the house, showing at least two ways out of every room. Also, open a window and put the screen and storm window up so that the sitter can see how the windows work. And remind the babysitter to get the kids out of the house first and then call 911 before trying to fight a fire.

DO A QUICK COOKING COURSE. If you have an infant or toddler, remind your sitter that the child needs to be in the high chair away from the cooking area, not roaming or crawling around. "You should go over safe cooking practices with the sitter," Stanley says. Even make sure that the sitter is wearing the right type of clothes—not long, loose sleeves that could catch on fire.

SPECIFY MEDICATION. "If the kids take medication, the babysitter needs to know where the medication is," says Stanley. Review the dosage with the sitter, and write out the instructions if they aren't legible on the container.

REVIEW THE LOCKS AND LATCHES. "If there are little ones, the babysitter needs to know how to work the gates at the top and the bottom of the stairs," says Stanley. For toddlers, it is good policy to have safety locks on drawers and cabinets, but even if you have taken this precaution, ask the babysitter never to leave a small child in a room by himself.

No-Fall Insurance

Many home injuries can be avoided with some practical fix-ups such as installing grab bars, handrails, and rubber matting. (For more information, see "A Fall-Safe Checklist" on page 13.) In addition, you can take a number of other precautions. These are particularly important if you are in the over-65 age group, among those who are most at risk of being injured in a fall.

WORK OUT TO STAY UP. At our bodies' peak, muscle

A Fall-Safe Checklist

Falls are a serious threat to the elderly. For people ages 65 to 84, falls are the second leading cause of injury-related death, responsible for more than 11,000 deaths every year in the United States. But no matter what your age, every year you run the risk of being the 1 person in 20 who receives emergency medical treatment for a fall-related injury. From the Nationwide Insurance Company, here is a checklist of some important precautions that you can take to avoid a tumble.

- Make sure that there is a light switch at the top and the bottom of every staircase.
- Install handrails on both sides of the stairs.
- Improve tread on stairs and steps.
- Never keep anything on a stairway.
- Put double-faced adhesive carpet tape or rubber matting on the backs of rugs.
- In the shower, install grab bars, textured strips, or a nonskid mat.
- Purchase a step stool that has a handrail.

---

accounts for 45 percent of our total weight. As we age and become inactive, we lose muscle and coordination, so falls become more common. Studies show that elderly people who exercise regularly fall less often. Probably the best way to avoid falls later in life is to maintain a good level of physical activity throughout life, says Bruce McClenaghan, a physical trainer who holds his doctorate in physical education and is director of the physical therapy program and Motor Rehabilitation Laboratory at the University of South Carolina in Columbia. An elderly person who is in relatively good health should participate in individual and supervised programs of physical activity designed to maintain muscular strength, endurance, and aerobic fitness, he advises.

GET SOME BALANCE. Gaining and maintaining balance is a very effective way to prevent falls. Tai chi, a fitness program practiced in Eastern cultures, provides good balance training for older individuals because of the slow, controlled movements that are used, says Dr. McClenaghan. To find a class in your area, look in the Yellow Pages under "Martial Arts."

Fire Away

The two leading causes of home fires are cooking equipment and heating equipment, says Julie Reynolds, director of public affairs for the National Fire Protection Association in Quincy, Massachusetts. Most of these fires aren't caused by the equipment, she adds; they are the result of people making safety mistakes while using that equipment. So, for better fire protection, check this list.

SLEEPERS, AWAKE. If you are in the habit of cooking up a little midnight snack, that nosh could cost you dearly. "One of the most lethal mistakes," says Reynolds, "is when a person gets up in the middle of the night, turns on the stove, and then falls back to sleep." If you are heating something up, don't get too comfortable while you are waiting, she advises.

DON'T TURN YOUR BACK. Too often, people walk away from the stove for a second to answer the phone or take care of the baby. A home fire can start when you turn your back even for a few seconds, Reynolds cautions.

"If the phone rings or there is some other interruption, turn off the burner and take something with you—a great big wooden spoon or ladle or a hot pad—so that you have a constant reminder with you," suggests Reynolds.

That way, even if you are distracted for a few minutes, the reminder in your hand will prompt you to get right back to the stove.

PUT A LID ON IT. Using a fire extinguisher is not the best way to stop a fire in a pan, Reynolds cautions. "Have a lid nearby that fits the pan you are using or another pan or lid that could slide over the top of the pan you are using." And always use a sturdy, fire-resistant oven mitt that protects your entire forearm, says Reynolds.

If you have a fire in the pan, put on the oven mitt to slide the lid over the top of the pan—coming at it from the side. When the lid is on, turn off the burner. Leave the lid in place until the pan is completely cooled. Though you may be tempted to peek, that simply introduces more oxygen, which can cause the fire to flare up again, Reynolds cautions.

The mitt-and-lid is safer than a fire extinguisher because the fire extinguisher is meant to be used 8 to 10 feet away from a fire, Reynolds points out. Often, you can't get that far from the stove, and if you use it up close, the pressurized spray could actually spread the fire. "You could actually shoot the burning contents of the pan around the kitchen," she notes.

HEED THE HOT SPOTS. Be careful with auxiliary heating equipment. "With heating equipment, the biggest problem is the way people use auxiliary heaters like portable and space heaters, either electric or kerosene, and woodstoves and fireplaces," says Reynolds. No matter what the source of extra heat, you need to take precautions, she says. "Make sure to keep anything that can burn at least three feet away from the heating equipment. Don't pull your chair up to a space heater or pile Sunday newspapers next to the fireplace."

Of course, you never want to leave an auxiliary heater on when you are out of the house, and it is also dangerous to have an auxiliary heater turned on while you are asleep.

Stop on the Gas

Carbon monoxide is a colorless, odorless gas that causes the unintentional death of 1,500 Americans every year. Nine hundred of these deaths occur in the home. Some warning signs may let you know that this substance may be invading your living quarters, symptoms that include dizziness, fatigue, headache, confusion, nausea, irregular breathing, or vomiting.

Carbon monoxide comes from many innocent-looking sources: heating appliances fueled by gas, oil, kerosene, or wood; cars, motorcycles, and lawn mowers; and blocked chimneys and flues. Normally, it disperses into the open air, doing no harm. But it can build up in enclosed spaces. Even a charcoal grill or hibachi can cause carbon monoxide poisoning if it is fired up in the house or in the enclosed confines of a recreational vehicle.

To prevent poisoning, experts at Nationwide Insurance advise homeowners to never keep a car, motorcycle, generator, or lawn mower running in a closed or attached garage. Make sure that your heating appliances, including water heaters and gas dryers, have been installed properly and checked by a service technician annually. Keep doors and windows open when you are using a kerosene or gas space heater that doesn't emit its fumes outdoors.

Be sure to install a carbon monoxide detector on each occupied level of your home, advises Rose Ann Soloway, R.N., administrator of the American Association of Poison Control Centers in Washington, D.C. And if you use a fireplace or wood-burning stove, have your chimney flue checked annually to make sure that it is intact and clear of obstructions.

Apart from certain wood-burning stoves that are designed to heat a room all night, any extra heating equipment should be turned off when you are feeling sleepy or when you go to bed, Reynolds says.

ATTEND TO THE BUTTS. "Make sure that the smokers in your household have access to deep, sturdy ashtrays," says Reynolds. "The leading cause of home fire deaths is lighted tobacco products." Any cigarette that is perched on the edge of an ashtray can easily fall out. Reynolds advises smokers to pour water in used ashtrays to make sure that nothing is smoldering in there, or flush the contents of ashtrays down the toilet. "If you have had a party or people over to your house and there was smoking, before you go to bed search behind and under the cushions of furniture to make sure that there are no smoldering cigarettes," Reynolds adds.

CELEBRATE WITH A DETECTOR CHECK. Check smoke detector batteries at least once a year, advises Yuwiler. But how do you remember when you last checked the detector? Do it when the time changes in the spring and fall, she advises. "Or choose a family member's birthday."

Out of Arms Way

Don't go gunning for trouble. About 34,000 people in the United States die each year from gunshot wounds and about 100,000 people are treated in emergency rooms.

Preventing these deaths should be simple. "No firearms should be stored with bullets in the firearm," says Linda Tate, R.N., a health education specialist located in Denver and author of the booklet *Gun Safety in the Home*.

That goes for pellet guns as well. "Pellet guns can do a lot of damage," Tate says. "Many parents consider pellet guns safe because they don't have bullets. But if they are loaded, you never know when they are going to go off. And the pellet can put out an eye."

The ammunition should be stored in a separate locked cabinet, she says. And, adds Thorson, that storage place for both ammunition and guns should be too high for children to reach.

TELL THE KIDS, "HANDS OFF." All children need to be educated about gun safety, not just the children of gun owners, says Tate. Often, the gun is an object of curiosity. "Parents sometimes think that they have hidden their firearms well, but many times children find guns. Harmless, curious play often results in accidents," says Tate. "Children should be told to never touch a gun."

SAFETY ON FIRST. Always keep the gun's safety on, even if the gun is unloaded, says Tate.

No More Crash Courses

When most people think "accident," they think "car accident," and the reason is obvious. In the United States, motor vehicle crashes are the leading cause of death among men and women between the ages of 15 and 24. Some 45,000 people a year are killed in car accidents, and another 4 million are injured badly enough to require an emergency room visit.

The mixture of alcohol and automobile is particularly lethal. "Whether you think you can hold your liquor or not isn't the point. The point is that your senses are dulled, and your reaction time is slowed," says Anthony Scotti, president of the Scotti School of Defensive Driving in Medford, Massachusetts.

The alternatives? "Call a cab. Use a designated driver. Don't get into a car when somebody else has been drinking," says Thorson. And she questions the usual "safety" rule that stipulates if you have had two drinks over a two-hour period, you can drive. "That's not always true," she points out. "Have those two drinks been beer or straight alcohol?

Are you a person with a smaller body, so that less alcohol affects you more?" These are factors that can affect the way you react to alcohol.

But alcohol isn't the only danger. Here are some other precautions that can help keep you safe on the road.

CINCH 'EM UP. If you have an accident, it is better to be held in than thrown out. "Everybody should be seatbelted," says Thorson. "Some people don't wear their seat belts because they think, 'If my car goes into water or catches on fire, how do I get out?' But less than 1 percent of car crashes have anything to do with water or fire."

With a seat belt on, you have a better chance of staying conscious in a car crash, Thorson points out. And you are less likely to be thrown from the car. "Ejection is a major cause of injury and death, and that's one reason that seat belts are so important," she says.

GET OFF THE CHAT LINE. If you talk on a cellular phone while you are driving, you quadruple your risk of colliding with another vehicle, according to a study in *The New England Journal of Medicine*.

"The motor activity of dialing or holding the phone to your ear demands a portion of your attention, and the conversation with another person also demands your attention," says John Violanti, Ph.D., professor of preventive medicine at the University of Buffalo and professor of criminal justice at the Rochester Institute of Technology in Rochester, both in New York. In a study that Dr. Violanti conducted with James R. Marshall, Ph.D., professor of public health at the University of Arizona in Tucson, he found that folks who talk on a cellular phone more often than the average (50 minutes a month) were five times more likely to have an accident than those who either talked less or did not own a car phone. Because you give most of your attention to the conversation, you lose track of what you are doing, notes Dr. Violanti. "And in that split second of being inattentive, you may hit somebody."

His advice? "If you need to make a call, especially an intense business call, pull over in a safe place, maybe a rest area."

GIVE THEM SOME SPACE. At a speed of 40 miles per hour, you travel approximately 60 feet in one second. "If you blink, that's one-tenth of a second—you have traveled 6 feet," notes Scotti.

An easy way to judge how far you are traveling behind the vehicle in front of you—when you are both traveling about 40 miles per hour—is the two-second rule. "If you are on a road and the car in front of you drives by an object, let's say a light pole, you count two seconds and you should reach the same light pole," explains Scotti. That leaves a distance of 120 feet, enough time to stop if the car ahead of you slams on the brakes.

GO WITH THE FLOW. Not too slow, not too fast. "Drive with the flow of traffic," says Scotti. "What is dangerous is driving either faster than or slower than the flow of traffic. Because if you close up on something quickly while driving fast, it is hard to judge distances, speed, and the spaces around you." If you drive too slowly, you are on the opposite end of this hazard. Driving 40 miles an hour in the middle lane of a highway with a speed limit of 65 miles an hour can create scenarios for unsafe passing, says Scotti.

FAVOR A LIMO. Drive a big car, advises Scotti. It is a statistical fact that people are safer in bigger cars. "My daughter's first car was the biggest thing I could find," says Scotti.

UPGRADE TO ABS. An antilock braking system (ABS) is "the greatest invention since the wheel," says Scotti. Instead of locking when you slam on the brakes, the so-called ABS brakes deliver rapid-fire lock-and-release that helps prevent skidding. "With an ABS car, you can stop the car as quickly as you can and still have the ability to steer out of trouble," says Scotti.

TAKE CARE WITH SUVS. Sports utility vehicles are not

cars, Scotti reminds drivers. "They can't do some of the things that cars can do, like make a quick lane change."

Are they unsafe? "No," says Scotti. "It's just that you have to remember what you are driving."

LIGHT UP THE DAY. Turn on your headlights during the day as well as the night, suggests Scotti. "Driving with your headlights on is a must," he notes. "Other people see you better, so there is less chance of an accident. It should be a law."

TAKE A TRAINING CLASS. Adults as well as teens need driver training, notes Scotti. "Driver training creates emergencies for kids and grown-ups in a controlled manner that is beneficial. For instance, you learn where your eyes should focus." If someone cruises through a stop sign as you enter an intersection, "you should be looking for an opening, not concentrating on the bozo who went through the stop sign," says Scotti. "To learn that, you have to practice."

Playing Safe

"There are two big mistakes people make when engaging in recreational activities," says Arthur Mittelstaedt, Ed.D., executive director of the Recreation Safety Institute in Ronkonkoma, New York. "One is overconfidence. People think that they can do something in which they have had no instruction or practice, and they end up injuring themselves. The other big mistake in recreational activity is discourtesy, disregard of others and not accepting responsibilities," he says.

In other words, take precautions, play fair, and everyone will be safe, advises Dr. Mittelstaedt. Here are some specific ways to do all three.

DON'T DIVE RIGHT IN. The water may look fine, but that doesn't mean it is safe for diving or even swimming. "Drowning can occur in any depth of water," cautions Dr.

Mittelstaedt. Unless you are in the diving end of a well-marked pool, you have no way of knowing what lies beneath the surface of the water. "I have been personally involved in diving accidents where water became too shallow because of tides, or where there was a submerged wreck, weed growth, or construction debris," he says. "Diving, in particular, should only be engaged in when that area is clearly marked and permitted."

MAINTAIN LAW AND ORDER. Trampolines and other recreational toys are potential hazards, especially if children aren't closely supervised. In order to ensure that kids play fair, make sure the rules of using recreational toys are written, says Thorson. Every child, family member, or friend and neighbor who participates in game playing must understand the rules and then play by them, she says. Most important, adults must be willing to enforce rules if they are not followed, she states.

KNOW THE SLOPES. It is best to know and accept your skills and limitations in an activity, says Dr. Mittelstaedt. When skiing, don't go for that steep slope if you are not taught or experienced in how to handle a fast run, he advises. Whether you are a skier, a tuber, or a tobogganer, you should always stick to marked trails or hills at your ability level. Accidents often happen when people get themselves into a situation where they have no idea what to expect, he explains.

GRAB A BUD. Don't engage in an activity without a buddy or without telling someone where you are going, suggests Dr. Mittelstaedt. Never go surfing, swimming, hiking, or scuba diving alone. "Fatalities occur when rescuers don't know where to look," he states. If you can't take a buddy along or tell a friend or relative where you will be, check in with local authorities who have an emergency routine plan for rescue, he advises.

HEAD FOR A HELMET. "For bicycling, in-line skating, skateboarding, horseback riding, and skiing, you need to wear a helmet," says Thorson. And parents need to set an example. "How many times have you seen a child with a helmet on and a parent with no helmet on? It doesn't make sense."

A helmet is particularly important for bicycling. "In the United States, more than 800 people a year are killed in bicycle crashes, a lot of them involving head injuries," says Randy Swart, director of the Bicycle Helmet Safety Institute in Arlington, Virginia. "A good bicycle helmet will prevent 85 percent of those injuries."

CHECK THE FIT. When you are putting on a bike helmet, take the time to make sure that it fits your head, says Swart. "When a helmet doesn't fit, it can come off in a crash," he says.

Make sure that the straps are adjusted so that the helmet is level and the straps meet just below your ear. The chin strap should be loose enough so that it doesn't chafe or irritate, but it shouldn't be so loose that you can see daylight underneath it.

To test whether the helmet has the right fit, "put the helmet on, adjust it, and try to tear it off," says Swart. "If it doesn't come off in the store, it won't come off when you hit something else."

ADULT ACNE
Zits *Again?*

What a relief to not be a teen. If you were, you would have to deal with rap music. Tattoos. Piercings in odd places. Clothes that look like they are about to fall off.

But even if you're mostly free from general teen worries, one may still haunt you. Many of us still get an annoying dose of that main bane of teenage years: acne. And even if it is called, technically, adult acne, it still looks like the same darn thing that we had when we hit adolescence.

"In the 1980s, doctors didn't talk about adult acne," says Kathy Fields, M.D., a clinical instructor of dermatology at the University of California Medical Center at San Francisco. "It was just glossed over. But now dermatologists do recognize it as a very real problem, particularly in women. It can come and go with hormone cycles and can last well into postmenopause."

"The prevention of adult acne is an everyday thing," adds Esta Kronberg, M.D., a dermatologist in private practice in Houston. "It's not that you clear up the problem and

Revealing the Inner You

"A persistent skin symptom can be a message from your inner self, a call for help," says Ted Grossbart, Ph.D., an instructor in the department of psychiatry at Harvard Medical School, senior associate and clinical supervisor for the department of psychiatry at Beth Israel Hospltal, a clinical psychologist in Boston, and author of *Skin Deep: A Mind/Body Program for Healthy Skin*.

"I have detected a familiar psychological pattern with adult acne, a problem that is especially common in hard-driving, high-powered, and perfectionistic women in their twenties and thirties," says Dr. Grossbart. If people are grappling with old adolescent issues and impasses, it seems more than a coincidence that their skin is also struggling with an adolescent concern.

Many family and personal issues can trigger acne outbreaks. "I find that as people get into therapy and chip away at the conflicts, they experience improvements in their skin," says Dr. Grossbart. "The therapy helps resolve the adult acne, and the new psychological health acts as a kind of insurance policy against its return."

then you're cured. For adult acne, prevention is about *control*." And here is what the experts have to say about controlling it.

START MILD. Start your acne prevention program by washing your face once a day with a mild, 2.5 percent form of benzoyl peroxide wash, suggests Dr. Kronberg. This over-the-counter medication kills the bacteria that cause acne, but you need to apply it properly. The trick, she says, is to "get the medicine all over your face and on any other areas where you have acne, like your arms, chest, and upper back. If you use it only on the bumps, you won't get results."

Turn Treatment into Prevention

If you visit a dermatologist for treatment of acne, you may wonder whether prescription drugs are effective for *prevention* as well.

All the standard dermatological treatments for adult acne should also be used for prevention, says Kathy Fields, M.D., a clinical instructor of dermatology at the University of California Medical Center at San Francisco.

Because acne has so many causes, Dr. Fields advocates that dermatologists use a combination approach when treating it. "Acne begins with an excess of oil on your skin," she explains. "That oil causes a stickiness of the cells that line a pore, creating a plug. Bacteria forms around the plug. And the body's immune system responds to the bacteria. The end result is a big pimple. To prevent that, you need to work on all the factors that create acne."

Depending upon the type of acne, elements of a combination approach, she notes, might include these treatments.

Even if you don't get results right away, stay with this mild treatment, Dr. Kronberg advises. "It takes a couple of months for this topical medicine to work. You need to be patient."

PLAY OUT THE PREVENTION. Pimples are forming inside the skin two weeks before you see them on the surface. Even when they disappear, you're not done, Dr. Fields says. Endorsing the 2.5 percent benzoyl peroxide treatment, she stresses allover coverage rather than spot treatment, adding, "When you look gorgeous, don't quit, or your acne will be back the next month."

BE A DUBIOUS MOISTURIZER. Skin moisturizers aren't

- Topical antibiotics, which kill the bacteria. Examples include benzoyl peroxide (Benzac), clindamycin (Cleocin), and erythromycin (Emgel).
- Tretinoin (Retin-A) or adapalene (Differin), powerful drugs that unplug pores.
- A cream containing azelaic acid (Azelex) that prevents oiliness, unplugs pores, and helps to fade spots.

If topical combination therapy is unsuccessful, then your dermatologist may suggest that you begin taking oral antibiotics such as tetracycline (Achromycin), erythromycin (Em-Tab), or minocycline (Dynacin) while using topical creams. Finally, if these oral antibiotics don't prove effective, then isotretinoin (Accutane) may be prescribed for a five-month period, says Dr. Fields. "Accutane, while not a cure, is the most effective remedy for extremely resistant, severe acne, but it is used as a last resort because there are many possible side effects and precautions associated with it."

Your dermatologist may recommend other medications as well, both prescription and over-the-counter. "Work with your dermatologist to find a combination approach," Dr. Fields advises.

for everyone, even though advertisers would like you to think so, observes Dr. Kronberg. "Skin-care companies want to sell everybody a moisturizer—even if you have the oiliest skin in the world," she says. "But if your skin isn't dry, you shouldn't use a moisturizer. It can cause acne."

CLEANSE GENTLY. If your skin care includes soap, scrub, toner, and moisturizer, maybe your complexion will do better with somewhat less attention. "Most women use a lot of skin-care steps, and they should use fewer," says Dr. Kronberg. "You want a gentle cleanser and, if you feel dry, a light moisturizer. That's *two* steps." All the additional steps can actually cause an outbreak of adult acne. "You are overmanipulating your skin and clogging your pores," she says.

GO AGAINST THE "GRAINIES." The grainy scrubs that are supposed to help cleanse your skin may actually be doing a lot of harm, according to Dr. Kronberg. "They spread infections. They inflame pimples. They also make little cuts in your skin. You think that you are scrubbing bad things out, but you are actually irritating your skin and then spreading the bacteria all over it." Her advice is simple: Don't use them.

ADOPT A SUMMER CLEANSING SCHEDULE. Summer's heat and humidity invite flare-ups of acne. "People sweat a lot more, and that seems to clog up the pores," says Dr. Kronberg. But even though you should try to cleanse your skin a little bit more often in the summer, don't wash too much, she advises. "Typically, clean twice a day, unless you are getting hot and sweaty—then a third time is fine."

FREE YOURSELF FROM OIL. Cosmetics can cause acne, especially if they are laden with oils, according to Robert M. Peppercorn, M.D., a dermatologist and cosmetic surgeon in private practice in Yuba City, California. "If people have a tendency to develop acne, I advise them to avoid all oil-containing facial products and to use only oil-free makeup, oil-free lotions, and oil-free sunscreen."

DON'T RELY ON RABBIT EARS. Cosmetic products labeled "noncomedogenic" claim that they won't give you a comedo, or pimple. But the way scientists determine if a product is noncomedogenic is less than foolproof, says Dr. Peppercorn. They put the product on a rabbit's ear and see if the rabbit develops blackheads. If a rabbit's ear stays smooth as a baby's bottom, does that mean your face will, too? "There's no saying for sure," he says.

SLUMBER MAKEUP-FREE. Even if your makeup is oil-free and noncomedogenic, you should never exercise or sleep with it on, cautions Lia Schorr, a skin-care expert in New York City. "It is a sure way to clog the hair follicles in

Beware the Cook's Hazard

As occupational hazards go, it is not on a par with riveting girders on the 89th story of a skyscraper or removing deadly asbestos from old school buildings. But even so, restaurant-caused acne is a face-threatening hazard.

"If you work in a restaurant, the oil and grease coming off the french-fry maker and the frying pan can clog the skin and cause acne," says Robert M. Peppercorn, M.D., a dermatologist and cosmetic surgeon in private practice in Yuba City, California.

Dr. Peppercorn's recipe for a clearer-complexioned cook goes like this: In the morning before setting off to work, wash your face with a 2.5 percent benzoyl peroxide solution. Then gently wash your skin every two to three hours with a nondrying, mild soap such as Dove or Aveeno or a cleansing lotion such as Cetaphil, while working at the restaurant. "This will prevent restaurant acne," he says.

your skin—and clogged follicles are one major part of the acne-causing process."

SPRAY WITH CARE. Hair products can have a "plugging" effect on your skin so that you develop pimples along your hairline, says Dr. Peppercorn. To prevent that, he advises using as little hair spray as possible.

And protect your forehead when you do use it. "Put a towel over your face and then spray," says Dr. Kronberg.

HANDS OFF! Constantly touching your face with your hands can cause adult acne, says Dr. Peppercorn, probably because of the combination of acne-causing oils and bacteria that people have on their hands. For instance, if you are on the telephone a lot, you might develop acne where your hand touches your cheek. Or maybe you instinctively brush back your hair. "A woman who has hair over her forehead and is constantly touching her fingers to her forehead may develop pimples on her forehead," he observes.

THROW IN THE TOWEL—AND THE PILLOWCASE. "People should change their towels and pillowcases more frequently—a few times a week," says Schorr. "That helps keep blemish-causing bacteria off your face."

AVOID IODINE OVERDOSE. Excess iodine can "make people break out like crazy," observes Lindy J. Batis, an aesthetician and owner of Lindy's Healing Facials in Los Angeles and Ojai, California.

Iodine is found naturally in some foods, like fish, but many multivitamins have excess iodine. So if you are taking a multivitamin and you are prone to adult acne, read the label to find a brand that doesn't have iodine, Dr. Peppercorn advises.

OKAY A. "A daily dose of vitamin A—between 10,000 and 15,000 IU (international units)—may also offer some help in improving acne," says Dr. Fields. If, however, you are pregnant or planning on becoming pregnant, speak to your doctor first before supplementing your diet with vitamin A.

LOOK FOR THE ACID INGREDIENT. Many nonprescription facial treatments contain glycolic acid, which Batis recommends as an acne treatment. "Glycolic acid comes from the family of AHAs, or alpha hydroxy acids," she says. "The reason I choose glycolic acid for acne treatment and prevention is that the molecules are small enough to penetrate the skin. Glycolic acid makes your skin more resistant to acne by unplugging pores. It also brings all of the impurities under the skin up and out."

In-salon glycolic acid peels are available in varying degrees of concentration as are over-the-counter glycolic acid creams and lotions. Some people actually have a breakout of acne during the first few weeks of glycolic acid treatment, says Batis. "But once the impurities come up and out completely, the pores appear to close."

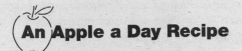

An Apple a Day Recipe

A-Plus Stew

Lean kielbasa lends a rich, smoky flavor to this sweet potato stew. The sweet potatoes are loaded with skin-enhancing vitamin A.

¼ pound lean turkey kielbasa, chopped
1½ pounds sweet potatoes, peeled and chopped
1 cup sliced celery
1 cup chopped onions
1 cup chopped carrots
2 cans (14½ ounces each) diced tomatoes
1 cup water
¼ teaspoon ground black pepper

Coat a large pot with nonstick spray. Add the kielbasa and cook over medium-high heat for 3 minutes, or until browned.

Add the potatoes, celery, onions, carrots, tomatoes (with juice), water, and pepper. Bring to a boil. Reduce the heat to low. Cover and cook, stirring occasionally, for 25 to 30 minutes, or until the vegetables are tender.

Makes 4 servings. Per serving: 269 calories, 3 g. fat, 500% of Daily Value of vitamin A

Glycolic acid exfoliates dead skin cells and unplugs pores. It makes pores appear smaller because they are not impacted, says Dr. Fields.

TAKE OFF SOME STRESSES. "My typical patient is a

woman in her thirties or forties," Dr. Kronberg says. Her explanation? Women of this age are often under a lot of stress. "And stress definitely causes acne."

One way to reduce the stress level is by saying no more often, Dr. Kronberg observes. "I tell my patients, 'When your plate is full, don't put more on it. And find some quiet time for yourself. And try to pamper yourself occasionally.' "

LOOK ON THE YOUNG SIDE. In many cases, people who have adult acne actually have *younger* skin, says Schorr. "If you have adult acne, it means that your skin won't age as fast—the skin is still oily and productive. Look at your acne positively: It is slowing the process of aging."

AGE SPOTS
The Rewards of Sun-Full Living

Liver spots—sounds bad enough. Worse: senile lentigo. But to those of us who hate signs of aging, the most sinister name of all for those unsightly brown skin patches is . . . age spots.

In fact, the third name rings truest because these spots have a lot more to do with aging than with livers or senility. As you get along in years, age spots can colonize the backs of your hands, your forearms, your shoulders, your face, your forehead—just about anywhere there is skin. The only reason they were ever called liver spots is that a pathologist observed that the brown color of these spots roughly matches the color of the liver.

But even though age spots occur mostly in people over 55, they are not caused by aging. In fact, their originator comes from outer space: It's that seething, yellow orb that so many of us bask under all summer long.

"An age spot is the result of many years of sun exposure that damages the melanin, or the color-producing cells of the skin, which are called melanocytes," says Robert M. Peppercorn, M.D., a dermatologist and cosmetic surgeon in private practice in Yuba City, California. "After years of sun exposure, something happens to the ability of the melanocytes, and they produce too much color. That creates the brown spots."

So the biggest prevention steps are obvious. Put the sun back in its place. Here's how.

SCREEN OUT THE BURN. "Age spots can absolutely be prevented by using sunscreen in the early years of life," says Dr. Peppercorn. Noting that most of us get the largest dose of sun exposure before we are 20, he speculates: "If, from the age of 0 to the age of 20, people used sunscreen every day, they would not get a large number of these spots."

Look for two important factors when you are shopping for sunscreen, suggests Dr. Peppercorn. First, it should have a sun protection factor (SPF) rating of 15 or higher. "If you have the option of a higher number than 15, why not use it?" he says.

Second, your sunscreen should block both ultraviolet type A *and* ultraviolet type B rays from reaching your skin. Many brands don't block both, so it is particularly important to check the label. A sunscreen called Shade UVA-Guard protects against both ultraviolet A and ultraviolet B rays, adds Dr. Peppercorn, noting that few other brands meet these criteria.

SCREEN FOR THE FUTURE. "If you are starting to get age spots, you can decrease the number of new ones you get by using sunscreen," says Dr. Peppercorn. You can't stop them entirely, he adds, because the sun damage to your skin has accumulated for many years. But if you continue to use sunscreen, you might get fewer new age spots.

GO UNDERCOVER. Most undercover agents don't think about skin protection, but you can protect your skin if

Prevent Worse, Too

As long as you are trying to prevent age spots, you should also be on the lookout for a far more serious problem—a brown blotch that resembles an age spot, but isn't.

Age spots are *benign*—that is, they never become cancerous, says Robert M. Peppercorn, M.D., a dermatologist and cosmetic surgeon in private practice in Yuba City, California. But as long as you are taking sun-protection measures to avoid age spots, you are also helping to prevent sun-caused spots that *can* become cancerous.

The potentially cancerous blotches are called actinic keratosis. And they do look quite different from age spots, says Laura E. Skellchock, M.D., associate clinical professor of dermatology at the University of California, San Francisco, School of Medicine; senior physician at Kaiser Permanente Medical Center in South San Francisco; and editor in chief of *Skin Care Today*. "They are scaly and can be pink, reddish, or whitish," she says. "Sometimes they itch and bleed. And they feel weird when you run a finger across them—a sort of hurting, bad feeling. Frequently, these spots will fade in four to six weeks after they first appear. But if they stay more than six weeks, they may not go away—and about 15 percent of them can eventually become a skin cancer."

Your doctor definitely needs to look at and keep track of these suspicious-looking spots, says Dr. Skellchock.

you dress like one. "Definitely put sunscreen on your face and your hands, but also cover up with sun-protective clothing," advises Laura E. Skellchock, M.D., associate clinical professor of dermatology at the University of California, San Francisco, School of Medicine; senior physician at Kaiser Permanente Medical Center in South San Francisco; and editor in chief of *Skin Care Today*.

The ideal apparel? "Wear a hat and large sunglasses," says Dr. Skellchock. In addition, "walk on the shady side of the street; get out of the sun every possible time you can," she advises.

TINT YOUR WINDOWS. Even the sun that streams through your car window can be calling up age spots. "When I talk to a husband and wife, I can tell who is usually the driver and who is the passenger because the driver has age spots on the left side of the face, and the passenger has age spots on the right," says Dr. Peppercorn. "Window glass does not shield you from ultraviolet A. It is unlikely that you will get a sunburn, but you are certainly getting sun damage."

To avoid skin damage while you are driving, he says to make sure that you are wearing sunscreen even when you are in the car with the windows rolled up. If state laws allow you to tint the windows of your car, consider having it done on both the driver's and passenger's sides, suggests Dr. Peppercorn.

TRY CELLEX-C. The inventors of the skin-care product Cellex-C, a 10 percent vitamin C solution, call it skin food, and they say it may deliver 20 times more vitamin C to your skin than you would get from your own diet. If your skin is sun-damaged, the capillaries in the dermal layer are unable to properly feed nutrients to the skin. Cellex-C provides the nutrients the skin needs to repair sun-damaged collagen. "Cellex-C will definitely help prevent the appearance of new age spots due to sun exposure," says Lorraine Faxon Meisner, Ph.D., professor of preventive medicine at the University of Wisconsin in Madison and one of the creators of Cellex-C.

"When you are exposed to the sun, your skin's reservoir of vitamin C goes down, and unlike most animals, humans cannot make vitamin C," Dr. Meisner explains.

Therefore, if you don't replenish the vitamin C and you are exposed again, your skin loses some of its ability to inhibit the damage caused by the sun's ultraviolet radiation, she adds. Cellex-C is available through dermatologists, spas, and aestheticians and by mail order.

AIDS
Keeping the Faith and Taking the Tests

Though the government's Centers for Disease Control and Prevention (CDC) in Atlanta has heralded a decrease in the incidence of deaths from AIDS—the deadly disease caused by an infection with HIV—it remains a huge public health problem. According to preliminary data from the CDC, AIDS is now the second-leading cause of death for all Americans ages 25 to 44 and hits all demographic groups—gay, straight, male, female, young, old. In all, between 650,000 and 900,000 Americans are HIV-positive. Most important, AIDS is communicable. Every person who has it has the potential to pass it along.

You get HIV infection by intimate contact with the bodily fluids of a person who has it. The two most common ways of transmission are through the sharing of intravenous needles and through sexual contact and exposure to the fluids that carry the virus. The first problem is easy to deal with: Don't share needles. But the sexual method of transmission, which according to the American Medical

Association accounts for 65 percent of the AIDS cases in the United States, is more complex. HIV can be transmitted from infected semen, vaginal secretions, or blood that comes in contact with an uninfected person. Although HIV has been transmitted by mouth-to-semen contact, this rate is very low when compared with other penetrative sexual acts.

High Fidelity

There is no question that the single best way to prevent HIV is not to have sex with someone who has it, says an HIV/AIDS prevention report from the Centers for Disease Control and Prevention.

But, alas, this is the real world, complete with human beings. People stray from Monogamy Road. And fairly often, according to the General Social Survey conducted by the National Opinion Research Center at the University of Chicago. In this survey, 22 percent of married men and 14 percent of married women reported that they have been unfaithful to the person for whom they promised to forsake all others.

GET TESTED. "If there has been infidelity in a marriage or a committed relationship, one thing that both partners need to do is to talk about getting tested for HIV," says Gary Harper, Ph.D., assistant professor of psychology at DePaul University in Chicago and an expert in AIDS prevention.

But one HIV test probably isn't enough. That's because, says Dr. Harper, it can take up to six months after the infective incident for the presence of the virus to show itself on the standard HIV test. "I always encourage multiple testings. The first test should take place three to four weeks after the incident, and then a follow-up test should occur after six months to make sure that a person doesn't have HIV," he says.

Protecting the Unborn: Why Every Pregnant Woman Should Take an HIV Test

The government's Centers for Disease Control and Prevention (CDC) in Atlanta recommends that all pregnant women take an HIV test as soon as they know they are pregnant. Why? Because a report on HIV and pregnancy has shown that pregnant women who are infected with HIV can reduce the risk of transmitting the virus to their babies from 25 percent to 8 percent if they take the antiviral drug AZT during pregnancy, labor, and delivery and if the newborns are also given AZT.

"This is one of the bigger medical breakthroughs in the prevention of HIV infection," explains R. J. Simonds, M.D., a medical epidemiologist in the division of HIV/AIDS prevention at the CDC. "Before 1994, each year 7,000 pregnant women infected with the virus had babies, and 2,800 of those newborns were infected with the virus. That number is now being drastically reduced. Every year, we can now prevent 2,000 babies from getting AIDS."

Sex and the Single Girl (or Boy)

Of course, not everybody is in a steady relationship. What if you are out there in the dating world, still searching for Mr. or Ms. Right? How do you protect yourself from HIV infection? Here are some strategies you should keep in mind.

BEFORE YOU HAVE SEX, *TALK* ABOUT AIDS. Sure, nobody likes to talk about it. A deadly disease isn't exactly the stuff of courtship and romance. "People make a lot of dangerous assumptions," says Ariane van der Straten, Ph.D., a research scientist at the Center for AIDS Prevention Studies at the University of California, San Francisco. "I've heard women say, 'My partner didn't use a condom, so he must have known that he didn't have AIDS.' Don't make assumptions like this."

MAKE SURE YOU HAVE NEGATIVE TESTS. Talk is very cheap. Okay, both you and your new partner *say* that you are not infected with the virus, but there is only one way to be certain: taking an HIV test. "Two individuals with HIV-negative test results who have not sustained risk exposure within the six months prior to testing can be reasonably certain that neither partner is HIV-infected," according to the American Medical Association.

BECOME A CONDOM-MANIAC. Although it is the safest method, waiting six months before having sex may not be realistic. Your other options are to correctly and consistently use latex, not lambskin, condoms when you do have sex or to engage only in nonpenetrative sex when condoms aren't used, says Dr. van der Straten. "The safest scenario for preventing HIV infection in a new relationship," she adds, "would be to say, 'Let's start our sex life using a condom all the time until we have our test results six months from now.'" Deciding to give up condoms, she points out, is a safe choice *only* if both partners stay committed to being mutually monogamous.

Condoms: Deployment Secrets

Though they may seem like simple enough devices, condoms aren't always used correctly. In the heat of some moments, people can make foolish mistakes. Here is the prophylactic primer for the male condom, according to the CDC.

PUT IT ON EARLY. Semen isn't the only fluid that can carry HIV. So can pre-ejaculate and vaginal secretions. Don't wait until you are about to climax to don the protection.

BOYCOTT OIL. *Don't* use an oil-based lubricant like petroleum jelly, cold cream, hand lotion, or baby oil. They can weaken the latex. Instead, use water-based lubricants like glycerine or lubricating jellies.

GET IT ON RIGHT. Here are directions from the American Medical Association for the best way to put on a condom.

1. Carefully open the condom package and remove the condom.
2. Place the condom against the head of the erect penis, leaving about ½ inch of space at the end by gently squeezing the end of the condom to remove air from the tip.
3. Hold the tip of the condom and unroll it to the base of the penis.
4. If uncircumcised, pull back the foreskin before unrolling the condom.
5. Check the condom frequently during sex to make sure that it hasn't slipped off or broken.
6. After ejaculation, hold the base of the condom to keep it from coming off while removing the penis from the partner's vagina, mouth, or anus.
7. Dispose of the condom. Never use a condom more than once.

If a male condom cannot be used, a female condom may be used as a last resort. Although the female condom serves as a barrier to most viruses, further research is needed to determine its effectiveness in preventing HIV transmission, according to the CDC.

Teach Your Children Well

Lots of parents worry that talking to their kids about HIV will make them more promiscuous. It appears that just the opposite is true. A report sponsored by the National Campaign to Prevent Teen Pregnancy shows that educational programs that focus on sexuality do not increase sexual activity. In fact, some programs made teens less likely to engage in sex, and those who did have sex had it less often and were more likely to use contraception.

"It is important for parents to begin talking with their children about sexuality while their children are young. If you wait until your child asks you questions about sexuality, then you have probably waited too long," says Douglas Kirby, Ph.D., co-author of the report and a senior research scientist at ETR Associates, a nonprofit health education organization in Santa Cruz, California. Rather than having a single large discussion, he suggests taking many opportunities to talk about sexuality so that it becomes a normal topic of conversation and not taboo.

When you do talk to your children, you should convey your knowledge of HIV along with your values and beliefs on sexuality, advises Dr. Kirby. If you feel that you need to brush up on your knowledge, visit your local library, family doctor, or family planning clinic for information. "Use any opportunity as a springboard to discuss sex, such as situations that arise on television or sex education classes in school," he says.

But one of the most important things that parents can do to help their children not contract HIV is to develop a close relationship, adds Dr. Kirby. Research has shown that children who feel connected to their families and schools are less likely to engage in risk-taking behavior.

ALCOHOL ABUSE
Saving Yourself–And Others

Burying your troubles in a bottle will do more than damage *your* health; it may make you a health hazard for your loved ones and other people who cross your path. Alcohol use is involved in almost half of all fatal automobile accidents and in one-third of all drowning, boating, and aviation fatalities.

Alcohol can wreak havoc on your liver, central nervous system, gastrointestinal tract, immune system, and heart. It can also impair sexual function. Abusing alcohol can cut your life expectancy by 10 to 15 years.

All those figures add up to a very good reason to prevent getting attached to alcohol. Yet the National Institute on Alcohol Abuse and Alcoholism says that more than one-half of all Americans claim that one or more of their relatives has a drinking problem. In fact, it is estimated that one in every 13 adults—that is 14 million Americans—are problem drinkers. But you do not have to become one of them.

Do You Drink Too Much?

"Alcohol problems are not an either/or phenomena," says Robert Westermeyer, Ph.D., a psychologist in private practice in San Diego, California. "People vary tremendously in terms of how much they drink, when they drink, and how drinking affects their lives. Some people drink a relatively small amount of alcohol, yet it is enough to cause significant problems in their lives. Others drink more than average and do not find important aspects of their lives to be impaired." But remember that under any circumstances, heavy drinking can take a serious toll on your physical health.

If you're unsure whether your drinking is social, Dr. Westermeyer says to consider the guidelines for moderation accepted by many counselors: If you don't drink every day—and you never have more than three drinks per day, or one per hour—you are within the guidelines. But moderation means you don't have more than 12 drinks per week. And you never drive after drinking alcohol.

"Alcohol misuse grows out of a chosen pattern of living," says Martin B. Spray, Ph.D., executive director of the Victoria Life Enrichment Society in British Columbia, Canada, which specializes in working with people who have alcohol and drug problems. "Nobody sets out to become a problem drinker, and no one really knows exactly what causes alcoholism, but some lifestyle choices are more likely than others to lead people in that direction. That does not mean, however, that it is easy for individuals to prevent themselves from misusing alcohol. Still, making different choices can help."

"To prevent abuse of or addiction to alcohol, the first and most important thing a person must do is know the difference between reasonable and unreasonable use," says Bruce S. Liese, Ph.D., professor of family medicine and psychiatry at Kansas University Medical Center in Kansas City and editor of *The Addictions Newsletter*.

Usually, the process of crossing the line from reasonable to unreasonable use of alcohol happens without the person being aware of it, Dr. Liese explains. If you understand when your drinking habits are out of control, you may be able to prevent alcohol abuse.

For some people, any amount of alcohol may raise the risk of alcohol abuse to unacceptable levels. "Some of the people who are at the greatest risk for alcohol abuse are those with a family history of alcoholism," says Michael Schiks, executive vice president of Recovery Services for the Hazelden Foundation, a nonprofit organization in Center City, Minnesota, that handles treatment of alcohol and drug problems.

No one knows exactly why it runs in families, but many scientists think that there may be a genetic component. "I can't tell you the number of people I've talked with who have alcoholism in their families who said, 'I was an alcoholic from the moment I had my first drink,'" says Schiks. Look at your family tree. If you think that you may be at high risk or if you are the child of an alcoholic, your best prevention policy may be abstinence.

Taking Control

To keep your alcohol use in check, consider these recommendations.

MAKE A MATRIX. Dr. Liese says that people who suspect that they have an alcohol problem should draw a matrix, a square with four equal-size squares inside it. Above the top left square write "not drinking." Above the top right square write "drinking." To the left side of the top left square write "advantages." To the left side of the bottom left square write "disadvantages."

Now, make lists inside the respective squares of the advantages and disadvantages of using and not using alcohol. "If you do this exercise and if you share it with others who are close to you, you will gain some real perspective on your use of alcohol and be much less likely to move into unreasonable use," says Dr. Liese.

BE HONEST WITH YOURSELF. "Only the rarest of people is able to say honestly, 'I have a problem,' and *not* be willing to do something about it," says Dr. Liese. If you are willing to admit to yourself that you may be crossing the line into unreasonable drinking, you are much less likely to do so.

BELIEVE WHAT OTHERS ARE TELLING YOU ABOUT YOUR DRINKING. "If somebody close to you complains or expresses concern about your drinking, their concern is probably valid," says Dr. Liese. It is very likely that you are drinking too much.

TACKLE THE NEGATIVES. Are you bored? Depressed? Angry a lot of the time? If you are, then you are at a greater risk for unreasonable alcohol use, says Dr. Liese, and you need to find constructive ways to deal with your emotional difficulties. As hard as it may seem, you need to make some changes in your life. "If you drink because you are depressed, have your depression treated by a doctor. If your job is lousy and you go home every night and drink, look into getting a better job," he says.

LOOK FOR SOMETHING NEW TO DO. Find people, places, and things other than drinking to entertain yourself, says Dr. Liese. Instead of going to a bar, go to a gym.

FIND FRIENDS SOMEPLACE ELSE. Most people who use alcohol unreasonably are lonely. In fact, they may be using alcohol because it provides them access to a whole network of friendships and relationships. Try taking adult-education classes or become a volunteer. Whatever you choose, figure out how to spend more time with people in nondrinking situations.

DISCOVER SPIRITUALITY. "I believe that one of the most important things that a person can do to prevent unreasonable use of alcohol is to have a strong spiritual life," says Dr. Liese. "I counsel all of my patients to have faith in something bigger than themselves. You need to find meaning in your life that is bigger than the bottle."

SEEK HELP. If you think that you have a problem and you want to prevent it from going any further, get help. Dr. Liese recommends 12-step programs such as Alcoholics Anonymous. For alternatives to the 12-step model, he suggests trying SMART (Self-Management and Recovery Training) or Rational Recovery. Look in your local phone directory for Alcoholics Anonymous. If SMART is not listed in your local phone directory, you can write to the national office at 24000 Mercantile Road, Suite 11, Beachwood, OH 44122, to get local contact information. For information on attending a Rational Recovery meeting in your area, write to the organization at P. O. Box 800, Lotus, CA 95651. There are also in-patient treatment programs all over the United States that are willing to provide information and help for people who have problems with alcohol.

Recognizing Trouble

Use this checklist to learn what constitutes alcohol abuse.
Ask yourself the following questions.

1. Do you find that you are drinking more than you
   used to?
2. Are you drinking because of difficult circumstances,
   such as stress at home or at work?
3. Are you developing a tolerance to alcohol so that you
   need to drink more to get the same effect?
4. Have you tried to cut down on drinking, but can't?
5. Do you feel guilty about drinking?
6. Do you feel angry at people who are trying to get you
   to drink less?
7. Do you drink alone?
8. Do you forget what you did while you were drinking?

Answering yes to any of these questions is an
indication that your drinking has become unreasonable
and that you may need to seek outside help to prevent
yourself from developing a more serious drinking problem,
says Bruce S. Liese, Ph.D., professor of family medicine
and psychiatry at Kansas University Medical Center in
Kansas City and editor of *The Addictions Newsletter*.

ALLERGIES
Avoid the Invaders

Xenophobia is the fear of foreigners or strangers, and the immune system of a person with an allergy is very xenophobic. It regards the miniature driftwood of everyday life—house dust, animal dander, pollen, mold—as outsiders that are sure to do some dreadful damage.

To recognize and capture these strangers, the immune system first assembles a vigilante committee of antibodies, chemicals that gang up on the strangers. Then it gathers a mob of inflammatory substances (like histamines) that try to do away with the evil intruders. If you have a common allergy with symptoms of sneezing, wheezing, watery eyes, and a clogged or runny nose, all your symptoms are the end result of your cells overreacting to the invaders.

Many medications can treat allergy symptoms, but maybe you won't need any medication if you can prevent your xenophobic immune system from freaking out in the first place. To do that, you have to keep the foreigners away from your body. Here's how.

Snagging the Villains

The first step in preventing contact with your allergens, the substances to which you are allergic, is to figure out what they are, says Robert Plancey, M.D., assistant clinical professor of medicine at the University of Southern California in Los Angeles and an internist and allergist in Arcadia.

Sometimes, common sense will tell you what is causing your allergies, says Dr. Plancey.

"Patients will say to me, 'When I'm around a cat or I touch a cat, I sneeze, my eyes itch and water, or I develop asthma, or I get hives.' Or they say, 'When I eat anything with soy in it, I get an immediate reaction. Within 30 minutes, I'm having stomach upset and diarrhea.' So, sometimes the person just knows his allergy," says Dr. Plancey.

On the other hand, maybe you don't know the cause. "Inside a house, there may be feathers and pets and house dust—and a person could be allergic to any one of those or to all three. That's when an allergy test can yield a lot of useful information," says Dr. Plancey.

"If a person is having persistent allergic symptoms, but he cannot isolate the allergen, it is a good idea to see an allergist, get tested, and find out what the allergens are," says Dr. Plancey. If you get a skin test, a tiny bit of allergen is put on your skin, and the doctor sees whether or not there is a reaction. Or you can get a blood test, called the Radioallergosorbent (RAST) test. That test is less sensitive, he says, but on the other hand, you don't have to put up with the skin reaction that you get from the skin test. Once you have the results of the test, you can plan a well-targeted strategy for prevention.

Declare War on Dust Mites

House dust is a strange recipe, a mix of castoffs from fabrics, pets, plants, and insects. But the worst component in that brew—the one most responsible for runny noses, sneezing and watery eyes—are dust mites. These microscopic, spiderlike animals are so plentiful that the population in one gram of dust—about 1/33 of an ounce—can be in the thousands. And many of us are allergic to them.

Dust mites like to hang out in bedding, carpeting, and upholstered furniture, feasting on leftover skin scales shed by people. There, they chow down and defecate. The miniature mite feces are so light that they waft into the air anytime you walk on the carpet, roll over in bed, or sit in an upholstered chair. If you have an allergic reaction to dust, it is usually the dust mite feces that are causing the problem. Unfortunately, there are no pooper-scoopers for these microscopic sneeze inducers, but you can banish dust mites from your house with the following tips.

GET ALL WASHED UP. Hot water works wonders when it comes to flushing out dust mites and their leavings. "You should change the sheets once or twice a week," recommends Dr. Plancey. "Have a washable blanket, and wash it once or twice a month. And have a washable bedspread, and wash it once a week."

He recommends washing all bedding in water over 130°F, which means that you will probably have to turn up the thermostat on your water heater. (But warn other members of the household when you do so that they don't get an unexpected scalding next time they use the hot water.)

Use chlorine bleach, which is another effective mite-killer, recommends Dr. Plancey. "Also," he says, "be sure that the sheets are really dry when you put them back on the bed because dampness fosters the growth of dust mites."

KEEP THAT SPREAD ON YOUR BED. For dust control, Dr. Plancey says that the bedspread should always be over the bed when the bed isn't being used. And when you lift off the bedspread, raise it carefully and fold it up so that you don't shake a lot of dust around the room.

MAKE WAY FOR A NEW MATTRESS. Old mattresses and

box springs are a happy home for settled-in mites. "If you have a really old mattress and box spring, it is better to just get rid of them and purchase new material," says Dr. Plancey. "When the new bedding arrives, remove the plastic carefully so that you don't introduce a lot of dust. Then enclose the bedding in plastic mattress and box spring covers." Some department stores carry the plastic covers, or you can order them from a medical supply store.

WAVE THEM OFF. "A waterbed can be an excellent way of avoiding the dust problem," says Dr. Plancey. But he cautions against letting dust collect in the frame around the waterbed or between the mattress and the frame. And be sure to wash the mattress pad frequently since dust mite colonies tend to form there, he says.

FORGO FEATHERS. Use polyester or fiberfill, rather than feather pillows, Dr. Plancey advises. Mites like to live on the detritus, or miniature layer of debris created by feathers, and the feathers themselves can be an allergen. He recommends that you don't use feather-filled quilted bedspreads for the same reason. If you want to use a quilted bedspread, choose one filled with polyester fiber.

MOVE OUT MEMENTOS. Bedding isn't the only bedroom hangout for dust mites. "You should remove everything from the bedroom that tends to collect dust," says Paul Ratner, M.D., an allergist in private practice in San Antonio. That includes stuffed animals, knickknacks, and even books.

"DE-FURNISH" YOUR ROOM. Any excess furnishings can provide landing places for mites. "I would not put heavy curtains on my windows," Dr. Ratner notes. "I would use wood shutters or venetian blinds that would be easier to clean." He also recommends taking out excess furniture that doesn't need to be in the bedroom, especially if it is upholstered. "And make sure that you clean the tops of ceiling fans," he cautions.

SWAP CLOTH FOR VINYL. Cloth lampshades are a

problem because they act as a magnet and reservoir for dust. "Vinyl is much better," says Dr. Plancey.

SHOP FOR SLICK SURFACES. When you are buying furniture, you are better off with an impervious surface, such as leather or Naugahyde, notes Dr. Plancey. These surfaces can be easily cleaned.

SCRAP THAT CARPET—OR GO FOR A TIGHT WEAVE. Choose to have hardwood floors with washable area rugs or have linoleum or tile, rather than carpet, says Dr. Plancey. "Carpets are basically condominiums for dust mites."

Any carpeting should be low-pile, and Dr. Plancey recommends replacing it every five years. "Berber carpet is much better than loose-pile carpet," he adds. "Berber has a very tight weave and very short curled pieces, whereas a cut-pile carpet is softer and higher. And the softer and higher the carpet, the more dust can fit into the spaces and be trapped at the lower levels."

CLEAR THE AIR. "The heating and air-conditioning system in the house can be very important in reducing the dust mite population," says Dr. Plancey. Baseboard radiant heat is an excellent choice because it doesn't blow dust around, he says. If you have a forced-air system, however, he recommends installing a high-efficiency particulate air (HEPA) filter on the air intake to reduce the amount of dust that enters your house.

"A HEPA filter removes 99.97 percent of the particulate matter in the size that causes allergic symptoms—down to 0.3 microns in size. They were originally designed to remove radioactive dust from Strategic Air Command shelters, so those people would be protected in case of a nuclear war. Later, this technology was released for use in manufacturing and hospitals, and ultimately became available to people in their homes. All you have to do is replace the filter every 6 to 12 months as needed, depending on usage and air quality, to keep the efficiency," Dr. Plancey says. The people who service your heating and air-conditioning should be able to install the filter.

DRY THE ATMOSPHERE. Dust mites depend on moisture for growth, so people with a dust mite allergy should keep the humidity a little lower—somewhere between 20 and 30 percent, says Dr. Plancey. Hygrometers are the devices used to measure humidity. They are usually sold at clock stores. Sometimes, you can find hygrometers at electronic supply shops at the mall, but their accuracy may not be as precise as the ones sold at clock shops. Using a dehumidifier is one way to keep humidity down. In addition, "make sure that moisture from showers and baths is exhausted to the outside with fans," says Dr. Plancey. He also advises people to use kitchen fans to make sure that steam from cooking is exhausted rather than distributed into the home.

Air-conditioning is also very helpful in reducing humidity, Dr. Plancey says. But he advises against the evaporative air coolers (also called swamp coolers) that are commonly used in the southwestern states because they can encourage the growth of invisible organisms, including dust mites.

VACATE DURING CLEAN-UP. "Vacuuming can be very effective in controlling dust mites," says Dr. Plancey, but he points out that most vacuum cleaners are inefficient and just blow dust around the house. If you have dust sensitivity, it is worthwhile to invest in a vacuum cleaner with a HEPA filter or have a central vacuum system installed, he says.

In a central system, you hook up the vacuum attachment to intake pipes in the walls, and a powerful vacuum sucks the dust into a central disposal area, usually located outdoors. But even if you have this central system, Dr. Plancey says that the house should be vacuumed by a member of the family who does not have allergies. "I also suggest that the person with allergies not be present in the house while it is being vacuumed," he adds.

WIPE UP—AND TOSS. "When you dust hard surfaces, you should use some kind of agent on the rag—Endust, furniture polish, or another dusting product that picks up the dust," says Dr. Plancey. Use a disposable rag, he advises, and when that rag is dirty, go on to the next. "You are really removing dust from the house, and not just moving it around."

DUST THE HARD-TO-REACH PLACES. "Think of the areas you normally don't think of," Dr. Plancey says. Among the hard-to-reach areas are tops of fixtures, tops of breakfronts, and the tops of grandfather clocks. Also, be sure that you do the blades of ceiling fans, or they will swirl dust around when you turn them on.

DECIMATE MITES WITH MITICIDE. "There are a variety of safe, natural substances called acarosides, such as Acarosan—made from benzoates—which are used for cutting down on dust mite growth," says Dr. Ratner. These miticides help control dust mite population, but they are not a substitute for the other precautions, he notes.

If you are using one of these products, "simply sprinkle it on your carpeting or upholstered furniture, leave it on for several hours, and then vacuum it up," says Dr. Ratner. You can purchase miticides at some large discount retailers.

When Pets Bring You to Your Sneeze

Whiskers may be a lovable cat, but he belongs to an allergy-inducing club. In fact, cats generally cause more sniffles, sneezes, and rashes than their other pet counterparts. But dogs, hamsters, and other furred pets can also wreak havoc. In fact, 15 percent of Americans are allergic to dogs or cats.

It is the proteins in the animal's dander (flakes of dead skin), saliva, or urine that are the culprits. These proteins are spread all over the house as the pet roams. Unfortunately, many people don't discover they are allergic to animals until after they have brought a pet into the home. And no one wants to part from Whiskers once the lovable cat has moved in.

"My mother, for example, would gladly have discarded her allergist before she got rid of her cats, even though she was allergic to them," Dr. Plancey says. From a medical perspective, he notes, the ideal step is to get rid of the pet. But many families just won't make that choice, he acknowledges. So here is what you can do to reduce exposure to the animal's allergens.

CLOSE OUT THE ALLERGEN. Keep the pet outdoors if you live in a part of the country where it remains reasonably warm year-round, suggests Dr. Plancey. But, he adds, if the pet is outside, anybody who touches that pet should remove their clothing before they enter the house. That way, they are not bringing the allergen into the house. And the clothing should stay out of the house until it is washed, he adds.

EXILE THE LITTER BOX. A cat's litter box is a very significant source of allergens, says Dr. Plancey. He suggests that it be put in the garage or in some other area that is separated from the rest of the house.

CREATE A RESTRICTED AREA. Another alternative, says Dr. Plancey, is to confine the pet to a certain area of the house where there is linoleum rather than carpet and where the pet doesn't have access to upholstered furniture. As long as the pet stays there, the allergen will be trapped and will be easy to remove.

SAVE THE BEDROOM FOR PEOPLE. Keep your pet off the bedding and out of the bedroom. After all, you spend six to eight hours a day there. If you keep the pets out, at least you will have an allergy-reduced environment in your home—and certainly increase your chances of sleeping better.

DON'T COUNT ON SWAPPING. "I often find that people who are sensitive to one furry animal become sensitized to another furry animal," says Dr. Plancey. "If you are sensitive to cats, you aren't likely to gain much by getting a dog, hamster, or gerbil instead. You are likely to become sensitive to those allergens with time," he notes.

FISH FOR A SOLUTION. Fish are the safest pet, says Dr. Plancey, because the only thing that a person with allergies needs to be concerned about is the growth of mold in the aquarium. Turtles, lizards, and snakes are also unlikely to be a source of allergies, although a person with allergies can become sensitized to their urine and feces.

DITCH THE PESTS THAT AREN'T PETS. Rodents can be a very significant source of allergens in older dwellings, says Dr. Plancey, so you want to get rid of mice and rats. Cockroaches, too, can cause terrible symptoms such as breathing difficulty, hay fever, itching, sneezing, nausea, and diarrhea in people who live or work in cockroach-infested buildings. Professional extermination is a very good way to approach these problems, according to Dr. Plancey.

Break the Mold

Mold might be in the refrigerator on the cheese. Mold might be in the foyer on the arrangement of dried flowers. Mold might be in the bathroom in the cracks between the tiles. Wherever it is found, mold launches tiny reproductive spores that dance on the air right into your nostrils. And those spores can cause an allergic reaction in many people. The best way to control it is to figure out ways to put mold on hold.

DRY OUT. "Avoidance of excessive moisture is probably one of the most important measures to control mold growth," says Dr. Plancey. Use dehumidifiers and keep water leaks and dampness to a minimum, he advises. If your roof springs a leak, you should not only repair the roof but also replace the wet materials as soon as possible. A major flood will mean that you have to replace all carpet and dry the damp areas as soon as possible. "In a house that has been terribly flooded," Dr. Plancey observes, "the mold contamination may reach a point where the levels are so high that a person with allergies can't live in the dwelling."

CLEAN IT RIGHT. Products containing chlorine or sodium hypochloride are very effective in killing mold spores and discouraging future growth, says Dr. Plancey. Use them on bathroom tiles and grouting and even on kitchen counters. Just make sure that a person without allergies does the cleaning and follow the label instructions when you are using strong cleaning products.

GET YOUR DUCTS SCOURED. One study showed that when people hired professionals to clean the air ducts of the heating, ventilating, and air-conditioning systems in their homes, there was a 92 percent decrease in airborne molds during the winter and an 84 percent decrease during the summer. This indicates dramatically that air-duct cleaning by a qualified commercial firm does indeed provide relief from airborne molds, one of the most common aeroallergens, says Dr. Ratner.

LET SOMEONE ELSE DO THE COMPOST. "You want to avoid compost heaps and decaying vegetation," says Dr. Plancey. "These are all sources of mold." For the same reason, he says that you should avoid going outside during and shortly after rainstorms, when mold levels are higher.

For information on preventing allergic contact dermatitis, please see Dermatitis and Eczema on page 252. For information on preventing allergic reactions to stinging insects, please see Bites and Stings on page 123. For information on preventing allergies to foods, please see Food Allergies on page 328.

ALTITUDE ILLNESS
How to Go Up without Feeling Down

Ah, adventure travel—the new style of active vacationing, where you trek in Nepalese yak pastures at the hem of a 28,000-foot peak or mountain bike over the 16,000-foot Punta Olimpica Pass in Peru.

Not your cup of exotic tea? Well, even so, there is a chance that you may want to ski at 10,000 feet in the Rockies. Clearly, high-altitude locations have their attractions and their vistas: blue skies, clear air, exhilarating views of peaks and valleys.

Once there, however, you may encounter a mountain menace that you didn't anticipate, attacking you with headache, fatigue, loss of appetite, dizziness, and insomnia. These are just a few of the symptoms of a very common (and very preventable) health problem called altitude illness.

Going Up

You don't have to be a professional mountaineer or alpine skier to get high-altitude illness. Any lowlander who travels—by plane, car, bike, ski lift, or hiking shoe—to 8,000 feet or more above sea level is at risk for the problem. In fact, some casual visitors to high altitudes might get one of the extreme forms of altitude illness, high-altitude pulmonary edema (HAPE), which is a potentially deadly accumulation of fluid in the lungs. Far from a peak experience, HAPE can attack people when they are no higher than 8,000 feet—less than two miles above sea level.

People get sick at higher altitudes for one very simple reason: The body can't get enough oxygen. That is not because there is less oxygen up there. It is because there is less *air pressure* (or barometric pressure), which usually helps move oxygen from your lungs to your blood. Standing at sea level, your blood is 95 percent saturated with oxygen. At 18,000 feet, saturation drops to 71 percent.

Some people acclimatize quickly to the lack of oxygen, but others don't. Anybody can get altitude illness, says David R. Shlim, M.D., medical director of the CIWEC Clinic Travel Medicine Center in Kathmandu, Nepal. It can happen whether you are young, old, male, female, fit, unfit, a first-time skier, or a mountaineering veteran. So if you are planning any kind of trip to the peaks, you simply need to take some basic precautions to avoid altitude sickness. Here is how not to be buried under an avalanche of physical problems when you are above 8,000 feet.

STOP HALFWAY. Let's suppose you are a sea-level dweller heading to Aspen for your ski vacation. Eager to make the most of your vacation, you go straight to Aspen, spend the next day on the slopes, eat a big dinner at a great restaurant, have a couple of drinks, stay up late dancing, and fall asleep ready for more skiing. When you wake up the next morning feeling as though you have a hangover with symptoms such as headache, loss of appetite, and nausea, it is probably not the booze that is making you want to dive back under the covers. It is likely that you have altitude illness, says Dr. Shlim. An estimated 25 percent of those who fly from sea level one day to altitudes between 6,300 and 9,700 feet the next will get the problem, according to one study.

"A good way to prevent this would be to spend one night in an intermediate elevation, like Denver, to let your body acclimatize to a higher altitude," says Tod Schimelpfenig, Rocky Mountain School director of the National Outdoor Leadership School in Lander, Wyoming. But what if you just don't have the time or patience for that? "The next best thing is to make sure that you are drinking a lot of fluids, avoiding alcohol, and taking it easy the first day on the slopes." He recommends drinking three to four quarts of water a day to prevent altitude illness.

BE WARNED BY WARNING SIGNS. Whatever your eagerness to ski, Schimelpfenig cautions, you should always be aware of the symptoms of HAPE, the accumulation of fluid in the lungs that can threaten your life. "If you have shortness of breath, tightness in your chest, and a cough and you feel very weak and tired, you should immediately seek medical care," he says. "Some skiers who ski hard the first day, feel kind of lousy, ski hard the second day, then develop some fatigue and shortness of breath from the accumulating fluid in their lungs, have died from HAPE."

GET AN ALTITUDE ADJUSTMENT. If you are a trekker on mountain trails, experts offer other cautions to help you avoid acute mountain sickness—another name for altitude illness. "Make a rational ascent that gives your body time to acclimatize," says Dr. Shlim. In other words, take your time; don't try to make it to the summit in one day.

Though different people adapt to altitude at different rates, the CIWEC Center gives this general rule: Above

10,000 feet, average no more than 1,000 feet of ascent per day.

PLAN EXTRA SLEEP-OVERS. Spending some nights at intermediate altitudes helps your body acclimatize, says Schimelpfenig. Start out your trip in the mountains by sleeping two to three nights at or below altitudes of 10,000 feet, he advises. Sleep *an extra night* at a new altitude for every 2,000 to 3,000 feet you have gained. In other words, if you walked from 10,000 to 11,000 feet on Wednesday and from 11,000 to 12,000 feet on Thursday, you would spend Thursday night *and* Friday night sleeping at a campsite near 12,000 feet.

GO WITH A GOOD GROUP. "Over the past 10 years, 80 percent of altitude sickness deaths in Nepal occurred in organized trekking groups, even though only 40 percent of people trekked in an organized group," says Dr. Shlim.

Those deaths were from HAPE and from a condition called high-altitude cerebral edema (HACE), which is caused by diffused water leaking into the brain. Trekkers in these groups may not reveal their symptoms because they don't want to be left behind, especially on the "trip of a lifetime," Dr. Shlim explains. Or, he says, an inexperienced trek leader may minimize the importance of the symptoms of altitude illness because he doesn't want to have to split up the group. If you are enrolling in a group for an adventure vacation, make sure that the leader has a strategy for those who develop altitude sickness, he advises. If you develop telltale symptoms and need to stay behind, you want to make sure that the group has the resources to split off porters and guides to get you back safely. "It's not an issue of saving your vacation," he says.

BE REALISTIC. Although it is not clear why exertion at a high altitude contributes to the development of altitude illness, preliminary data suggests that certain substances are released into your body after heavy exertion that may contribute to the condition. Factors such as carrying a heavy pack; tackling a steep trail; walking over snow, ice, or unsteady ground; and being out of shape may all work together in one way or another to trigger altitude illness in some people, says Dr. Shlim. Knowing yourself and your limitations is the key to preventing its onset.

CONSIDER MEDS CAREFULLY. A prescription medication called acetazolamide (Diamox) speeds the process of altitude adjustment. Although you should always avoid taking medications when possible, acetazolamide is a remarkably safe drug to use, says Dr. Shlim. It does have side effects, however, which consist of tingling in the hands, feet, and sometimes lips. Increased urination has also been noted in people taking the drug. Since acetazolamide is a sulfa drug, it should be avoided by those who are allergic to sulfa medications.

Dr. Shlim recommends acetazolamide as a preventive medication for people who have had altitude sickness in the past. It can also help if you have to make a rapid forced ascent into high altitudes, like flying into the city of Lhasa in Tibet, which is at 12,000 feet.

STOP WHEN YOU SEE SYMPTOMS. "In every instance of severe altitude illness that I've treated, this rule was violated. Stay at the same altitude until your symptoms completely go away. Once your symptoms are completely gone, you have acclimatized and it is okay to continue ascending. If your symptoms are getting worse while resting at the same altitude, then it is mandatory to descend, whether it is day or night," says Dr. Shlim.

And it is *always* okay to head down if you have symptoms, he notes. In fact, as soon as you descend, you will get better faster. Above 8,000 feet, the first sign to watch out for is headache, says Dr. Shlim. The next symptoms signaling danger include fatigue, loss of appetite, and nausea, which then progresses to vomiting.

If you are hiking with someone who seems confused and starts to stagger, assume that person is in considerable danger and should receive care immediately. And it is always important to remember that if any of your hiking companions complain of these symptoms, stop the ascent until that person recovers, warns Dr. Shlim.

ALZHEIMER'S DISEASE
Brain Maintenance Is the Key

The heartbreaking mental deterioration of Alzheimer's is all too familiar to many of us. It starts with small memory lapses and can progress to an inability to recognize the images of familiar human faces. It is a cruel end.

But isn't Alzheimer's an inevitability for some people? No, say some scientists—prevention is possible. There are a number of practical and simple ways—many of them discovered in just the last few years—to lower your risk of developing Alzheimer's disease.

Cherish Your Brain

The anti-Alzheimer's plan takes care of the old gray matter. Objective number one is to prevent mini-strokes. "Strokes seem to put people at risk for Alzheimer's," says David Snowdon, M.D., director of the Nun Study at the Sanders-Brown Center on Aging at the University of Kentucky in Lexington.

Are Anti-Inflammatories Anti-Alzheimer's?

In a 15-year investigation of 1,686 people, those who took for two years nonsteroidal anti-inflammatory drugs (NSAIDs), such as ibuprofen, naproxen (Aleve), and other drugs used to treat pain, had a 50 percent lower risk of developing Alzheimer's than people who didn't take the drugs. And those who took them for longer than two years had an even lower level of risk. Why do NSAIDs help prevent Alzheimer's?

According to the study, protein plaques found in the brains of people with Alzheimer's are there because of an inflammatory response of some kind. The study's researchers at the National Institute on Aging and Johns Hopkins University recognize that inflammation may play a heavy role in the Alzheimer's disease process. That is why anti-inflammatory medication shows so much promise in preventing, or at least slowing, the progression of the disease.

That's the good news. The bad news is that daily use of NSAIDs is not without risk. They can cause ulcers and impair kidney function, so you must talk with your doctor before taking them to help prevent Alzheimer's.

Dr. Snowdon isn't talking about the devastating kind of stroke that causes paralysis and speech problems, but the small, silent mini-stroke that can occur without a person even knowing it has happened. Dr. Snowdon and his colleagues studied 102 nuns, ages 76 to 100, tracking their mental abilities while they were alive and conducting autopsies on their brains after they died. The researchers discovered that the women who'd had mini-strokes, as revealed in the brain autopsies, were 11 times more likely to have had symptoms of dementia than those who had no strokes.

"Taking the proper measures to reduce the risk of stroke is something we can all do now," says Dr. Snowdon. First, you will want to eat low-fat foods and exercise regularly, measures that also reduce your risk of Alzheimer's. Also, here are some other tactics that are targeted at avoiding stroke.

CONSIDER TAKING A LOW-DOSE BABY ASPIRIN DAILY. There is powerful evidence that this can help keep the blood flowing freely, says Dharma Singh Khalsa, M.D., president and medical director of the Alzheimer's Prevention Foundation in Tucson, Arizona, and author of *Brain Longevity*. But before you get on a regular dose of aspirin, consult your doctor, especially if you have any stomach-related problems, he cautions. Aspirin can sometimes irritate the stomach and aggravate an ulcer.

REDUCE BLOOD PRESSURE. Lowering blood pressure can also decrease the risk of stroke. Researchers tracked the blood pressure of nearly 400 men and women beginning at age 70. Fifteen years after the study began, only a few in the study had developed Alzheimer's disease. But those who did had higher diastolic blood pressure (that's the bottom number) than those who didn't.

While it is too early to say for sure that high blood pressure causes Alzheimer's disease, it is never too early to keep your blood pressure in check. Your doctor can tell you whether your blood pressure is in the healthy range. If you need to put a lid on it, here is how, according to Dr. Khalsa.

- Maintain a healthy weight.
- Exercise regularly, with a little aerobic exercise and a little weight training.
- Ask your doctor if you should reduce your sodium intake.
- Be faithful about taking your high blood pressure medication.

Why Alzheimer's Is Like Heart Disease

Alzheimer's disease is like heart disease in one very important way: It is affected by lifestyle, according to Dr. Khalsa. In his book *Brain Longevity,* he offers some self-care commandments for maintaining maximum mental function.

CONSUME A LOW-FAT DIET. One study reviewed World Health Organization literature on Alzheimer's and diet and found that countries with the highest fat intake also had the highest incidence of Alzheimer's, said Dr. Khalsa. You should limit the percentage of fat in your diet to approximately 20 percent of total calories. Cut back on red meat and high-cholesterol foods, but chicken and fish are okay. "And certain fish like tuna, trout, mackerel, and salmon are rich in omega-3 fatty acids," he says. "They are good for the brain because they insulate nerve fibers."

TRY VITAMIN E. Research suggests that moderate Alzheimer's disease can be reversed with supplemental doses of vitamin E. Dr. Khalsa recommends 400 to 800 IU (international units) per day. If you are considering taking amounts above 200 IU, discuss this with your doctor first. One study using low-dose vitamin E supplements showed an increased risk of hemorrhagic stroke.

TRY COENZYME Q₁₀. Dr. Khalsa suggests taking 100 milligrams a day of this supplement, which he calls a neuroprotector of brain cells. "It also adds energy to the brain because it works in the 'power plants' of the cell, the mitochondria," he says.

GO WITH GINKGO. Ginkgo improves memory because it increases circulation throughout the body, including the brain, says Dr. Khalsa. He recommends 120 to 240 milligrams per day. Check with your health-care practitioner before taking ginkgo if you are taking any MAO-inhibiting drugs (depression or anxiety medication) because of possible interactions.

TRY SERENITY. "Stress produces a chemical in the blood called cortisol, which is toxic to the memory center of the brain. It is like battery acid; it eats away at it," says Dr. Khalsa. "That's why I recommend taking some time for peace in the morning." He feels that the best way to do this is to meditate, read the Bible, or pray, depending on your religious or spiritual orientation. "When we are talking about maintaining optimal levels of brain health and preventing our brains from deteriorating as we age, there is nothing better than stress management or meditation," he says.

GIVE YOUR BRAIN REGULAR WORKOUTS. Dr. Khalsa offers three different kinds of exercises in his brain-boosting program.

1. Mental exercise. Research has shown that older people can create new connections between brain cells by keeping their minds active. In one study, one group of seniors rode stationary bikes while reading, and another group simply rode. Interestingly, the reading group showed improved memory that the nonreading group didn't, says Dr. Khalsa. The type of mental stimulation doesn't matter. "Reading, learning a musical instrument, learning the computer, doing jigsaw puzzles—whatever you want to do," he says.

2. Aerobic exercise. Even if you just take a walk for 20 minutes, three or four times a week, you are getting enough aerobic exercise to make a difference. "This increases positive brain chemicals and helps people maintain high levels of emotional wellness, which is very important because depression can lead to memory loss," Dr. Khalsa says.

3. Breathing and flexing exercises. Dr. Khalsa believes that these can help with the ancient art of brain regeneration. "Simple breathing and

flexing exercises, such as those found in yoga, improve attention and increase what is called global brain energy," he says. The most basic breathing and flexing exercise is to straighten the spine while you slowly inhale (mildly arching) and then round the back while you slowly exhale. As you do this, pick up the pace so that you are exerting yourself. You can do this in a chair or while sitting on the floor.

ANAL FISSURES
Avoid the Strain and Pain

The pain was so bad that I told my wife I was going to the emergency room. . . ."

"We all know about the pain and humiliation. I found myself delaying treatment for years. When I finally did get treated, turns out it didn't work. . . ."

"The pain and bleeding grew more and more bothersome, appearing with every daunting trip to the bathroom. . . ."

Those are the words of three people who are part of an anal fissure self-help group on the Internet and who are intensely familiar with the mental and physical costs of this condition. Given the pain explicit in their words, it is easy to understand why they would never wish this condition on anyone, not even their worst enemy.

An anal fissure is a painful and sometimes hard-to-heal tear in the lining of the anal canal, the cylindrical tube at the end of the rectum.

While women over 60 and children under 10 are

the most common victims of anal fissures, anyone can get this condition.

Why do they happen? The cause of chronic anal fissures and the reasons for their failure to heal remain unclear, says one scientific report. But there are doctors who think that the cause is obvious. "Most patients who develop anal fissures also have chronic constipation," says William B. Ruderman, M.D., a practicing physician at Gastroenterology Associates of Central Florida in Orlando.

Since constipation is easy for most people to prevent, why not do so if it might also prevent this painful condition? Here are some suggestions.

FIBER UP TO FIGHT FISSURES. "Constipation is the most common cause of anal fissures," agrees Randolph Steinhagen, M.D., associate professor of surgery at Mount Sinai Medical Center and a colon and rectal surgeon in New York City. He recommends a high-fiber diet, which, besides bran, includes lots of fruits, vegetables, beans, and grains.

A Danish study lends support to the high-fiber recommendation. In the study, Danish doctors divided 75 patients who had a history of the condition into three groups. The doctors gave high-fiber supplements to the people in the first group; the second group received medium-fiber supplements; while the third, the control group, received a placebo—a dose that looked like a fiber supplement, but wasn't. Only 16 percent of the high-fiber group got anal fissures again. In the medium-fiber and placebo groups, however, about 60 percent of the patients got fissures.

GULP DOWN THE WATER. "When you are eating more fiber, it is also very important to drink lots of liquids," says Dr. Steinhagen. "Without sufficient water, the fiber can become very thick and make constipation worse." He recommends eight eight-ounce glasses a day.

TRY A FIBER SUPPLEMENT. If you have been eating a lot of fiber and drinking plenty of water but you are still

An Apple a Day Recipe

High-Fiber Chili

Beans are an outstanding source of fiber, which helps to relieve constipation. This simple vegetarian chili has 10 grams of fiber per serving—that's almost half of the recommended daily amount. Dried seasonings make it flavorful and quick.

2 tablespoons olive oil
1 large onion, chopped
1 clove garlic, diced
2 red bell peppers, chopped
1 small fresh or canned jalapeño chile pepper, seeded and finely chopped (wear plastic gloves when handling)
1 can (28 ounces) crushed tomatoes

½ cup vegetable broth or water
½ cup bottled salsa
2½ teaspoons chili powder
1 teaspoon ground cumin
½ teaspoon dried basil or oregano
1 can (19 ounces) kidney beans, rinsed and drained
1½ cups corn

Warm the oil in a large saucepan over medium heat. Add the onion and garlic. Cook for 3 minutes, or until soft. Add the bell peppers and chile pepper. Cook for 4 minutes, or until soft.

Add the tomatoes, broth or water, salsa, chili powder, cumin, basil or oregano, and beans. Bring to a boil. Reduce the heat to medium-low and simmer, stirring occasionally, for 10 minutes, or until the mixture has thickened slightly. Add the corn and simmer for 8 minutes.

Makes 4 servings. Per serving: 410 calories, 5 g. fat, 10 g. fiber constipated, maybe you need some extra help in the fiber department. "When a patient tells me, 'I eat a lot of fiber, but I'm still constipated,' I suggest a fiber supplement," says Dr. Steinhagen.

Among his recommendations are Metamucil or Konsyl—both of which are psyllium-based high-fiber supplements—or Citrucel, which uses methylcellulose as its source of fiber.

"If you take a spoonful of, say, Metamucil every day, and you find that your stool is softer and your bowels move more easily, that is an indication that you are not getting enough high-fiber food," says Dr. Steinhagen. As for taking the supplements daily, they are safe if you follow the directions, he says. "They are not laxatives or stimulants, which can damage your digestive tract. They just add more fiber into your system."

GET THE FIBER WITHOUT THE GASES. To avoid one possible side effect of fiber supplements, extra gas, Dr. Steinhagen says to start with small amounts of the supplement and gradually work up to the recommended amount. Some of his patients have told him that they prefer Citrucel because it produces less gas than the rival psyllium-based supplements.

DON'T LET THE FIBER THICKEN. If you do need a fiber supplement, make sure that it doesn't get clogged up inside your digestive tract. Dr. Steinhagen tells his patients to take the fiber supplement by mixing a heaping spoonful in a glass of water or juice. He also tells them to drink a full glass of water right afterward. "This ensures that there is enough water so that the fiber doesn't thicken," he says.

CHOOSE AN EASY WAY. If you don't like the taste of powdered fiber supplements, you may be tempted to take fiber pills instead, but Dr. Steinhagen doesn't think the pills work as well. For those who can't stand the taste of the supplements, he recommends the product Perdiem Fiber. "You don't have to mix this product with water," he says. "You just put a spoonful of the granules in your mouth and swallow them with a full glass of water, and that tends to go down easier. It doesn't have the sawdust consistency of the fiber supplements."

Noting that the Perdiem product comes in two forms, Perdiem and Perdiem Fiber, Dr. Steinhagen recommends the latter because it doesn't contain senna, which is a laxative.

Get a softer stool. If his patients prefer to prevent constipation with a stool softener, even though the fiber supplement is likely to be more effective, Dr. Steinhagen suggests Colace. This over-the-counter product keeps more water in the stool, making it softer.

For some people, a stool softener is easier to take than fiber supplements, Dr. Steinhagen acknowledges. "If people tell me that they just can't take Metamucil or another fiber supplement and Colace works for them, that's fine."

Prevent a fissure encore. Fissures heal, but they also tend to come back again. To prevent a fissure from returning, be sure to maintain your high-fiber diet, says Dr. Steinhagen.

ANAL ITCHING
Toward a Better Ending

Doctors call it pruritis ani. It is a fiendishly irritating itch, usually worse at night, in one of the body's most tender and hard-to-scratch spots. Large, protruding hemorrhoids—the kind called prolapsing—can sometimes cause the itching, and so can a yeast infection. But anal itching can be prompted by nothing more serious than irritating foods or tiny cracks in the anal skin.

To make sure that the itching is a minor-league problem, first have a medical examination to be certain that there aren't any significant health problems. A doctor can quickly rule out a prolapsed hemorrhoid or an anal fissure (a tear in the anal canal), says Randolph Steinhagen, M.D., associate professor of surgery at Mount Sinai Medical Center and a colon and rectal surgeon in New York City. But even after those problems are ruled out, you are still left with the threat of future itching.

DON'T PASS THE HOT SAUCE. "A common dietary cause of anal itching is hot, spicy foods," says Dr. Steinhagen.

A spice like cayenne pepper is an irritant, as you probably realized if you have ever felt that hot, burning sensation all around your mouth. Red pepper and mustard are also major offenders. Such spices are not digested, and since the lining of your anal canal is similar to the lining of your mouth, the spices perform an encore before they exit. Or, as Dr. Steinhagen puts it, "If it's irritating in, it's irritating out."

CANCEL THE COFFEE. It is the caffeine that is the culprit, according to Dr. Steinhagen. So while you are skipping the coffee, also consider a boycott on tea, chocolate, and any other beverage or food with a lot of caffeine. Any caffeine-containing substance can cause anal itching.

FIND OUT WHAT IS BEHIND IT ALL. To discover which foods are bothering you, Dr. Steinhagen says to pay careful attention to what you eat—perhaps by keeping a food diary—and to what the effect is a day or two later. Once you have a suspect, eliminate it from your diet and see if the itching stops. In addition to spicy irritants and caffeinated beverages, other possible culprits are acidic foods like tomatoes and alcohol. But the list is much longer. "Anal itching can be caused by almost any food," he says.

SKIP THE TOILET PAPER. For someone who has a tendency to develop anal itching, dry toilet paper is like sandpaper, says Dr. Steinhagen. It can easily cause the anal irritation that leads to the itching. Instead, he suggests cleaning yourself with soap and water. "Of course, that is not always practical," he says. "So use baby wipes, like Huggies Natural Care, instead of toilet paper."

Embarrassed about hauling a big box of wipes with you to the bathroom? Not to worry. Dr. Steinhagen suggests buying a pocket dispenser so that you don't have to carry around a big box. "Refill it every morning and take it with you," he suggests.

One caution: Some of these moistened wipes may contain alcohol, which can further irritate the skin of the anus. So check the ingredient list to make sure that the product you buy is alcohol-free.

WASH UP BEFORE BED. Anal itching is often worse at night. You can prevent that problem, however, by washing your anus with soap and water at the end of the day, even if you haven't moved your bowels since the morning. "A lot of sweat and moisture accumulates in that area, and sometimes a little bit of fecal residue, all of which can be very irritating, especially if there are small cracks in the skin," says Dr. Steinhagen.

ANEMIA
Take Care of Those Red Blood Cells

Your red blood cells are your body's transit system for oxygen, shipping that crucial component to every cell. When you have anemia, you have too few of these oxygen shippers, and you are likely to feel very tired. In effect, you are being suffocated from the inside out. Even when the symptoms aren't dramatic, too little oxygen pumping throughout your body undermines your health in countless ways.

Anemia has many causes, and sometimes there is nothing you can do to prevent it. Some types of anemia, like sickle-cell, are genetic. Others are a consequence of another disease. But the most common types of anemia are caused by a factor that you *can* control: your diet. You need to get iron, protein, and other vitamins and minerals to help support the function of red blood cells that carry oxygen to your tissues. Iron is especially important—but you also need other nutrients to make sure your cells *absorb* the iron.

An Apple a Day Recipe

Vitality Pasta

Clams are a rich source of blood-building iron. Plus, they are low in fat and easy to fix. Here, clams and a fresh tomato sauce jazz up pasta.

1 tablespoon olive oil
2 pounds tomatoes, chopped
1 onion, chopped
3 cloves garlic, thinly sliced
2 tablespoons tomato paste
8 ounces rigatoni, ziti, or penne pasta
1½ cups fat-free chicken broth
½ cup chopped fresh basil or parsley
2 teaspoons dried oregano
½ teaspoon hot-pepper sauce
3½ dozen littleneck clams, scrubbed

Warm the oil in a large nonstick skillet over medium heat. Add the tomatoes, onion, garlic, and tomato paste. Simmer over medium heat, stirring occasionally, for 20 to 30 minutes.

Meanwhile, cook the pasta in a large pot of boiling water, according to the package directions. Drain.

Stir the broth, basil or parsley, oregano, and hot-pepper sauce into the tomato sauce. Set the clams atop the sauce. Cover, increase the heat to high, and cook for 6 minutes, or until the clams open. Discard any unopened clams.

Serve the clams and sauce over the pasta. If desired, remove the clams from their shells first.

Makes 4 servings. Per serving: 357 calories, 6 g. fat, 70% of Daily Value of iron

The Anti-Anemia Menu

Here is how to keep your red blood cells booming by properly consuming.

PUMP ENOUGH IRON. "The best source of dietary iron is red meat," says M. T. Atallah, Ph.D., associate professor of nutrition in the department of nutrition at the University of Massachusetts in Amherst. But if you are trying to cut back on red meat, emphasize spinach, potatoes, tofu, grain products, and beans in your diet. They are iron-rich foods.

DRINK AN ABSORBER. Have a glass of orange juice along with your meals, recommends Dr. Atallah. "The vitamin C in the juice will increase your body's absorption of iron from plant foods."

BEWARE OF THE BLOCKERS. A number of dietary factors can block the absorption of iron, says Bessie Jo Tillman, M.D., a doctor specializing in wellness and preventive medicine with a private practice in Redding, California, and author of *The Natural Healing Cookbook*. Calcium is one, so she says not to take your iron supplement with milk, which is high in calcium, whether it is whole, low-fat, or skim. Coffee and tea, with their high concentrations of caffeine, can also block iron absorption.

PUT FOLATE ON YOUR PLATE. Folate, a B vitamin, is another nutrient necessary for the production of healthy red blood cells. And not everybody gets enough. "Folate is found primarily in fresh fruits and vegetables, and people who eat a lot of canned or prepackaged foods can become deficient," says Louise Schneider, M.D., medical director of Brigham and Women's Primary Care Associates in Norwood, Massachusetts. Elderly people who live alone and don't want to cook for one person and college students who eat a lot of junk food are two groups especially at risk for anemia caused by folate deficiency.

This type of anemia doesn't take long to develop— about six months of poor eating can set the stage. Dr.

Schneider suggests that a few servings of fresh fruits and vegetables every day is the best bet for prevention. If you can't bear brussels sprouts, consider taking a daily nutritional supplement with 400 micrograms, the Daily Value of folic acid (the supplemental form of folate).

BE ALERT ABOUT B$_{12}$. Your body needs vitamin B$_{12}$ to create red blood cells. B$_{12}$ is found in red meat, chicken, fish, eggs, and dairy products, but not in plant foods. Most of us get plenty, but super-strict vegetarians who don't eat any nonvegetable foods are at risk for a deficiency of vitamin B$_{12}$—and for anemia. The solution is to take a daily nutritional supplement that contains at least six micrograms, the Daily Value of B$_{12}$, says Dr. Atallah.

DON'T OVERDO THE COCKTAILS. "People who drink alcohol in excess are at risk of developing anemia," says Dr. Schneider. Alcohol, she explains, is a direct toxin to the bone marrow, the factory for red blood cells, and can shut off production. How much alcohol is too much? "Moderate drinking is one or two drinks a day," she says. If you are beyond that, cut back on the booze, she suggests.

PAUSE IN YOUR POUNDING. Oddly enough, repeated pounding on the body—on the feet of a marathoner or the hands of a musician who plays the bongo drums for hours a day—can destroy red blood cells and cause anemia. "All of the tiny red blood cells in the tiniest blood vessels of the body, the capillaries, can get ruptured from repeated contact," says Dr. Schneider. A nutritional supplement with 18 milligrams of iron, the Daily Value, will supply enough of the mineral to guarantee an adequate level of new red blood cells to replace those that are destroyed, she says.

Managing Menstrual Loss

"Iron-deficiency anemia is most commonly caused by menstrual blood loss," says Louise Schneider, M.D., medical director of Brigham and Women's Primary Care Associates in Norwood, Massachusetts. "Menstruating women develop anemia if they don't have an adequate iron intake to replace the iron in the blood they are losing every month."

Here are some tips to help compensate for monthly iron loss.

GET SOME EXTRA. Food is the best source of iron, but Dr. Schneider also suggests that every menstruating woman take a daily nutritional supplement that contains between 18 and 25 milligrams of iron. Don't take large amounts without your doctor's supervision because iron overload may be a problem for some individuals. And be sure to keep iron supplements out of the reach of children, she warns.

HAVE A WITH YOUR IRON. To help reduce heavy menstrual flow and the risk of iron-deficiency anemia, load up on vitamin A, says Bessie Jo Tillman, M.D., a doctor specializing in wellness and preventive medicine with a private practice in Redding, California, and author of *The Natural Healing Cookbook*. She suggests this regimen: 60,000 IU (international units) of vitamin A per day for one month; 30,000 IU per day for the second month; and 10,000 IU per day for a month after that. Following the third month, she recommends staying on a maintenance dosage of 10,000 IU every other day. If a heavy flow returns, repeat the rotational routine starting back with 60,000 IU.

Caution: Since levels of vitamin A over 15,000 IU can be toxic, Dr. Tillman strongly advises that you check with your doctor before you begin this regimen.

ANKLE SPRAINS
Pain Preventers for People at Play

Whether it is your ankle, knee, wrist, finger, shoulder, or some other joint, it only takes a sudden twist or overextension to cause a sprain. From this momentary action, ligaments can stretch or tear, causing swelling, tenderness, black-and-blue coloring, and most notably, terrific pain. In more severe forms, sprains can put you out of commission for two months or more.

The ankle is the most common location for a sprain, with good reason. It can move in almost any direction, which makes it simultaneously a great asset to human mobility and an easy joint to injure. Because your ankle can move in so many angles, it takes many muscles, tendons, and ligaments to make it work, says Peter Bruno, M.D., associate professor at New York University School of Medicine in New York City and team doctor for the New York Knicks.

"Mother Nature made just a few errors in the construction of the human body, one of which is that the strongest ligaments in the ankle are on the inside, and the weaker ones are on the outside," says William Roberts, M.D., co-director of MinnHealth SportsCare in White Bear Lake, Minnesota. That is why it doesn't take much to sprain your ankle.

To combat this design dilemma, Dr. Roberts and Dr. Bruno offer the following tips.

KEEP FIT. Being in good shape is like taking out sprain insurance, says Dr. Roberts. Fit muscles respond better in situations that can lead to sprains—like when you have a bad landing while stepping off a curb. A physically fit person also generally reacts faster in these kinds of situations, many times heading off a sprain at the pass, he explains.

TAKE STRENGTHENING TO THE EDGE. You don't need to invest in barbells to get stronger ankles, says Dr. Bruno. "Stand with both heels off the edge of the bottom step of a flight of stairs, using a rail or wall to balance. Slowly let your heels drop below the level of the step and then slowly rise up on the balls of your feet." Your own body weight will provide an ample workout for the leg muscles that keep your ankles on course.

GO IN CIRCLES. Ankles that are flexible have an increased range of motion, which can contribute to your overall sprain-prevention plan, says Dr. Bruno. To give your ankles a good stretch, take turns rotating each foot in small circles, he says.

PRACTICE YOUR ABCs. For another ankle-challenging stretch, Dr. Bruno recommends alphabet writing. "I have patients write the alphabet on the floor with each big toe, keeping the writing leg as stationary as possible to really get the ankles moving in all kinds of angles," he says. It is as effective as the circle exercise and a little more challenging.

DON'T WORK OUT WHEN YOU ARE WEARY. Getting in shape lowers your sprain risk, but give yourself a chance to learn the right way to play the game, Dr. Roberts advises.

What to Do If You Get a Sprain

No matter how hard you try to avoid it, you can still end up with a sprained ankle. Here is the standard first-aid procedure to help prevent the pain and swelling. It is known as the RICE treatment plan, says William Roberts, M.D., co-director of MinnHealth SportsCare in White Bear Lake, Minnesota.

Rest. Completely rest the affected joint area for at least the first 24 hours.

Ice. Apply an ice pack wrapped in a towel to the injured area for 20 to 30 minute sessions, three to four times daily, for as long as you have swelling. (When all swelling is gone, you can switch to a heating pad for 20 to 30 minute sessions, three to four times daily, until the pain is gone.)

Compression. Wrap the joint area with a compression bandage, being careful not to cut off the circulation.

Elevation. Rest the joint in a raised position until the pain and swelling begin to lessen.

Over-the-counter analgesics, like Tylenol, can help ease some of the initial pain, says Dr. Roberts. If your doctor recommends them, over-the-counter anti-inflammatory medications may be in order after two or three days. Your doctor may also fit you with a brace or clamshell case (also called a functional splint).

Getting back into exercise slowly is an important part of sprain recovery, and it can help you avoid reinjuring the joint. With a mild sprain, you can probably go on a stationary bike or swim in a pool once the pain and swelling begin to diminish, says Dr. Roberts. But it is best to consult your doctor before you take up energetic exercise again.

"Beginners in any sport shouldn't learn or practice when they are tired. You will only get sloppy with your form, which will increase your chances of getting a sprain," he says. Instead, go into each training session fresh and attentive. Your ligaments will thank you for it.

AVOID THE OBVIOUS PITFALLS. Running at night or on bumpy ground is asking for trouble, says Dr. Roberts. Run during the day and stay on level surfaces, with obstacles that you can see clearly.

DRESS YOUR FEET FOR THE OCCASION. To some degree, high-top athletic shoes can be helpful in protecting against ankle sprains. Hikers in rough terrain, for example, can benefit from boots that support the ankle, says Dr. Roberts. Basketball players with troublesome ankles might also find high-top sneakers helpful. Some studies have even shown that "low-top" sneakers worn with protective or support braces can reduce the risk of ankle sprains. Dr. Roberts recommends the lace-up ankle braces available at most sporting goods stores.

ARTHRITIS
Invest in Joint Protection

Your bones hang out in a lot of joints. Knee joints. Hip joints. The joints in your fingers and the joints in your toes.

Wherever bones meet, there is also cartilage, a rubbery, protective layer that ensures your joints bend smoothly and painlessly. But even cartilage cannot do this tremendous job alone. A thin membrane called the synovium provides fluid that lubricates the moving parts of the joint. When the cartilage wears out or the synovium becomes inflamed, the result is generally a case of osteoarthritis or rheumatoid arthritis.

In osteoarthritis, the cartilage can be eroded so much that bone does rub on bone. This type of arthritis develops gradually over a lifetime as a simple result of the wear and tear placed on your joints over the years. Very few people escape some degree of osteoarthritis, though the severity varies a great deal. As a matter of fact, if you are over the age of 50, you are likely to have at least one joint affected by osteoarthritis. Osteoarthritis affects men and women almost equally and is by far the most common type of arthritis—16 million Americans have it.

In rheumatoid arthritis, damage to the synovium is at the source of trouble. Doctors and researchers are not absolutely sure what causes it, but most think that rheumatoid arthritis is a disease in which the immune system actually attacks certain tissues in the body, including those that connect the joints and the synovium.

Rheumatoid arthritis begins with swollen, red, stiff, and painful joints, but it may progress until scar tissue forms in the joint or, in extreme cases, until the bones actually fuse together. Seventy-five percent of the two million people with rheumatoid arthritis in the United States are women. The disease can hit as early as the teen years.

Shielding Joints from Pain

Preventing arthritis is not an exact science, but physicians have discovered a few ways to lower your risk. Here's how.

DON'T WEIGHT AROUND. "The single most important measure anyone can take to prevent osteoarthritis of the knee is to lose weight if they are overweight," says James M. Fox, M.D., an orthopedic surgeon and knee specialist with the Southern California Orthopedic Institute in Van Nuys and author of *Save Your Knees*.

Extra weight puts extra stress on your knees. If you are 10 pounds overweight, for example, you put 60 pounds per square inch of extra pressure on your knees every time you take a step. "That extra pressure can slowly but surely erode the cartilage in your knees, leading to arthritis," cautions Dr. Fox.

A study has clearly supported the theory that weight loss weighs in on the side of prevention. In the study, overweight women who lost 11 pounds or more over a 10-year period decreased their risk of developing osteoarthritis of

Exercising Your Prevention Options

Investing a little time in developing a good weight-bearing, low-impact exercise and stretching plan can add up to great results when it comes to staving off arthritis pain. Strong muscles help protect the joints from wear and tear, and the movement keeps joints flexible.

Any kind of stretching is good as long as you do not bounce, which can lead to a muscle pull, says Emil Pascarelli, M.D., professor of clinical medicine at Columbia-Presbyterian Medical Center in New York City. Try to hold a slow, steady stretch for 15 to 20 seconds, then relax and repeat. It is best to limber up by stretching before any exercise, especially running and walking. But it is also a good idea to stretch each day. Ask your doctor to teach you stretches that focus on potential arthritis trouble spots, such as the knees or the lower back.

Take a good, long walk at least three times a week or participate in a step-aerobics or low-impact exercise routine for maximum results, recommends Dr. Pascarelli. There is no proof that running is bad for the joints, but remember, it may aggravate an injury if you already have one. Remember to check with your doctor before starting a new exercise program.

the knee by 50 percent. (For tips on managing your weight, see Overweight on page 593.)

PUT ON THE BRAKES WITH VITAMIN C. Vitamin C may not be able to prevent osteoarthritis, but research shows that it may help prevent the rapid progression of the disease. In a Boston University study of 640 people with and without knee osteoarthritis, those participants eating the most vitamin C had three times less disease progression than the people eating the least amounts of that vitamin, the least being about 120 milligrams (the equivalent of two oranges) per day. These results suggest that the people eating more vitamin C lost less cartilage and were likely to develop less pain during the eight years of the study than did those people who didn't get as much of the nutrient.

Study leader Tim McAlindon, M.D., assistant professor of medicine at the Boston University School of Medicine, theorizes that an antioxidant vitamin like vitamin C provides important protection when the inflammation from arthritis is in full swing.

Vitamin C and other antioxidants earn their name by helping to prevent the aging process, which is accelerated by cell-attacking free radicals that come from oxygen molecules. Inflammation is believed to release cell-attacking free radicals that do more damage to the joint, unless antioxidant vitamins are there to stop the radicals from doing harm. So while antioxidant vitamins may not stop you from getting arthritis, they may prevent the disease from becoming severe.

FILL UP ON FISH. Research conducted in Seattle found that 324 women eating two or more servings of baked or broiled fish a week (mostly salmon) had a lower risk of developing rheumatoid arthritis. Researchers believe that it is the omega-3 fatty acids that help make the difference. Other fish high in omega-3's include anchovies, bluefin tuna, bluefish, canned white (albacore) tuna, herring, mackerel, rainbow trout, sablefish, sardines, and swordfish.

DON'T HURT—TRY HRT. If you are a postmenopausal woman, you probably already know that taking estrogen during hormone-replacement therapy (HRT) helps protect you from osteoporosis, the bone-thinning disease that can shatter hips and spines. Researchers at the University of California, San Francisco, have discovered that estrogen may help protect bones from another disabling bone disease—osteoarthritis. The scientists, who were led by Michael C. Nevitt, Ph.D., assistant adjunct professor of epidemiology and biostatistics, examined the hip x-rays of

4,366 women. All of the women were age 65 and older. They discovered that the women taking estrogen had a 38 percent lower risk of developing any osteoarthritis in their hips than women who weren't taking the hormone. Even better, estrogen-takers had a 46 percent lower risk of developing moderate to severe hip arthritis.

ASTHMA
Keeping Your Airways Open

Asthma is a disease on the rise. Since the early 1980s, the number of Americans with asthma has increased by a whopping 61 percent. Why this is so isn't exactly clear. Doctors can only agree that there are many causes, ranging from air pollution to allergies.

Asthma, which may appear in childhood or develop in adults, is a chronic inflammatory disease that affects the lungs and bronchial tubes (the body's airways). When an asthma attack is under way, the muscles around the bronchial tubes tighten, causing them to narrow as they become inflamed and swollen. The overworked glands within the tubes then begin to produce mucus, which begins to clog the body's breathing apparatus. Attacks can be mild, limited to a shortness of breath, or life-threatening if the person experiences suffocation.

The first and most important step to protecting yourself from asthma and keeping your lungs in good shape is steering clear of potential lung irritants. Common culprits are indoor pollutants such as dust mites, fumes from cleaning products, mold, cockroaches, and animal dander, especially from cats and dogs. Seasonal allergen exposure, as well as air pollution, can worsen asthma, according to Stuart Stoloff, M.D., clinical associate professor of family and community medicine at the University of Nevada School of Medicine and a physician in Reno.

Putting together an effective prevention plan means taking a good look at your environment—inside and out—and finding ways to clear the air.

An Anti-Pollution Solution

In 1977 and again in 1992, scientists from Loma Linda University in California, the University of Arizona in Tucson, and the U.S. Environmental Protection Agency gave more than 3,000 nonsmokers a questionnaire about their respiratory health. During those 15 years, 106 of those people developed asthma. The scientists then calculated the amount of air pollution that each person in the study had been exposed to during that time period. They concluded, "Ambient air pollution exposure was significantly related to the development of asthma in adults." In other words, the more pollution you are exposed to, the more likely it is that you will get asthma.

So what do you do? Don a gas mask whenever you go outside? Or just hold your breath? Well, protecting yourself can be a lot easier than that. Here are some clues that could make for breezier travel through your airways.

COUNT ON E AND C. Recent research has found that adults with asthma who take daily supplements of vitamins E and C were able to prevent some breathing difficulties. These findings are significant because both vitamins are antioxidants—that is, they help prevent damage to living cells. "Our results show that a combination of antioxidant vitamins can benefit people with asthma who are sensitive to air pollutants," concluded Carol Trenga, Ph.D., lead author of the study that was conducted at the University of Washington School of Public Health and Community Medicine in Seattle.

In this preliminary study, 17 people who were prone to asthma attacks took 400 IU (international units) of vitamin E and 500 milligrams of vitamin C every day for five weeks. The researchers believe that these vitamins help reduce lung damage from air pollution and that the vitamins work better together than they do on their own. Taking them could help you breathe a lot easier, according to this study. A few of the fruits and vegetables high in vitamin C include oranges, kiwifruit, grapefruit juice, and broccoli. Food sources highest in vitamin E are nuts and vegetable oils, including wheat germ oil, soybean oil, and corn oil. If you are considering taking amounts of vitamin E above 200 IU, discuss this with your doctor first. One study using low-dose vitamin E supplements showed an increased risk of hemorrhagic stroke.

WATCH OUT AT WORK. The American Lung Association estimates that about 15 percent of all cases of adult-onset asthma are occupational—that is, they are caused by something you encounter at work. What causes occupational asthma? All kinds of substances can do it, from grain dust to the waste of laboratory rats. The asthma develops as a reaction to irritants like chemicals, gases, or fumes in the workplace. If you are at risk for this kind of exposure, your best prevention is to eliminate the asthma-causing substance from your area. Talk to your supervisor about taking steps to create a safer work space and consider wearing a breathing mask (available at most hardware stores) while on the job, Dr. Stoloff says. You can also reduce exposure by increasing ventilation. If none of these methods work, call your local office of the U.S. Occupational Safety and Health Administration (listed in the blue pages of your telephone directory) for further information.

STAY SMOKE-FREE. Exposure to cigarette smoke, whether it is firsthand or secondhand, can worsen asthma, says Dr. Stoloff.

You can even help protect unborn children from developing asthma later in life. "Children whose mothers smoke throughout their pregnancy and during the first year of life are at a much greater risk for becoming asthmatic," says Dr. Stoloff.

Turn Off the Triggers

Shutting out air pollution is only part of the battle. Unfortunately, there are lots of other common household items that also lead to lung trouble. Here are some steps that may help to prevent future attacks.

ELIMINATE EVERYDAY ALLERGENS. According to researchers Thomas Platts-Mills, M.D., Ph.D., and Melody C. Carter, M.D., children who develop allergies to "foreign proteins" in their homes are at an increased risk of asthma. Among the most common sources of indoor allergens—foreign proteins—are house dust mites, which are most often found on bedding, stuffed toys, and carpets; cat and dog dander; cockroach droppings; and fungus. (To avoid exposure to these allergens, see Allergies on page 50.)

MONITOR YOUR MUNCHIES. Doctors who treat asthma warn that the aggravation of food allergies can also set off an asthma alarm. Among the foods likely to cause problems are nuts, chocolate, and eggs, along with foods that contain sulfites, such as beer, wine, and some salad bar items. So read labels, check with restaurant managers, and most important, pay attention to your body so that you know when you are getting a reaction to a certain food. Then you can eliminate it from your diet.

CLEAN WITH CARE. Even though it is important to keep household dust and dirt to a minimum, doctors recommend that you proceed with caution when using household chemicals or solvents. Some common products known to cause asthma problems include paints and paint thinner, bleach, spray starch, spray furniture polish, and room deodorizers. Wear a mask while cleaning, be sure your rooms are well-ventilated, and minimize your exposure.

ATHLETE'S FOOT
Keep 'Em Dry

The fungi that cause athlete's foot are moisture-lovers. They hang out in the shower, by the swimming pool, and on the locker room floor. If they hitch a ride on your feet, they get very comfy in the damp, airless spaces between your toes—though they will settle for settling on the bottoms and sides of your feet. The infection of athlete's foot can be rough. On top of intense itching, the skin may turn white and soggy and may peel, or be raw, red, and inflamed. Sometimes you will even see cracking and oozing.

Athlete's foot is quite common, but there is no reason that it should be. Here is how to prevent the infection.

WASH YOUR DOGS. "Wash your feet at least once a day," says Jerome Z. Litt, M.D., assistant clinical professor of dermatology at Case Western Reserve University School of Medicine in Cleveland and author of *Your Skin: From Acne to Zits*. Every time you wash well, you are flushing away some of those itch-producing fungi. "When you bathe, get in the toe webs and make sure that they are clean," he advises.

USE A TOUGH SOAP. Sometimes the bacteria on your feet, coupled with the fungus, will start athlete's foot more readily. Try an antibacterial soap instead of a perfumed kind, says Dr. Litt.

DRY FROM WEB TO TOE. This may be the most important anti–athlete's foot strategy, according to Dr. Litt. Dry the whole foot. Toe webs, too. Think Sahara desert.

CHOOSE THE RIGHT SHOES. Wearing light, ventilated footwear in the summer—when hot, moist weather increases the risk for athlete's foot—can help prevent the problem, according to Thomas Helm, M.D., assistant clinical professor of dermatology and pathology at the State University of New York at Buffalo and director of the Buffalo Medical Group Dermatopathology Laboratory in Williamsville. He recommends wearing canvas boat shoes or sandals.

BE SHOD IN THE LOCKER ROOM. Wearing sandals in the locker room can help shield you from an infection, says Dr. Helm.

STAY AWAY FROM PLASTIC SHOES. "They are very bad for you because they don't breathe and the moisture just sits in them," Dr. Helm says. Kids, in particular, need to be careful about their choice of shoes: "I'm seeing a lot more athlete's foot in kids now that everybody is wearing high-top sneakers that don't allow the air to circulate."

GO NATIVE. Sometimes the best strategy is no shoes at all. "Walking barefoot can be very helpful in preventing athlete's foot," says Dr. Helm. Unlike the locker room, where your bare feet are at risk, a clean environment like your home is a perfect place to air your toes. "Heat, sweat, and moisture aggravate the problem, and a cool, dry environment is helpful," he points out. "Obviously, you don't want to walk around outside in your bare feet because of rusty nails and other risks. But around the house—absolutely."

DIVIDE TO CONQUER. "To prevent and cure athlete's

Don't Let One Fungus Lead to Another

Often athlete's foot can be caused by an obnoxious neighbor—fungal infections in the toenail beds. "The way you can think of it is this: If your neighbor has dandelions all over his lawn, you will have dandelions, too, because their seeds will come over into your yard," says Thomas Helm, M.D., assistant clinical professor of dermatology and pathology at the State University of New York at Buffalo and director of the Buffalo Medical Group Dermatopathology Laboratory in Williamsville.

According to Dr. Helm, a fungal nail infection can seed the surrounding skin of your feet with the fungus. Fungal nails are often yellowed, crumbly, thick, brittle nails, he explains. If you have this symptom, see your doctor—he will prescribe either oral or topical medications to cure the infection. Once the fungal infection is cured, you will cut your chances of getting athlete's foot, says Dr. Helm, because your nails will no longer be a constant reservoir for new infections.

---

foot, keep your toe webs separated, particularly the web of the little toe (where athlete's foot is prominent)," says Dr. Litt. To do that, he suggests putting lamb's wool or any cotton material—"not cotton batting, but an old piece of linen shirting or sheeting cut into one-inch squares"—between the toes. "You can also use small corks and cut them in half," he says. "If you keep your toe webs open, you can't be tripped up by athlete's foot."

POWDER THOSE PUPPIES. "Using an antifungal foot powder every day is the best thing that you can do to prevent athlete's foot from recurring," says Dr. Helm. "One brand that I recommend is Zeasorb AF, if it's not on your drugstore shelf, ask your pharmacist to order it. It absorbs the moisture and has an antifungal ingredient that kills the organisms. After your morning shower, dry your feet carefully, sprinkle a little on your feet, put your socks on, and you're ready to go."

SLATHER ON A LOTION. "People who are prone to athlete's foot might also want to use a good medicated foot lotion or cream containing micronazole or clotrimazole. Check the product labels. These antifungals work very well to stop the itching and burning sensations that accompany athlete's foot," says Dr. Helm. To help prevent flare-ups of fungal activity, he recommends that you ask your doctor about a lotion called Lac-Hydrin, which is available in prescription form. The lotion contains alpha hydroxy acids (AHAs), which remove the dead skin that is a perfect medium for the growth of the fungus.

BACK PAIN
Don't Damage Your Disks

A healthy back is pain-free and allows you to do your work, your daily activities, and your recreational activities without any discomfort."

That's the definition of a healthy back provided by Kenneth Light, M.D., medical director of the San Francisco Spine Center. But many Americans won't find that definition in their personal health dictionary—their backs *hurt*. Every year, six million Americans see a doctor because of back pain. That puts back pain at number three on the ailment list, behind colds and respiratory problems. Dr. Light estimates that 90 percent of all Americans will have back pain at some time in their lives.

What's the reason for all that pain? Its source is the spine, which is a stack of bones called vertebrae and, between them, cushions of cartilage called disks. Disk problems cause 99 percent of all back pain, says Dr. Light. When the disks are damaged, they develop rips, and little sections of the disk pop out and press on nerves. Or a disk can collapse, causing the vertebrae to shift.

Disks inevitably suffer some wear and tear as you age, and there is nothing you can do about that. But there is a lot of potential damage to disks that you can avoid. Many backaches are triggered by lifestyle factors like being overweight and having poor posture, so many such backaches are preventable, according to Dr. Light. Try these tips to keep your back in shipshape.

DON'T PLAY HERCULES. If an object seems too heavy or awkward, don't lift it alone, get help. Listen to your body's intuition about what you should and shouldn't lift, says Dr. Light. "Sometimes, when you are about to lift a heavy object, a fleeting thought may cross your mind that your back is too weak. Respect that hunch. In general, if you already have back pain, never lift anything over 40 pounds."

LIFT IT RIGHT. Once you have decided that you can lift an object, move as close to it as possible. Bend at your knees. "Keep your back straight as if you have a broomstick attached to your spine," says Dr. Light. Lift with your leg muscles, while tightening your stomach muscles. Breathe normally. Maintain a balanced position throughout the lift by keeping your feet shoulder-width apart. And don't twist your spine during the lift. "Keep your body squared to the object at all times," he says.

BELT UP FOR SAFETY. If your job requires frequent lifting, Dr. Light suggests that you wear an abdominal belt: "It pulls in the abdomen, helps support the spine, and reminds you to lift correctly." Weight lifters wear these belts to protect their backs during exercise. The belts are available at sporting goods stores and most drugstores.

KEEP YOUR ABDOMINAL MUSCLES STRONG. "The stronger your abdominal muscles, the less likely you are to injure your spine," says Dr. Light. When your abs are strong, they push up the abdominal contents, forming a cylinder of fluid that lifts and takes weight off the spine.

To strengthen your abdominal muscles, Dr. Light suggests abdominal crunches, a special kind of no-stress situp. To do a crunch, lie on your back on a carpeted floor or an exercise mat with your knees bent, feet flat on the floor, fingertips lightly touching the sides of your head, and elbows out to the sides. Tilt your pelvis so that your lower back stays flat on the floor, and then curl your body up so that your head and shoulders come off the floor. Keep the crunch slow— take three seconds to lift your head and shoulders, pause for a second with your abs fully contracted, and then take three seconds to lower your body. Dr. Light suggests that you do these crunches for a 10-minute session every day.

USE A STOOL WHEN YOU STAND. "If you are standing a lot, it is best to bend one knee and put it on a stool—that helps relax your back," says Dr. Light.

BE A GOOD-TO-YOUR-BACK DRIVER. Don't lean forward with your upper body when you are driving, cautions Hope Gillerman, a board-certified teacher of the Alexander Technique in New York City. The Alexander Technique is a method for improving movement and posture. "You want your neck, shoulders, and back to be as free of tension as possible," she says. Slide your hips all the way into the back of the car seat and lean into the seat back. And position your seat so that you can hold the steering wheel comfortably. If you are too close, you will have to hunch your shoulders to hold the wheel. If you are too far away, you will have to round your upper back to reach it.

DO A SIDEWALK WINDOW-CHECK. "When you are walking by a shop window, look at your reflection and check out how you are moving," says Gillerman. "If you are leaning forward, stop walking. Then bring your weight back on to the heels of your feet and feel the ground solidly underneath your whole foot."

THEN WATCH YOUR STRIDE. After you have checked out your reflection, continue to pay attention to your posture as you start walking again. If you are slumping and tucking your hips forward, let your hips shift slightly backward and unlock your knees. While you are moving, think about lengthening your spine, like an arrow pointing up away from the ground, says Gillerman.

WEAR WELL-CUSHIONED SHOES. "Any shoe with a cushioned sole and good arch support can help prevent back pain," says Dr. Light. But high heels are the worst shoe for your back. "They exaggerate the lumbar curve—the curve in the lower part of your back—and that can cause back pain," he says.

PICK THE RIGHT CHAIR FOR PROLONGED SITTING. "Sitting for prolonged periods can aggravate your back," says Dr. Light. "You should find a chair with a firm cushion on the seat and with armrests. Both of these will help support the spine."

GIVE YOUR BACK SWEET DREAMS. Choose a firm mattress that supports your spine, says Dr. Light. He recommends two possible sleeping positions to prevent back pain. Either sleep on your back, with pillows under your knees, or turn on your side, with your knees curled up and a pillow between your legs. Both positions help to ease back pain by taking the pressure off the vertebrae, he explains.

BONE UP ON SUPPLEMENTS. "If you are a woman over the age of 40, you should consider taking calcium supplements," says Dr. Light. He recommends that women take a 150-milligram supplement every day. Calcium helps protect your spine and the rest of your skeleton from osteoporosis, the disease of eroding and weakening bones. In older women especially, there is the risk that vertebrae may fracture if they are weakened by osteoporosis. But calcium can help prevent the disease.

If you have a family history of osteoporosis, Dr.

Light suggests talking to your physician about hormone-replacement therapy, which can also help protect the spine.

DON'T SMOKE. "Smoking decreases circulation to the disks and causes them to degenerate sooner," says Dr. Light.

BAD BREATH
The Trouble Is on Your Tongue

The most common fixes offered for bad breath just don't work. Why? The most familiar preventives fail for a simple reason: They don't treat the real cause, says Harold Katz, D.D.S., director of the California Breath Clinic, which is based in Los Angeles.

"Bad breath has nothing to do with digestive problems or poor oral hygiene," says Dr. Katz. "It's caused by anaerobic bacteria that thrive in a low-oxygen environment and live within the papilla, or fibers, of your tongue." These bacteria will sometimes extract the sulfur out of the amino acids in proteins and convert it into odorous sulfur compounds, like hydrogen sulfide.

Some people are prone to bad breath. If you are genetically equipped with heroic papilla, also known as large tongue fibers, the bacteria have more space to live. And frequently, older people produce less oxygen-rich saliva, thereby creating the more-anaerobic atmosphere that the bad bacteria love. But anybody can get blighted by bad breath, says Dr. Katz.

The Best Ways to Block the Ill Wind

The prevention trick is to minimize the buildup of the sulfur-leaching bacteria. Here's how.

BRUSH YOUR TONGUE. Not only should you keep a civil tongue, you should keep a clean one as well. Every time you brush your teeth, give your tongue a good bristling, too. You might consider trying a device called a tongue scraper, says Dr. Katz. Available at drugstores, the scraper cuts down on bacteria by doing just what its name suggests.

CLEANSE YOUR PALATE. "Make sure that you brush the roof of your mouth," says Dr. Katz. When you talk and eat, your tongue touches your palate, where it deposits the bad breath bacteria. Give the inside of your cheeks a good once-over while you are at it.

MINIMIZE MILK PRODUCTS. The more protein available to the bacteria, the worse the bad breath problem. According to Dr. Katz, the ideal anti–bad breath diet would have no high-protein foods, including meat and fish. "But people can't cut all of those foods out of their diets," he says. "So if they just cut down on dairy products, that will definitely help."

CUT COFFEE. The high acid levels in coffee, both caffeinated and decaffeinated, create more bacterial activity. "If you can reduce your coffee intake by half," says Dr. Katz, "you will definitely prevent some degree of breath odor."

KEEP POSTNASAL DRIP UNDER CONTROL. Another way to thwart the bad breath bacteria is to cut off their food supply, which you do when you block postnasal drip. Mucus has the exact same amino acids that are found in high-protein foods, explains Dr. Katz. "In people who have postnasal drip, the mucus settles in the back of the throat, which touches the back of the tongue, and provides a food source for the bacteria. Controlling allergic reactions and other causes of postnasal drip will help keep bad breath under control."

A Backhanded Test

You cannot smell your own breath, says Harold Katz, D.D.S., director of the California Breath Clinic, which is based in Los Angeles. "Physiologically, humans are designed that way," he says, "because if we could smell our breath, we would not be able to smell anything else since our mouths are close to our noses."

He points out that when your breath seems to smell sweet to you—after you have chewed on a breath mint, for instance—it might not smell sweet to someone else. That's because you are not really smelling your breath, you are tasting it. And smell and taste are two different senses. So your breath may *taste* sweet to you but smell sour to everybody else.

Here's how to assess your breath. "Lick the back of your hand, let it dry for a few seconds, and then smell that," says Dr. Katz. "You can smell the salts that comprise the sulfur compounds on the back of your hand. Smell the hand you licked, and you are smelling your own breath."

SKIP THE BREATH MINTS. "Breath mints and chlorophyll tablets do not work. They may even make your breath smell worse," says Dr. Katz. Most breath mints contain sugar, and the anaerobic bacteria use that sugar for energy. Sugar-containing gum does the same, he says.

DRINK PLENTY OF WATER DURING THE DAY. Dr. Katz tells his patients to drink 8 to 10 eight-ounce glasses of water a day because it thins out the saliva. When your saliva is thicker, he says, the bacteria harbored there have a richer food source. But if you really want to thin out that saliva, says Dr. Katz, you have to drink *water*—not soda or some other type of liquid, which won't have the same effect.

DON'T USE MOUTHWASH. Standard mouthwashes are full of alcohol, says Dr. Katz, and that dries up the saliva in your mouth, making your breath worse. "Saliva is rich in oxygen, which keeps your mouth healthy and fresh," he explains. "Anaerobic bacteria thrive in a dry, low-oxygen environment and produce more sulfur compounds. Commercial mouthwashes dry your mouth and definitely don't help your breath. In fact, they make it worse." Instead, if you want to freshen your breath, rinse your mouth out with water, he says.

SIDESTEP STRESS. When you are under stress, your bad breath becomes worse, says Dr. Katz. That's because the body's fight-or-flight response to stress rushes blood to the large muscle groups and away from your mouth, making your mouth drier, which, in turn, leads to bad breath. Deep breathing—slowly inhaling and exhaling—can help control that stress by calming your body, Dr. Katz says. But you have to inhale through your nose and exhale through your mouth. "If you use deep breathing to control stress and you inhale through your mouth, you dry off the surface of your tongue, which will worsen the bad breath."

BEDSORES
Ease the Pressure, Ease the Pain

No one wants to sit or lie in one place all the time, but some people don't have a choice. Like a victim of a spinal cord injury who is confined to a wheelchair. Or a person with arthritis so severe that he can't get out of bed.

More than two million of those immobilized Americans have another kind of injury to deal with: bedsores. Also known as pressure ulcers, bedsores are the result of a bone pressing constantly against some part of the body that's on a mattress or a wheelchair. That bone could be the sacrum (located at the base of the spine) or the hipbone. It could even be the heelbone. But almost all bedsores can be prevented, says Carol Jones, R.N., a board-certified enterostomal therapy nurse and a member of the ostomy-wound team at the Methodist Hospital of Indiana in Indianapolis. If you or someone you love is confined to a bed or a wheelchair, here is what to do.

ADD AN EXTRA LAYER. Cover the bed mattress with an air mattress or foam padding that is dense and at least four inches thick. "There are a lot of mattress overlay devices that put cushioning between the bony surface and the bed surface," says Jones. "And these devices can help prevent pressure ulcers." For people in wheelchairs, she suggests an air or gel cushion.

The egg crate paddings that were once used to prevent bedsores are not effective, she says. "These are not dense enough, so the bone would still lie on the surface of the mattress, and there would be tissue destruction."

TURN EVERY TWO. Reposition the person in bed every two hours, says Jones. That way, you ensure that the pressure isn't always on one area.

HELP OUT THE HIPS. One problem with repositioning—for example, turning a person from his back onto his side—is that a person lying on his side can get a pressure ulcer from his hipbones. To prevent this, turn the person on his back partway toward his side, say, 30 degrees (a full turn onto the side would be 90 degrees). Then support his back with pillows so that he stays in the new position. This way, the pillow takes some of the weight.

SEPARATE THE KNEES AND ANKLES. Pressure sores can also form when an ankle is pressing on an ankle, or a knee on a knee. Use pillows to keep them separated, says Jones.

LOWER THE HEAD OF THE BED. People who are propped up in bed tend to slide down, says Jones. And if the person is older, the skin on the back and the buttocks can stretch and tear, creating an ulcer. This phenomenon is called shearing, and it can be prevented by keeping the head of the bed at the lowest angle possible and limiting the time it is elevated.

DO A "PUSHUP." People who are confined to wheelchairs but still have the use of their upper bodies should do a slight pushup every four to five minutes on the arms of the wheelchair to relieve the pressure, says Jones.

CLEAN WITH CARE. A person in bed should be cleaned

regularly, says Jones, since excess moisture—from elimination or perspiration—can weaken the skin. But clean gently, using a mild soap. And afterward, apply a moisturizer so that the skin doesn't become too dry. "Keep the skin lubricated, but not saturated," she says.

BELCHING
Stopping the Upwardly Mobile

When we are breathing just right, the air flows in and out of our lungs nicely and quietly. The soft intakes of nourishing breath are followed by gentle whispers of exhalation. Chronic belching, however, is a great big glitch in the system.

What causes those embarrassing blares? Too much air in our stomachs, says Gary Lichtenstein, M.D., associate professor of medicine and director of the inflammatory bowel diseases program at the University of Pennsylvania School of Medicine in Philadelphia. If we eat too fast, drink too fast, or just gulp air as we talk and breathe, too much air finds its way to our stomachs instead of to our lungs. Something has to give—and it does. The buildup of air in our stomachs is relieved by a less-than-charming expulsion of air.

An occasional belch after a savored meal is one of life's small pleasures. But chronic belching is both painful and frowned upon in polite society. Here is how to prevent the blares.

SWALLOW LESS. Most people who are chronic belchers are also chronic swallowers. Some people just swallow more than others—often because of anxiety. If you belch a lot, see if you can deliberately cut down on your swallowing frequency. Sometimes, the excessive swallowing habit is not hard to break. Just being aware of it will do the trick, says Dr. Lichtenstein.

PUT YOUR FORK IN LOW GEAR. Many chronic belchers get too much air in their stomachs because they gobble their food or drink liquids too fast, according to Dr. Lichtenstein. "Take your time, chew slowly—and don't talk while you are chewing," he says. Talking can escort even more air into your stomach.

DROP THAT SILVERWARE. To help yourself go slow at supper, put your fork down for a beat or two between bites, says Dr. Lichtenstein. By taking the time to put your utensil down, you are giving your mouth more time to chew the food properly. As a result, it is less likely that you will swallow the air that causes belching in the first place.

ENLIST YOUR CHILDREN. Ask your family members to point out if you are wolfing down your food, suggests Dr. Lichtenstein. If you have teenagers, they will be only too happy to criticize your behavior.

MAKE A HOME MOVIE. Dr. Lichtenstein says that it can be very instructive to have someone in your family videotape you while you are eating. Because once you *see* how fast you are eating, it will help you slow down. Most chronic belchers are surprised by how quickly they down a meal.

COMPARE YOURSELF TO OTHERS. Five minutes into dinner, compare how much food is left on your plate to how much is on other people's, suggests Dr. Lichtenstein. This will tell you if you are eating too quickly and will help you slow down.

BOYCOTT CARBONATION. Shake a can or bottle of carbonated beverage and open it, and you will get a very graphic idea of what happens in your stomach when you drink the stuff—the bubbles want out. If you battle belching, belay the effervescent soft drinks, says Dr. Lichtenstein.

BEWARE BEER. Suds have lots of bubbles. Beer can make you belch, especially if you drink it out of a can. But if you have to have your brew, Dr. Lichtenstein suggests pouring it into a glass beforehand.

AVOID AIRY FOODS. Any food that has lots of air in it may make you belch more. If you are troubled by belching, stay away from soufflés, ice cream, omelets, and whipped cream, says Dr. Lichtenstein.

TAKE CARE OF YOUR ESOPHAGEAL SPHINCTER. Didn't know you had one, did you? This particular sphincter is the little valve located at the bottom of your esophagus that keeps food and gas from backing up on you. Certain foods make it malfunction. If you are a chronic belcher, avoid these sphincter relaxers: fried foods, high-fat meats, caffeine, chocolate, and peppermint, to name a few, notes Dr. Lichtenstein.

LET IT COOL OFF. When you sip very hot liquids like coffee, you also swallow a lot of air, says Roger Gebhard, M.D., a gastroenterologist and professor of medicine at the University of Minnesota School of Medicine in Minneapolis. Instead of sipping while it is piping hot, let the beverage cool a bit first, and then drink it.

DON'T GUM UP YOUR WORKS. When you chew gum, you tend to swallow a lot of air, says Dr. Lichtenstein. So if you are a chronic belcher, you should try to kick the habit, he says.

RETIRE YOUR ASHTRAYS. Smoking causes belching, too. "Smoking is inhaling air," says Dr. Lichtenstein. And when you inhale a lot of air, you are sure to swallow a lot of it, leading to belching.

EASE YOUR ANXIETY. Some air swallowing is caused

by nerves. A relaxation technique like meditation can have a beneficial, calming effect, says Dr. Gebhard. Or if you are in a stressful situation, try holding a pencil between your teeth, he suggests. It is hard to swallow air when your mouth is partially open.

BINGE EATING
Beating Diets and Despair

Binge eating happens often but is a well-kept secret. Many people go on hidden eating binges, wolfing down thousands of calories several times a week. They usually binge in secret because they're ashamed of being out of control. Often, each binge leaves them feeling guilty and disgusted.

Psychologists say that binge-eating disorder can be prevented. Although it is best addressed with a psychiatrist or therapist, there are self-help steps that you can take to prevent the occasional indulgence in Rocky Road ice cream from turning into a pattern of overeating.

Ditching Deprivation Diets

"Binge eating is a reaction to dieting," says Paula Levine, Ph.D., director of the Anorexia and Bulimia Resource Center in Coral Gables, Florida. We habitually forgo food, get hungry, and start bingeing. "A lot of people with binge-eating disorder have a history of yo-yo dieting and have gained and lost their extra weight 10 times," she says.

Calorie restriction creates the exact physical and psychological conditions for a binge, according to Craig Johnson, Ph.D., professor of clinical psychology at the University of Tulsa and director of the eating disorders program at the Laureate Psychiatric Clinic and Hospital in Tulsa, Oklahoma. "That's why we always say to our patients, 'The best defense against binge eating is to *eat*.'"

But Dr. Johnson doesn't mean pigging out, of course. He is talking about reshaping our eating habits. And here's how.

MAKE A MEAL PLAN. "The first order of business for anyone who is binge eating is to normalize the eating behavior. Create a meal plan and stick with it," says Dr. Johnson. "Eat several times a day at very predictable times and at a calorie level that will guard against ever feeling too hungry."

LEGALIZE ALL FOODS. Binge-eaters have to get over the dieter's habit of thinking of some foods as good and others as bad, says Dr. Levine. "Most binge-eaters are 'good' during the day—eating things like salad and rice cakes—and 'bad' at night, bingeing on french fries and ice cream." To normalize their eating habits, she says, they have to see all foods as legal, as long as the foods are eaten in moderation.

START THE DAY WITH FLAKES AND FRUIT. Always have breakfast—no matter what. If you binge and still feel stuffed when you wake up in the morning, eat breakfast anyway. "No matter what you have done the night before, have a normal breakfast," says Dr. Levine. "That way, you start the day off on the right foot instead of continuing the deprivation/binge cycle."

The Eating-Emotion Nexus

Binge eating is rarely a reaction to physical hunger alone. It is also a way to deal with emotional emptiness, says Dr. Levine. "Bingeing is a comfort and an escape. Like alcohol or drugs, it is a way of dealing with unwanted emotions— loneliness, sadness, frustration, depression, anxiety, low self-esteem—by not feeling them." Dr. Levine and other psychologists often use cognitive-behavioral therapy techniques to replace negative beliefs with healthier thoughts and to short-circuit the binge cycle.

The therapeutic process is often complex and demanding. But here are a few simple tips that may help you help yourself.

SIT QUIETLY. Sometimes sitting and getting in touch with your feelings is the best coping skill, says Dr. Levine. "This is not the activity that is most appealing when someone is in the initial stages of controlling binge eating. But I talk to binge-eaters a lot about just sitting quietly in the room. You can sit with your feelings, be with your feelings, feel your feelings—instead of using the food to push them away." You learn that feelings are not that scary, that it is not so terrible to have negative feelings like frustration or confusion or jealousy or hatred.

REACH OUT AND TOUCH SOMEONE. "I tell people to do something that involves social interaction," says Dr. Levine. "Call a good friend or reach out to someone you haven't seen in a long time. Bingeing itself is such an isolating experience—it is done in secret, it produces the feeling that you are shameful and unlovable—that getting connected is one of the best ways to help stop bingeing. The more connected you become to people, the less connected you will need to be to food."

GET UP AND GO. Moderate exercise is a great antidote to the bingeing urge, says Dr. Levine. "Go to the gym. Go for a walk. Go for a swim." With the heart pumping and the lungs working, you are less likely to sink into a pre-binge gloomy mood.

REMEMBER YOUR STRENGTHS AND TALENTS. People who binge tend to *become* the binge-eating disorder, says Dr. Levine. "They say to themselves, 'There's nothing good about me.' They think binge eating is their whole identity. Well, that's not true. People who binge should remind themselves every day that they are interesting, talented, and lovable people." If you are a good parent, good friend, good bridge player, or good golfer, take pride in the pluses that are also part of you.

BITES AND STINGS
Beware of Bowser, Bees, and Serpents

On the way to Oz, Dorothy and her companions had to worry about lions and tigers, and bears—oh, my! In our daily lives, the most threatening creatures are dogs, insects, and snakes.

Beware those canine teeth. Every 40 seconds, someone in the United States seeks medical care because of a dog bite. In most cases, the attacking dog isn't some vicious stray. "You are most likely to be bitten by your own dog or a dog owned by a friend or neighbor," says Randall Lockwood, vice president of training initiatives for the Humane Society of the United States in Washington, D.C. Research shows that 85 percent of dogs that attack are neighborhood or family dogs and that fewer than 15 percent are dogs with unknown owners.

Because the villain is most often the neighborhood or household pooch, you can protect yourself and your kids from becoming victims. "Dog bites are almost 100 percent preventable," he says.

Canine safety requires two steps, says J. Michael Cornwell, D.V.M., a veterinarian at the Glencoe Animal Hospital and the department of veterinary preventive medicine at Ohio State University, both in Columbus, and the developer of a dog-bite-prevention program for children. First, teach your dog not to be a biter. Second, teach yourself and your kids how to avoid provoking a dog inadvertently. "Very few dogs will bite you without some provocation," he says. Here are hints from the experts on keeping your canine threats at bay.

DON'T PICK A FIGHTER. "If someone with kids called me and asked me what breed to purchase, there are certain breeds I would steer them away from—dogs that have been trained to be police dogs or guard dogs or fighting dogs," says Dr. Cornwell.

Stay away from dogs that are known to be aggressive, agrees Ron Berman, a forensic examiner and a canine behavioral consultant and trainer. Be careful when choosing any of the herding dogs, such as German shepherds, Australian shepherds, and Australian cattle dogs. They have a tendency to be more aggressive because they are bred to protect the flock. Also, be particularly careful with dogs bred for hunting or fighting, such as Akitas and Rhodesian Ridgebacks, or with any dogs bred for protection, including Rottweilers and komondors, he says.

CHOOSE A GENTLE BREED. If you have kids, select a breed that is easygoing. Labrador retrievers and golden retrievers have a steady temperament. Poodles make nice companions for kids, says Dr. Cornwell.

"SOCIALIZE" YOUR DOG. You want your dog to be familiar with touch and with people, says Berman. "When your dog is a puppy, touch it a lot, and touch it in all different places. Stick your hands where children will stick their hands," he says. "That really gets a dog used to people." If a dog has fun with kids as a puppy, he will be at ease with kids later on. But it is important to supervise those early interactions, according to Berman, because small children sometimes unwittingly do things to provoke dogs.

SEND YOUR POOCH TO SCHOOL. Obedience school is a good idea. "Though we call it obedience school, it is really about socialization," says Dr. Cornwell. "It teaches your puppy to respond favorably to human beings and to other dogs."

INCREASE THE EXERCISE. If a dog doesn't get enough physical activity, it builds up a lot of tension and may become aggressive. "Very often, a dog that bites is an underexercised dog," says Berman. You want to keep your dog as relaxed as possible, and the more exercise dogs get, the more relaxed they are, according to Berman.

IF THE DOG GROWLS, TAKE IT TO THE VET. If your puppy is under three months of age and growls threateningly, you should take him to a veterinarian for behavior counseling, says Dr. Cornwell. If your veterinarian doesn't do behavior counseling himself, he can steer you to people who do. "Any time a dog growls, that's a threat," says Berman. A canine behavioral consultant can work with the dog to help remedy the situation.

DON'T LET YOUR PET DO THE BABYSITTING. A child under the age of five should never be left alone with a full-grown dog, says Dr. Cornwell. And even when a child is older, it is risky to leave him alone with a dog that's the same size or larger. While a puppy might be all right, leaving a child alone with a dog is like leaving a toddler alone in a bathtub, according to Dr. Cornwell. It is an invitation to a life-threatening accident.

STAY AWAY FROM STRAYS. If a dog doesn't know you, there is more of a chance that he will feel threatened by you and bite. If you spot a stray dog, just call the animal control office and let them know, recommends Dr. Cornwell.

RESPECT TERRITORY. Recognize and respect a dog's territory, says Dr. Cornwell. Don't enter your neighbor's yard without permission, especially if his terrier is on watch over by the swing set. Always assume that a dog will feel uneasy when you approach his turf.

BE A TREE. "Dogs bite bodies and body parts that move," says Dr. Cornwell. "It's instinctive." If you fear that a dog is going to bite you, the best strategy is not to move, he advises. In fact, even if a dog appears friendly, it is good policy to hold still rather than flee. Never run from a dog because it may trigger his instinct to chase you as if you were prey.

"If you are approached by a dog, be a tree," says Dr. Cornwell. Stand with your feet together, fists folded under your chin, and arms and elbows against your chest and stomach. "Being a tree is a neutral, nonthreatening position that minimizes the antagonism of dogs," he explains. Then in a nice, soothing tone, say something like "Nice doggie, good boy" and wait for the dog to walk away. "You want to be boring to the dog," he says.

GO DOWN WITHOUT A FIGHT. Even if a big dog knocks you down or if you are already lying down, you can avoid being bitten. Dr. Cornwell advises acting like a log. "Roll over facedown, feet and legs together," he says. "Put your fists behind your neck in such a way that your forearms cover your ears. This is a nonthreatening, neutral posture."

Don't be afraid if the dog sniffs your body when you are in this position. "That's not a pre-attack mode. It is just one way the dog figures out if you are a threat or not. Just be patient and wait for the dog to finish sniffing you and walk away," he says.

SHOUT IT OUT. If a dog is charging you but is still some distance away, you might try a firm shout like "Go home!" or "Get out of here!" says Dr. Cornwell. Some dogs will shy away. But if the dog keeps coming, you had better stand like a tree.

AVOID EYE CONTACT. "If you watch dogs that are about to fight each other, you will see that they have a lot of eye contact," says Dr. Cornwell. Eye contact could possibly incite aggression. So never look directly into the eyes of a dog that you feel uneasy about.

PAT WITH CAUTION. Before you pat an unfamiliar dog, ask the owner if it is okay, says Dr. Cornwell. If the owner gives you clearance, don't put your hand on top of the dog's head. Some dogs are uncomfortable with that gesture because it says to them that you want to dominate them. Instead, extend your hand out toward the dog, but stop before you reach him. Your hand should be in a fist, palm-down. This keeps your fingers protected. Let the dog come to you. If he is friendly, he will move toward you. If not, make your peace with him some other day.

RESPECT THE DON'TS. Berman and Dr. Cornwell also add these commonsense cautions to take for bite prevention when around unfamiliar dogs.

- Don't step over a sleeping dog or try to wake him.
- Don't approach or bend over a dog if he is lying quietly.
- Don't try to take a bone or a toy away from a dog.
- Don't disturb a dog that is taking care of her puppies.
- Don't disturb any dog while he is eating.

Dodging Mosquitoes and Ticks

Bug bites vary in seriousness, from the mere annoyance of a garden-variety mosquito bite to a possibly fatal allergic reaction to a bee sting. Here are some tips to prevent insects from bugging you.

DRY OUT TO DISCOURAGE MOSQUITOES. The best way to avoid mosquito bites around your house is to get rid of their breeding grounds, says Art Antonelli, Ph.D., an extension entomologist at Washington State University at Puyallup.

"Mosquitoes are fantastic opportunists," he explains. Any collection of freshwater—no matter how small—provides a breeding site. And they breed very quickly. So, sweep puddles off your driveway. Be careful not to leave buckets or cups outside to catch rainwater. Try to landscape the area around your house so that you don't have pools and puddles on the property after a storm.

TRY ANTI-TICK FASHION. Tick bites can cause bacterial infections like Lyme disease, which can lead to arthritis and heart problems. They can also transmit Rocky Mountain spotted fever with its flulike symptoms. Ticks are usually found in woods, in bushy and grassy areas, and anywhere that deer roam. If you find a tick when you get back from a walk, remove it carefully before it can dig in. If you develop fever, muscle aches, headache, or a rash within three weeks, see a doctor, says David E. Johnson, M.D., medical director and president of Wilderness Medical Associates in Bryant Pond, Maine.

When you are in an open field or the woods, wear high boots and long pants tucked into your boots, says Dr. Johnson. Also wear a long-sleeved shirt, buttoned at the collar, and a hat.

DO A FULL-BODY SEARCH. When you come in from the great outdoors, do a body check, says Dr. Antonelli. Have your spouse check you out from head to toe. Check out your kids, too. Examine their skin, hair, and scalp. "A lot of times ticks will not settle down and actually bite you for many hours," he says, "so a tick check after being in tick country goes a long way in preventing tick bites."

Stop the Stings

For most of us, insect stings are painful but not life-threatening. We have a local reaction to the venom—swelling, redness, pain around the sting. But for some people, bee stings are far more serious. Some folks are allergic to the venom that a bee injects, and those people may also be allergic to wasp, hornet, or fire ant stings. When stung, people with allergies may have a systemic reaction. They may break out in hives all over their bodies or vomit or feel faint or have asthma attacks. They may even go into anaphylactic shock, an airway-constricting allergic reaction that can be fatal.

For ways to help prevent bee stings and their accompanying reactions, see the following advice from Robert Plancey, M.D., assistant clinical professor of medicine at the University of Southern California in Los Angeles and an internist and allergist in Arcadia.

GET SHOTS FOR PROTECTION. "If you have ever had a systemic reaction to an insect sting, you should see an allergist right away," says Dr. Plancey. It is vital that an allergist test you to find out which insect venom you are allergic to. You can be placed on a regimen of allergy shots to lessen the intensity of or prevent allergic reactions in the future.

CARRY A KIT. People who are allergic to insect venom should also carry a special medical kit to prevent anaphylactic shock. It includes a chewable antihistamine and injectable adrenaline, both of which will help stop the symptoms. Your allergist can prescribe a kit to carry with you at all times, especially outdoors, and demonstrate its correct use. If you need to use the kit, you should go to the nearest emergency room via paramedic ambulance in case the reaction recurs.

BE "NON-SCENTS-ICAL." Bees are attracted to floral smells. So don't use perfume, aftershave, or even scented deodorant when you are headed for woods or fields or raking leaves and cleaning the gutters.

CHOOSE PLAIN SOAP—FOR YOUR LAUNDRY, TOO. Use unscented soap and wash your clothes in unscented detergent. You don't want to smell like a daffodil.

Don't Git Snakebit

About 1,555 people a year get bitten by poisonous snakes. Most of the perpetrators are rattlesnakes, but copperheads, cottonmouths, and coral snakes are dangerous, too. Fortunately, very few of those bites prove fatal. In general, snakes want to stay out of your way. Here is how to stay out of theirs.

KNOW WHERE THEY LIVE. "You should know if there are poisonous snakes in your area and have a basic understanding of their habitats," says David E. Johnson, M.D., medical director and president of Wilderness Medical Associates in Bryant Pond, Maine. On a cool day, for example, rattlesnakes may be lying on a warm rock. On a hot day, they may be in the shade, tucked away in rocky outcroppings. And since snakes like it under rocks, don't go reaching blindly into crevices.

LIVE WITH YOUR BOOTS ON. If you are walking in an area where there are dangerous snakes—whether it's Grand Canyon National Park or a local game preserve—be sure to wear hiking boots, says Dr. Johnson. No sneakers or sandals if you are in rattlesnake country. And avoid walking at night in these areas.

BACK AWAY, SLOWLY. Snakes are most likely to strike when they are surprised and are not given the opportunity to make a safe exit. If you see a rattlesnake, copperhead, cottonmouth, or any snake you don't recognize, stop whatever you are doing and back away slowly, says Dr. Johnson. These types of snakes strike at fast movements, he says. They sense heat, odors, and vibration well, but their vision and hearing are not very well-developed.

BE SOMBER. Avoid brightly colored clothing—no reds, yellows, blues, violets, oranges, or pinks. And no floral patterns either. Bees may mistake you for a garden.

SIP NO BEVERAGE ON THE VERANDA. A stinging insect is attracted to any beverage. If you leave a can of soda untended, a bee can fly inside. Getting stung in the mouth or throat can cause swelling that could obstruct the airway, even to a nonallergic person, says Dr. Plancey.

DRIVE WITH YOUR WINDOWS CLOSED. If your car is air-conditioned, leave the windows up all summer long, even when the car is parked. You never know when a stinging insect will make a beeline for the warm interior.

ALWAYS WEAR SHOES. If you are allergic to bee stings, you can't risk a fancy-free barefoot amble through the meadow.

TRY TO STAY CALM. If a stinging insect approaches, walk calmly away. If you start flailing your arms and running away, the insect is more likely to sting.

BLISTERS
"Shoe" Them Away

When you think of a hot spot, you probably think of Las Vegas or New York City—glitz, glamour, and good food. When foot doctors think of a hot spot, they have somewhat tamer thoughts. They think of an about-to-form blister.

"Blisters are caused by heat, friction, and moisture," says Douglas Hale, D.P.M., a podiatrist at the Foot and Ankle Center of Washington in Seattle. To prevent those tender domes of pain on your feet, you have to minimize those three blister inducers. Your first step is into the right shoe. Here are some tips from podiatrists on choosing footwear.

SHOP FOR SHOES IN THE AFTERNOON. That is when your feet are most swollen, says Dr. Hale. If you pick your shoe early in the day, you may end up with a pair that is too small for your afternoon feet.

HAVE YOUR FEET MEASURED. Even if you think you know your shoe size, get your feet measured every time you buy shoes, Dr. Hale says. Sometimes, feet spread out over time.

REMEMBER YOUR WIDTH. People tend to take the width of shoes for granted. You may need a different width than the standard, explains Dr. Hale. Not all brands come in all widths. If a shoe feels too narrow, ask the salesclerk for the next widest size.

TEST IT WITH YOUR THUMB. "Make sure that there is a thumb-width between the end of your shoe and your big toe when you are standing up," says Dr. Hale.

DON'T FALL FOR THE "IT'LL STRETCH" SPIEL. "Don't let the shoe salesclerk tell you that the shoes will stretch out," says Lawrence Z. Huppin, D.P.M., a podiatrist at the Foot and Ankle Center of Washington. "If they feel tight in the store, they will feel tight in a couple of weeks."

AVOID LOOSENESS. A loose shoe can also cause blisters because of the friction the shoe creates as the foot moves around in it, says Arnold Ravick, D.P.M., a podiatrist at Capital Podiatry Associates in Washington, D.C.

SHOP WITH A SOCK. When you shop for shoes, slip on the type of sock that you actually plan to wear with your new shoes, says Dr. Hale.

TAKE A TEST-DRIVE INSIDE. Even if you follow all these tips, there is always a chance that your new shoes may not fit perfectly. That's why you should wear them around the house for an hour or two before you ever wear them outside. "If you do that, you will know very quickly if there is a hot spot in the shoes," says Martin Lynn, D.P.M., a podiatrist at the Foot and Ankle Center of Washington. "And if there are hot spots, you can still return them."

INVEST IN SOCK OPTIONS. To help prevent blisters during exercise, choose a sock with a synthetic material that wicks moisture away from the foot, such as Capilene, says Dr. Huppin. "The ideal sock is a Capilene/wool mixture. While the Capilene helps to keep the foot dry, the wool protects the foot from the shoe."

You might also consider wearing two pairs of socks. The inner one should be a thin synthetic sock that wicks

Beat Those Bunions

At first glance, bunions don't seem to have much in common with blisters. Unlike a foot blister, which is puffy and tender, a bunion is an enlargement of the bone at your big-toe joint. As it thickens or moves from its normal position, it starts to look like a big knob sticking out. Protective tissue develops around the bony protrusion, and that tissue can become inflamed and painful. Bunions come in all sizes, and the accompanying redness and swelling can strike at any time. They range from a slight bump on the side of your foot to a big toe that is so misshapen that it seems to be crashing like the Leaning Tower of Pisa onto its neighbor. When it is that big, you may have trouble fitting into a normal-shaped shoe.

Different though they are, both blisters and bunions can be aggravated by wearing shoes that are too small. So the first thing to do, if you happen to be prone to bunions, is to make sure that you buy shoes that fit. In addition, you might be able to beat the bunions if you follow these tips.

GET SOME SUPPORT. Pronation, the tendency of your foot to lean inward, is another contributor to bunion growth

moisture away from the foot. The outer sock should be thick to absorb friction. "This is an old trick used by runners and hikers to prevent blisters," says Dr. Lynn.

NIP IT IN THE BUD. If you feel or see a hot spot—the red, sore, inflamed area that announces a blister is on the way—stop the blister from developing by applying moleskin. This is a feltlike, synthetic padding with an adhesive backing, available at most drugstores and sporting goods stores. First clean the hot spot with rubbing alcohol to remove the oils on the skin so that the moleskin sticks better. Then cut a circle of moleskin slightly bigger than because it puts pressure on the big-toe joint and the first metatarsal bone. A prescription arch support is sometimes a good fix, explains Glenn Gastwirth, D.P.M., executive director of the American Podiatric Medical Association in Bethesda, Maryland. It may stop a bunion from beginning by keeping your foot from rolling inward. And if you already have a slight bunion, it can stop the bunion from progressing to a more serious and painful stage.

STRETCH YOUR TENDONS. A simple stretching exercise can prevent problems, too. "Sometimes pronation can be caused by a tight Achilles tendon," says Donald Baxter, M.D., an orthopedic surgeon and clinical professor of orthopedic surgery at the University of Texas Medical School at Houston. "A tight Achilles tends to flatten the arch of your foot, which leads to pressure on the big toe during the push-off phase of walking."

Stretching the Achilles several times a day can be very helpful, says Dr. Baxter. A simple calf stretch should do the trick. To stretch the calf, place the balls of your feet on a low step. Holding on to a railing, gradually lower your heels a little until you can feel the stretch in your calves. Just be sure not to bounce.

the hot spot and paste it on, following the directions on the package.

GIVE YOUR FEET A LUBE JOB. Runners and other athletes who are prone to blisters on their feet can try a variety of products, such as Skin-Lube or Runner's Lube, says Richard Braver, D.P.M., a sports podiatrist and director of the Active Foot and Ankle Care Center in Englewood and Fair Lawn, New Jersey. "They are ointments that reduce the friction and help prevent blisters." They work better than petroleum jelly, which has a tendency to melt inside the heat of a shoe.

How to Keep Your Hands Blister-Free

Jenny Stone *knows* hand blisters. She is a certified athletic trainer and the manager of clinical programs in the division of sports medicine for the U.S. Olympic Committee in Colorado Springs. Training gymnasts, discus throwers, and volleyball players, she sees hands that get a lot of punishment. Here are her tips to keep your hands blister-free.

EASE INTO NEW ACTIVITIES. "Start slowly. Don't go out and play 36 holes the first time you play golf in the spring. Play 9 holes instead," she says. "You don't want to jump into any activity that your body is unaccustomed to."

USE EQUIPMENT THAT IS RIGHT FOR YOU. Equipment that is inappropriately sized—for example, the grip of a tennis racket that is either too small or too large—will have a tendency to cause blisters on the hands. "Ask your local pros to check if you have the proper size," Stone advises.

PROTECT THE TENDER SPOTS. "If you know that you get blisters on your hands when you do certain things, like play tennis or shovel, put some athletic tape or moleskin over that area before the activity," she says.

WEAR GLOVES. "They will absorb the friction that normally would transfer to your hands," she explains.

KEEP YOUR HANDS DRY. "If your hands are damp, they are more likely to get blisters. Powder your hands before exercise," says Stone. "And if you have a problem with excessive sweating, use an antiperspirant on your hands."

TURN UP YOUR TOES AT MEDICATED PADS. People with corns and hammertoes sometimes use so-called medicated pads for relief. But if you do, you put yourself at risk for a blister. These pads contain an acid that burns the skin and causes blisters, says Dr. Hale.

BODY ODOR
Bye-Bye Bacteria

Body odor is caused by sweat and bacteria. There is not much that we can do about sweating. We need to perspire. It is one way our bodies get rid of toxins. But bacteria are another matter. Here is how bacteria can be beaten on the way to smelling sweet.

SUDS 'EM AWAY. Soap is your best hope. "Use a mild antibacterial soap," says Joseph P. Bark, M.D., chairman of the department of dermatology at Saint Joseph Hospital in Lexington, Kentucky, and author of *Your Skin: An Owner's Guide.*

TARGET THE PITS. Your underarms generate a particular kind of sweat, called apocrine sweat, that is especially hospitable to the body-odor bacteria. Scrub them well on a daily basis using a mild antibacterial soap, suggests Dr. Bark.

SCRUB YOUR GROIN. Sound painful? No need to get rough. But wash your crotch thoroughly every day with an antibacterial soap, says Dr. Bark. Apocrine sweat also thrives there.

GO NUCLEAR. If you have strong body odor, you should try a powerful antibacterial cleanser, such as Beta-dine, says Dr. Bark. He cautions that you should only use this in your armpits and crotch and that you need to rinse it off well. Since it is strong stuff, there is no reason to subject the rest of your body to a Betadine bath. It could dry out your skin.

FIGHT OFF FRAGRANCE. Even after you have taken all the antibacterial steps, you will probably need an antiper-spirant. Only a deodorant containing antiperspirant will cut down how much you sweat, which reduces the moisture-harboring bad-news bacteria. Deodorants without an an-tiperspirant don't prevent the problem, they only mask the odor, according to Dr. Bark.

SEEK ALUMINUM CHLOROHYDRATE. A deodorant that has this ingredient is a good sweat-controller, according to Dr. Bark.

BREAK OUT THE BAKING SODA. If you have an allergic reaction to the common ingredients in deodorants, Dr. Bark suggests using baking soda instead. "Baking soda is mild and won't irritate your skin. It creates a condition where the bacteria don't grow as well." To apply, just put some in your hand and rub it on.

APPLY AN ANTIBIOTIC. If your body odor is impossible to control using more conventional means, Dr. Bark suggests using an antibiotic product called Cleocin-T solution, which literally kills the odor-causing bacteria. Ask your doctor about it. You will need a prescription.

BOILS
Stay Cool, Pressure-Free, Dry, and Clean

The nastiness of boils is well-documented, beginning with the time when the Egyptians endured a plague of them and long-suffering Job, of Biblical fame, came down with a bad case. These bacterial infections of hair follicles—red, painful, and pus-filled—can pop up anywhere. The bacteria in a boil, which is usually staphylococcus, is highly contagious. It can plant a boil on somebody else.

But they can be prevented. The trick is to minimize the causative factors, according to Joseph P. Bark, M.D., chairman of the department of dermatology at Saint Joseph Hospital in Lexington, Kentucky, and author of *Your Skin: An Owner's Guide*. You have to avoid the boil-making four: heat, pressure, moisture, and bacteria.

Remember these prevention provisos.

CHILL OUT. Excessive heat in a hair follicle can make infection more likely. Tight pants and sweatbands, for instance, create hot zones where boils can get started. So wear looser clothing for a cooler skin temperature, says Dr. Bark.

DEPRESSURIZE. Heat can also be created by pressure. "I see lots of boils on the lower backs and buttocks of salespeople," says Dr. Bark. "They sit on car seats for hundreds of miles a week, and their skin is chronically compressed." He suggests that people who spend a lot of time driving get a seat pad made of woven wire and wooden beads. "It distributes the weight more effectively and lets air passage occur."

PICK A LITTLE COTTON. Since moisture leads to boils and cotton underwear helps wick away humidity, changing your polyester undies for all-natural ones may reduce your boil-risk, explains Dr. Bark.

TRY SHOWER POWER. Frequent showers with antibacterial soap may help by fighting the boil bacteria, according to Dr. Bark.

LOSE A LITTLE WEIGHT. Boils tend to occur in areas of the body where skin is touching skin, like between the thighs, in the cleft of the buttocks, and underneath women's breasts, says Dr. Bark. People who are overweight not only have more folds of skin, but these areas are particularly pressurized and moist.

"Losing weight is the most fundamental preventive measure in people who are overweight and get boils," says Guy F. Webster, M.D., Ph.D., professor of dermatology at the Jefferson Medical College of Thomas Jefferson University in Philadelphia.

TRY SOME TALC. If you are overweight, be sure to dust some talcum powder in areas where the skin chafes, suggests Dr. Webster. It reduces moisture and prevents breaks in the skin where the staph bacteria might enter. Women should avoid getting talcum powder in the genital area, however. Studies show that there may be an increased risk of ovarian cancer among women who routinely dust with talcum powder after bathing.

Don't Share That Sweater

Boils are not only painful but also contagious. "The most common way that boils are transmitted—particularly in teenagers—is by sharing clothing," says Guy F. Webster, M.D., Ph.D., professor of dermatology at the Jefferson Medical College of Thomas Jefferson University in Philadelphia. So if someone in the family has a boil, don't steal his sweatshirt at the game. Also, you should launder his towels and washcloths separately.

BREAST CANCER
Prevention Is Only a Meal Away

The statistics are no secret. One woman in eight will develop breast cancer in her lifetime. Approximately 180,000 American women will be diagnosed with the disease this year; another 43,500 will die from it. But what is still a secret to many American women is that there really are some ways to help prevent this dreaded disease. A healthy diet, research shows, is a powerful stay-well weapon.

Consider this evidence for dietary protection: In the United States, breast cancer rates are four to seven times higher than in Asia. But when Asian women move to the United States, their breast cancer risk doubles in 10 years. While scientists aren't absolutely certain about all of the causes of this huge change, diet is probably one factor, says Regina Ziegler, Ph.D., a nutritional epidemiologist at the National Cancer Institute in Bethesda, Maryland. Living in the United States, these women start ingesting more calories, including meat and other foods high in saturated fat. They also eat fewer vegetables, fruits, grains, and soy products than they did in Asia. Combining all those factors with less activity, they end up putting on more weight.

An anti-breast-cancer diet might not guarantee prevention, but it will probably offer women added protection. Here is how to get on that diet.

TURN YOUR KITCHEN INTO A CORNUCOPIA. Women who eat lots of fruits and vegetables are less likely to get breast cancer, research shows. In one study, women in New York State who ate more than five servings of vegetables daily had half the risk of breast cancer as women who ate fewer than three servings. And women who ate five servings of fruit lowered their risk by a third compared with those who ate fewer than two servings. Based on the study conclusions, try to eat a rainbow of produce for protection: tomatoes, spinach, greens, corn, carrots, summer squash, cucumbers, melons, berries, apples, pears, raisins, lemons, and limes.

FILL UP ON FIBER. Why do women in Finland have half the incidence of breast cancer as American women? Perhaps because they consume 30 grams of fiber daily, compared with the 14 grams that American women consume. "We have strong evidence that fiber is protective," says David Rose, M.D., associate director and chief of the division of nutrition and endocrinology at the American Health Foundation in Valhalla, New York. According to one of Dr. Rose's studies, 30 grams of fiber a day—half from food and half from added wheat bran—can lower women's estrogen levels by 20 percent. Since high levels of estrogen may be a risk factor in breast cancer, that drop suggests a lowering of breast cancer risk as well.

You can reach 30 grams of fiber with five servings of fruits and veggies, five servings of whole grains, one serving of a high-fiber wheat-bran cereal, and one serving of dried beans per day. A fiber-filled tip: Always pick whole-grain products when you can. Bread and pasta that are made with refined white flour should be the exception rather than the rule, says Dr. Rose.

Forgo the fat. Peter Greenwald, M.D., director of cancer prevention at the National Cancer Institute, points to research showing lower rates of breast cancer in countries where less fat is eaten. Even within the same country, like Japan, breast cancer rises when Japanese women begin eating more foods that get a larger proportion of calories from fat. How much fat is safe? No one knows for sure, but 20 percent of total calories from fat is the level currently being tested to prevent breast cancer in the Women's Health Initiative study sponsored by the National Institutes of Health.

Drizzle with olive oil. When you need to satisfy your "fat tooth," do it with olive oil instead of steak, says Walter Willett, M.D., head of nutrition at Harvard School of Public Health. Three scientific studies have shown that women who eat several servings of food daily with olive oil lowered their risk of breast cancer. So use olive oil instead of other fats whenever possible when cooking, as a salad dressing, and as a dip for bread.

Be moderate with red meat. A scientific study from Uruguay, South America, where people eat lots of meat, found that women who ate the most red meat had four times the risk of breast cancer as those eating the least. Scientists say that the best policy may be to eat red meat only rarely, concentrating on chicken, fish, and other seafood.

Invite the sea to supper. Some varieties of fish may help prevent breast cancer, not only because they are a healthy alternative to red meat but also because they contain a protective factor: the omega-3 fatty acids in fish oil. Diets high in omega-3's have been shown to slow the growth and spread of breast cancer tumors in laboratory animals. And in a study of women having breast cancer surgery, a higher amount of alpha-linolenic acid (which the body converts to omega-3) in the fat tissue around tumors was associated with a decreased spread of cancer. Good sources of omega-3's are any canned or fresh salmon (but not smoked

An Apple a Day Recipe

Omega Salmon

Certain fish, like salmon, are rich in omega-3 fatty acids, which may help prevent breast cancer. These simple broiled salmon steaks are marinated in a lively teriyaki sauce. Look for mirin (rice wine) in Asian markets or the international aisle of supermarkets.

⅓ cup reduced-sodium soy sauce

2 tablespoons mirin (rice wine) or apple juice

2 teaspoons grated fresh ginger

2 scallions, chopped

2 tablespoons honey

3 tablespoons lemon juice

4 salmon steaks (4 ounces each)

In a resealable plastic bag, combine the soy sauce, mirin or apple juice, ginger, scallions, honey, lemon juice, and salmon. Shake well. Refrigerate for 30 minutes or up to 24 hours. Turn occasionally.

Coat a broiler pan with nonstick spray. Preheat the broiler.

Place the salmon on the pan and broil about 4" from the heat for 10 to 12 minutes, or until the fish is just opaque. Turn once during cooking. Meanwhile, transfer the marinade to a medium saucepan. Bring to a boil over medium-high heat. Cook, stirring occasionally, for 8 minutes, or until reduced by half.

Spoon the sauce over the fish.

Makes 4 servings. Per serving: 183 calories, 4 g. fat, 2.9 g. omega-3 fatty acids salmon or lox). Or get your omega-3's from canned white (albacore) tuna.

CURB THE COCKTAILS. A major scientific review of the alcohol-and-breast-cancer connection found that, on average, women having one drink a day had an 11 percent higher risk of breast cancer. If you stay at two to three drinks per week, the risk of breast cancer from alcohol is minimal, says Dr. Willett.

ENJOY SOY. There are a few foods that may have special anti–breast cancer power. And soybeans are on the top of that list. "In Asian countries where soy's a staple, there is a marked lowering of breast cancer," notes soy expert Kenneth Setchell, Ph.D., professor of pediatrics at the University of Cincinnati School of Medicine. According to Dr. Setchell, it is compounds in soy called isoflavones that make the difference. Isoflavones act like weak estrogens in the body and block stronger, cancer-promoting estrogens from inhabiting breast cells, he says.

You can try soy milk in puddings or on cereal, blend tofu in fruit smoothies, or make a soy-butter-and-jelly sandwich for lunch. (Soy sauce and soybean oil have very little of the good isoflavones.)

FEAST ON FLAXSEED. In studies on laboratory animals, flaxseed helped stop breast cancer from starting and slowed the growth of tumors already under way. Researchers give the credit to a compound in flaxseed called lignan precursors. In the body, these compounds convert to weak estrogens that may have the same protective quality as soy's isoflavones.

To get these substances, on days that you don't have a serving of soy, try for one serving of flaxseed by sprinkling two heaping tablespoons of ground flaxseed on cereal or mixing that amount into juice, says Lilian U. Thompson, Ph.D., professor of nutritional sciences at the University of Toronto in Ontario.

GET INTO GARLIC. In laboratory studies at Memorial

Mammograms: Once a Year for Maximum Protection

Together with monthly breast self-exams and annual physician's exams, annual mammograms are an important weapon against breast cancer. "Scientific research overwhelmingly supports annual mammography screening beginning at age 40," says Daniel B. Kopans, M.D., associate professor of radiology at Harvard Medical School and director of the breast imaging division at Massachusetts General Hospital, both in Boston.

Although the mammogram is not a perfect test, with its help, a doctor can often detect breast cancer at an early stage, says Dr. Kopans.

Early detection increases the likelihood that cancer will be limited to one small well-defined lump, which can be successfully treated without removing the breast.

Sloan-Kettering Cancer Center in New York City, researchers have shown that four of garlic's pungent compounds stop cancerous human breast cells from multiplying rapidly. To get the benefits, include one-half to one clove of garlic in your diet several times a week, says John Pinto, Ph.D., associate professor of biochemistry at Cornell University Medical College and director of the nutrition research laboratory at Memorial Sloan-Kettering Cancer Center, both in New York City.

ASK YOUR DOCTOR ABOUT ASPIRIN. Women who take medications called nonsteroidal anti-inflammatory drugs (NSAIDs) three times a week have a one-third lower risk of breast cancer, according to a study performed at the Comprehensive Cancer Center at Ohio State University in Columbus. The women in the study were taking nonprescription aspirin, ibuprofen, naproxen (Naprosyn), or ketoprofen (Orudis), says Randall Harris, M.D., Ph.D., leader of the study, and director of the School of Public Health at Ohio State University. He warns women not to use these medications without first consulting with their doctors since these drugs can have side effects like serious bleeding and irritation of the stomach.

BREAST LUMPS AND TENDERNESS
Minimize the Monthly Pain

Lumps in your breasts. Cysts in your breasts. Breasts that are painfully tender. Doctors used to call these problems fibrocystic breast disease. But they have realized that this name was about as accurate as calling the cramps and heavy bleeding many women experience every month menstrual disease.

Breast lumps, cysts, and tenderness are most often not symptoms of a disease. They are an unfortunate side effect of the menstrual cycle, and they're experienced by an estimated 30 to 50 percent of all women at some time in their lives.

If a woman has these breast changes, it doesn't mean that she is at higher risk for breast cancer. They are simply what the new name of the condition describes: *fibrocystic change* in the tissues of the breast.

"The breast tissue goes through cyclic changes just like the uterus does," says Barbara Smith, M.D., Ph.D., assistant professor of surgery at Harvard Medical School and co-director of the Women's Cancers Program at Massachusetts General Hospital, both in Boston. Unlike the uterus, however, the breast can't clean things out and start fresh. Instead, every month the breast has to adapt to the changes in its structure—in its ducts and in its fibrous and fatty tissue—that occur during each menstrual cycle.

"We think that a lot of fibrocystic symptoms, including inflammation and tenderness, are caused when that adaptation process goes a little bit awry," says Dr. Smith. If a breast duct isn't working properly, fluid can get trapped, causing a cyst. Sometimes, a malfunctioning duct can also cause a collection of extra fibrous tissue to become a lump.

You can take steps to minimize the monthly pain, according to Marianne K. Lange, M.D., assistant professor of surgery at Michigan State University in East Lansing and a physician in Grand Rapids. Here are some tips to limit breast lumps and ease breast tenderness.

NIX THE METHYLXANTHINES. Methylxanthines (pronounced meth-ill-ZAN-theens) are chemicals that may trigger the body to increase production of stress hormones, which are linked to breast lumps and tenderness.

"Ninety to 95 percent of women who have fibrocystic changes will have some resolution of their problem if they minimize or eliminate their intake of methylxanthines," says Dr. Lange. To help prevent the onset of breast pain, steer clear of coffee, tea, cola, wine, and beer, she advises. All contain methylxanthines. Other common foods to avoid include chocolate, cheese, bananas, raisins, nuts, peanut butter, mushrooms, pickles, and sauerkraut.

STOP THE CIGS. "Cigarettes should be avoided at all costs," says Dr. Lange. "Not only do they cause a host of medical problems, they also cause fibrocystic breast pain." (Like cola and coffee, cigarettes also contain methylxanthines.)

HOLD THE SALT. Some women gain a lot of water weight during their periods, which causes their breasts to feel heavy and sensitive. To help prevent the problem, try cutting back on the salt in your diet, especially two weeks before the start of your period, suggests Theodore Tsangaris, M.D., chief of breast surgery at Georgetown University Medical Center in Washington, D.C.

SWITCH YOUR HORMONES. Birth control pills and hormone-replacement therapy (HRT) can aggravate fibrocystic changes, says Dr. Smith. Women on HRT who take estrogen 25 days a month and progesterone 10 days a month may experience breast pain, she says. But if they switch to a regimen where they take both medications every day, they may be able to help prevent the discomfort.

Don't readjust any medications yourself, Dr. Smith cautions. If you think that your birth control regimen or HRT might be linked to your breast pain, discuss it with your doctor. An alternative form of birth control or some readjustment in your HRT program might help relieve the pain, she says.

TRY EVENING PRIMROSE OIL. This essential oil is a distant cousin to the painkiller ibuprofen, says Dr. Smith, and may help prevent fibrocystic changes and breast pain if it is taken regularly. She recommends taking one capsule twice a day until the breast pain resolves. You can resume taking evening primrose oil whenever you experience breast pain as long as you don't exceed the dose that is recommended on the label.

After you have experienced a period or two without breast pain, you can stop taking the remedy, says Dr. Smith. Evening primrose oil is available at many drugstores, supermarkets, and health food stores.

BE HIP TO E AND B₆. There is some evidence that vitamins E and B_6 may help prevent breast pain. Barley, wheat germ, cherries, and asparagus are good sources of vitamin E. The best food sources of vitamin B_6 are plantains, poultry, and avocados. Other good sources are spinach and lean meats. Because it is hard to get the full recommended Daily Value of vitamin E from food sources, Dr. Smith recommends taking it in supplements of 400 IU (international units), up to 800 IU each day, together with supplements of

50 milligrams of vitamin B₆. "Vitamin E is pretty good taken alone, but vitamin B₆ works better in combination with vitamin E," she says.

Caution: Don't take any dose of vitamin B₆ larger than 50 milligrams per day for an extended period of time without consulting your doctor since it can have some side effects. If you are considering taking vitamin E in amounts above 200 IU, discuss this with your doctor first. A study using low-dose vitamin E supplements showed an increased risk of hemorrhagic stroke.

To prevent discomfort, take a walk. "I recommend exercise for women with fibrocystic changes," says Dr. Lange. Exercise decreases stress levels, protecting the breasts from the stress hormones that can play a role in fibrocystic changes, so it may help prevent the pain. "Do vigorous exercise 30 minutes a day," she recommends.

Follow other roads to relaxation. Anything that helps you ease up—meditation, music, massage—can cut those stress hormones and offer some protection from breast tenderness.

Wear a bra. Many women with large breasts experience breast tenderness during their periods, says Dr. Tsangaris. Wearing a bra, especially while active, can help prevent and relieve the tenderness. "It immobilizes the breasts and eliminates the feeling of tenderness and heaviness," he says. To help relieve the pain, you can apply a heating pad to sore breasts.

Try some OTCs. You can also help ease the pain by taking over-the-counter anti-inflammatory drugs such as Midol or ibuprofen, says Dr. Tsangaris. Take two 200-milligram tablets of either drug when breast pain becomes a nuisance, he suggests.

BRONCHITIS
Guard Your Cilia from Harm

Bronchitis comes in two brands: chronic and acute. The most common cause of chronic bronchitis is smoking—while shorter-term, acute bronchitis is the result of infection. Figuring out how to prevent almost all cases of chronic bronchitis is straightforward. Although avoiding the acute variety is tougher, there are some steps that you can take to dodge its hacking cough, fever, and fatigue as well.

Air Your Lungs

Ninety-five percent of all cases of chronic bronchitis have the same cause: smoking. Most of the remaining five percent come from environmental exposures to dust or fumes, usually in an industrial setting. Coal miners and grain handlers are two types of workers at risk for this disease.

Prolonged smoking and, possibly, exposure to second-hand smoke disables the protective cilia, the small hairlike

Emphysema: The Smoker's Disease

The lung diseases emphysema and chronic bronchitis are close companions, and it is smoking that makes them that way. That is, many people with chronic bronchitis also have emphysema, and both diseases are almost always caused by smoking.

While both *can* develop in nonsmokers, it's less likely. People who carry the highest risk of getting this life-threatening disease are, overwhelmingly, long-term smokers. "It is very rare to see someone with emphysema who has not smoked," says Harold Palevsky, M.D., medical co-director of the program in advanced lung disease and medical director of respiratory care services at the University of Pennsylvania Medical Center in Philadelphia.

Tobacco smoke causes emphysema by irritating your lungs, which sparks an inflammatory process similar to what happens when your body fights an infection. The problem is, if you are a smoker, that inflammatory

appendages along our airways whose movements get rid of mucus. Once this "muco-ciliary escalator" is broken, we can't get rid of mucus or the dust and bacteria it catches for us. The result is a terrible cough; inflamed, weakened airways; and an increased susceptibility to many respiratory tract infections, from the flu to pneumonia.

If you are a smoker with chronic bronchitis, you simply have to quit smoking to prevent the symptoms from starting up, says Loutfi Sami Aboussouan, M.D., a pulmonary disease specialist and assistant professor of medicine at Wayne State University in Detroit. Beyond that, it is essential to minimize your exposure to dust and other cilia-damaging substances.

BECOME A MASKED MAN. If you have to work in a job

response becomes chronic—it happens day after day, year after year, until it finally destroys your lung tissue and your ability to breathe.

But you can protect yourself from emphysema, even if you have been a smoker all your life. "The way to prevent emphysema is to stop smoking," says Dr. Palevsky. "There is no other preventive intervention that would have any impact on this disease." And the sooner a smoker quits, the better. Here is how to live smoke-free.

- If you don't smoke, don't start.
- Be gentle with yourself. Smokers hardly ever succeed at quitting on the first try. If you fail, have faith and try again.
- Seek out support. Get involved in a clinic or church-based smoking-cessation program in your area. To find out more, contact the American Lung Association by writing to them at 1740 Broadway, New York City, NY 10019-4374.

that has respiratory risks, wearing a disposable mask may help guard your airways, advises Dr. Aboussouan.

SUCK IN SOME SUCCOR. Try using an inhalant bronchodilator, the same type of device used by people with asthma to prevent an asthma attack. The medicine in these inhalers helps revive your battered cilia so that they can clear out more mucus. If you have less extra mucus in your airways, you won't be as likely to have an acute attack. And if you do have an attack, your symptoms are likely to be less severe.

You should use the inhaler between two and four times a day, according to Marc Peters-Golden, M.D., professor of internal medicine in the division of pulmonary and critical care medicine at the University of Michigan

Medical Center in Ann Arbor. Prescription inhalers are better and safer than over-the-counter versions, he says, and he urges people with chronic bronchitis to discuss this preventive option with their doctors.

Take a gulp of fresh water. Liquids make your mucus less thick and tenacious, says Dr. Peters-Golden. That makes it easier to cough up the mucus and less likely that you will have an acute attack. He suggests drinking six to eight eight-ounce glasses of water a day.

Get it out with a workout. Some people with chronic bronchitis can't exercise because their airways are just too weak. But if you can, you should, says Dr. Peters-Golden. Aerobic exercise helps mobilize the mucus in your airways.

Acute Bronchitis: Try Vigilant Avoidance

Acute bronchitis is a viral or bacterial infection of the airways that lasts a week or two. During those miserable days, you painfully cough up thick, yellow or green mucus, feel wiped out, and may have a fever. Your key strategy is to avoid germs in any way possible. Here are a few ways to ward them off.

Engage in hand-to-mouth combat. The viruses that cause acute bronchitis usually end up on your hand, which ends up ushering them to your mouth or your nose, says Dr. Aboussouan. He suggests keeping your hands away from your face and washing your hands frequently, particularly when you have been near someone with a cold.

Get off on the healthy floor. An elevator is another enclosed spot where viruses love to lurk. If you have touched the buttons, go straight to the bathroom and wash your hands, says Dr. Aboussouan.

Reach out but don't touch someone. After you

Drink and Wash to Stay Germ-Free

Airplanes are the perfect spot for viral ambush, says Loutfi Sami Aboussouan, M.D., a pulmonary disease specialist and assistant professor of medicine at Wayne State University in Detroit. The recirculated air is almost sure to carry viruses from at least one of the passengers. Further, the air in the cabin is usually so arid that it dries out your mucous membranes and makes them more susceptible to viruses.

Drink lots of fluids, suggests Dr. Aboussouan. A good rule of thumb is to drink eight ounces of fluid for every hour that you are on a plane, but stay away from alcoholic or caffeinated drinks because they can cause dehydration. And to avoid getting infected by other people's carry-on viruses, wash your hands right after you get off the plane.

use a pay phone, rinse off your hands. Better yet, carry alcohol wipes with you and give the receiver a quick wipe before using it, says Dr. Aboussouan.

HANG UP THE HANDKERCHIEF. You and everybody else in your family should use disposable tissues, particularly if somebody is sick. That way, the viruses or bacteria don't have as many opportunities to contaminate others, says Dr. Aboussouan. And teach your children to dispose of their own tissues. "If parents predisposed to bronchitis are touching a child's used tissues, then they must wash their hands afterward," he adds.

LOCK OUT TOBACCO TEMPTATIONS. Smoking—and breathing secondhand smoke—can increase the likelihood of acute bronchitis because even *one* exposure to cigarette smoke poisons the cilia, says Dr. Peters-Golden.

BURNOUT
Don't Get Singed

You are healthy and full of energy. You rarely get sick, and you are on the go almost all the time. You are sociable and outgoing. You like people, and they like you. You are smart and creative. You enjoy using your talents and capabilities. And at work, you're passionate about achievement.

That might sound like a perfect description of success on the job. Trouble is, that could also be a perfect description of someone who's headed for burnout.

"The personal qualities that create peak performance at work are also the qualities that may push a person into burnout," says Ruth Luban, a counselor and consultant in private practice in Laguna Beach, California, who specializes in preventing and treating burnout and is the author of the book and audiotape *Keeping the Fire: From Burnout to Balance*.

Those overachiever qualities, she says, cause a person to overdo and "overgive" on the job, that is, to inadvertently give more and more time and energy to work at the expense of self-nourishing activities that would provide balance. Month after month and year after year of constant stress, relentlessly pushing ahead, can lead to trouble. "Burnout is the gradual erosion of one's energy and spirit as the result of chronic, relentless long-term stress," says Luban.

Because burnout can build slowly over years, its early symptoms are easy to deny. They grow until you notice that you start to have trouble sleeping. You develop headaches, back pain, digestive upset, or frequent infections. You may notice that your energy fades to exhaustion. And your positive, outgoing personality turns into self-doubt and cynicism. When your enthusiasm for achievement is blackened by depression and hopelessness, you have reached the final stage of burnout.

But burnout is preventable. And the first step, says Luban, is acknowledging that it can happen to you.

KNOW YOUR ENEMY. People decide not to smoke because they have been educated about the consequences of chronic smoking, says Luban. In the same way, you need to be educated about the potential risks of chronic overwork. That way, you can decide not to let your job overwhelm you because you know the end result isn't worth it. "The number one way to prevent burnout is to be well-educated about what burnout is," she says.

REMEMBER THAT YOU ARE NOT YOUR JOB. One of the leading causes of burnout is overidentification with work, says Luban. If you believe that your career is the key to expressing and fulfilling yourself, you will overidentify with your professional role. At that point, your success at work becomes your primary source of self-worth. So you end up working harder and harder. It is a self-administered poison. What's the antidote? "You need to ask yourself who you are besides your role at work," she says. "You need to find out how to express and enjoy your individuality outside that role."

When the Sizzle Fizzles

The key to preventing burnout is recognizing it in the early stages, says Ruth Luban, a counselor and consultant in private practice in Laguna Beach, California, who specializes in preventing and treating burnout and is the author of the book and audiotape *Keeping the Fire: From Burnout to Balance.* Here is Luban's description of the five stages in the process of career burnout.

1. Honeymoon. This is the entry point of a career; your energy, enthusiasm, and expectations are high. There are no symptoms of burnout.
2. Disillusionment. You have a vague notion that your expectations of constant achievement and satisfaction might be unrealistic. You feel confused and a little impatient with the job. But everybody else at work seems to be functioning without a problem, so you decide that your sense that something isn't quite right is your imagination. And you tell yourself, "If I just try harder, everything will be okay." You go into denial about your feelings of disappointment and confusion, says Luban. If you continue to ignore them, you will progress to the next stage of burnout.
3. Brownout. The symptoms of burnout are starting to become evident. Your emotional fuel is running low. You feel tired and irritable a lot of the time. Your sleep may be disturbed. Maybe you are overeating

DON'T START YOUR DAY STARTLED. "Managing the early morning is critical for preventing burnout," says Luban. If you have a demanding job, you probably wake up to an alarm clock and leap into the day.

Change your routine. Instead of leaping into each day,

or overdrinking. You don't feel as decisive, but you carry on. If you don't do something about those symptoms, you enter the next stage.
4. Frustration. You feel angry and don't have any enthusiasm. You are cynical and pessimistic about yourself, your work, and your co-workers. You have less and less tolerance for the stress that was always part of the job. "If you don't take action at the frustration stage," says Luban, "you are likely to progress to the final stage."
5. Despair. You are hopeless and depressed. You feel like a failure, and you are full of self-doubt and loneliness. You want to run away from your work, your friends, and your family. You feel that you have nothing left to give. At this last stage of burnout, you are in danger of serious illness or clinical depression.

"Throughout all the stages—especially the final stage of burnout—instead of talking about their problem, people tend to withdraw socially because they are so exhausted," says Luban. "They feel increasingly misunderstood and really lonely." Often, you may start having physical complaints, such as infections, stomachaches, fatigue, and headaches. "When illness and depression are chronic, this is very often when people come in for therapy," says Luban, "because at this point their physical, mental, and emotional symptoms have gotten the better of them."

use the first 30 minutes or hour of your day for relaxation and reflection. Have a cup of tea in your garden. Write in a journal. Listen to music. "Do something self-nourishing to begin your day," suggests Luban. "That will help you cope with stress the rest of the day."

MAKE A "TO DO" LIST AND *DON'T* DO EVERYTHING ON IT. "People who are prone to burnout are usually perfectionistic strivers," says Luban. "They think that they have to do everything and do it just right." So make a "to do" list with eight items on it and give yourself permission to choose only three to complete in this day. This can teach you that you don't have to do everything completely or perfectly. "It will help you reduce the demands you impose on yourself," she says.

INTERNALIZE GOALS AT WORK. "The secret that keeps some people resilient, alert, productive, happy, and balanced at work is the ability to internalize corporate goals," says Jeff Davidson, a certified management consultant and executive director of the Breathing Space Institute in Chapel Hill, North Carolina, and author of *Breathing Space: Living and Working at a Comfortable Pace in a Sped-Up Society*. In other words, he says, take the goals given to you by your company and your boss and make them your own.

"The happiest and most productive people are able to see organizationally imposed goals as their own. They think, 'Yes, that will benefit me. Yes, I accept it. Yes, I am going for it.'" Unless you think in those terms, it is easy to feel resentful and get overwhelmed by work obligations.

GIVE YOURSELF GOOD BREAKS. Luban tells her clients who fear that they are headed for burnout to alternate work with rest and relaxation. "Take a 10-minute break every two hours. Even if you can't leave the office, put your feet up on your desk, close your eyes, and relax. The idea is to stop the constant mental activity and refresh your body and mind."

TAKE DEEP BREATHS. For instant stress release, Luban suggests taking three or four deep breaths, inhaling deeply into your abdomen rather than just into your upper chest. This relaxes the body, quiets the mind, and stimulates creativity and intuition.

HEAD FOR VACATIONLAND. If you find yourself uninterested in a vacation, you may be a good candidate for burnout, says Luban. It is important that you take a few days here and there to refresh yourself and see yourself outside of a work context. Go to some new place, see a few different sights, and hear a few different sounds.

MAKE TIME FOR LOVE. Healthy relationships are great stress-reducers, explains Luban. You are not just an account supervisor. You are also a spouse, a parent, a friend. Give yourself time to be with the people you love. Take a day off to go to a ball game with a child or to a museum with a friend.

WATCH YOUR WELLNESS. "Getting enough sleep, exercising regularly, and focusing on good nutrition are all important in preventing burnout," says Luban.

REDUCE STRESS—YOUR WAY. Most people already know what works for them to reduce stress, says Luban. The problem is that they don't take the time to do it. She recommends that you schedule a set time every day to practice your personal stress-reduction strategy.

"Try yoga, writing in a journal, or taking a walk by yourself or with a friend," says Luban. "Whatever helps you reduce stress, make sure it happens almost every day."

CREATE A DECOMPRESSION RITUAL. "To prevent burnout, compartmentalize work and separate it from the rest of your life," advises Luban. One way to do that is to create a decompression ritual between work and home—a way for you not to take work (or work worries) home with you.

"Identify a quiet place—a park or a beach—where you can park your car, turn off the engine, put your seat back, and just relax and breathe for a few minutes. This is particularly necessary for people with kids because they are going home to their second full-time job," she says.

THINK ABOUT CHANGING YOUR JOB. "The work environment can have a great deal to do with burnout," says Luban. Do you work for a slave-driving boss? Do you face constant deadlines and crises? Do you live in a work atmosphere that is tense and demanding with no room for humor or relaxation? If so, you may want to consider changing jobs.

"No matter what you do, a toxic work environment constantly creates more stress, and burnout-prevention strategies often don't work," points out Luban.

BURSITIS AND TENDINITIS
Staying in Play

A professional cook who chops vegetables—for dozens of meals, all night long. A "weekend warrior" who plays volleyball for hours, spiking the ball at the net every chance he gets. A mom who picks up and puts down her baby over and over again all day. A runner who decides to train for a marathon and suddenly increases her weekly miles from 20 to 30.

These folks have one thing in common: They are all at risk for developing bursitis or tendinitis, an inflammation of a bursa or tendon, two commonly injured parts of the musculoskeletal system. Bursae are fluid-filled, envelope-like sacs that lubricate areas throughout your body where there is friction directly on the skeleton. Tendons are fibrous bands that attach muscle to bone. Both body parts can incur what doctors call micro-trauma, a series of tiny tears in their structures that may culminate in pain. The sore shoulder. The aching elbow. The throbbing knee.

Doctors who specialize in sports medicine have discovered many ways to prevent bursitis and tendinitis. Here is how to avoid the aches.

CHANGE SLOWLY. Don't go suddenly from running one mile a day to running three. Increase your level of activity gradually, says John P. DiFiori, M.D., assistant professor of family medicine and a sports medicine specialist in the department of family medicine at the University of California, Los Angeles, and a team physician in the department of intercollegiate athletics. "Allow your body to become accustomed to the new demands. That will be very helpful in preventing bursitis and tendinitis."

PAY ATTENTION TO PAIN. If you begin to feel even some slight tenderness or soreness in a shoulder, elbow, or knee (the three most common sites for bursitis and tendinitis), don't ignore it, says Dr. DiFiori. People who try to work through pain often end up with chronic cases of bursitis or tendinitis. Instead, reduce your activity and apply ice to the area three or four times a day, for 10 to 20 minutes each time.

BE FLEXIBLE. Making sure that your muscles are well-stretched and flexible may help prevent bursitis or tendinitis, says Dr. DiFiori. He advises stretching all the extremities and the trunk once or twice a day. Because different activities place demands on different parts of the musculoskeletal system, it may be helpful to discuss the ideal flexibility program for your activity with a physician or certified personal trainer. It is important to avoid overstretching and to stretch at the right time.

Try this sequence, Dr. DiFiori suggests. Warm up a bit with a little walking or light jogging. Then, stretch a little. Only after that should you start your activity. You should also stretch immediately after any exercise, with a more-moderate-to-full stretch at that point. That greatly improves flexibility.

Hold each stretch from 15 to 30 seconds. Stretch

gradually—no bouncing. And repeat each stretch three or four times.

GET STRONG. "Developing muscular strength helps prevent bursitis and tendinitis," says Dr. DiFiori. That is why he recommends strength training, working out with weights at least twice a week.

Focus on large muscle groups: the abdominals and lower back, the biceps and the triceps in your arms, the chest and the upper back, the quadriceps and the hamstrings in your thighs, and the calves. Use a weight that you can lift comfortably at least 8 to 12 times. Do two sets, with 8 to 12 repetitions in each set. Your physician or personal trainer can suggest specific exercises for your activity.

Warning: Don't overdo strength training. You can actually develop bursitis or tendinitis if you use weights that are too heavy and lift them too many times or lift with improper technique.

DOUBLE-CHECK YOUR EQUIPMENT. Equipment that is not fitted properly for you can cause bursitis or tendinitis, says Dr. DiFiori. If the grip on a tennis racquet is too big, for example, you could develop a problem in your elbow. Check with a coach or pro to make sure that your equipment is well-suited.

TAKE A BREAK. "Incorporate rest into your work and training program," says Dr. DiFiori. "If you are sitting at a computer and typing all the time, take periodic breaks."

How often? "Take a five-minute break every hour," says David Jones, M.D., medical director of the Spine and Sport Medical Center in Orange, Texas. He also recommends that during those breaks you do forearm and wrist stretches to prevent carpal tunnel syndrome. Here's how.

Stretch your right arm out in front of you, keeping your elbow locked and your fingers pointing toward the floor. With your left hand, gently pull your fingers toward your body until you feel a stretch in your wrist and forearm. Hold the stretch for 30 seconds, then release.

Next, stretch out your right arm in the same locked-elbow position, but raise the palm to point your fingers toward the ceiling. Pull back on those fingers with your left hand, again holding the stretch for 30 seconds. Then switch arms and do the same two exercises on your left arm. Do one of each exercise on each arm every time you take a break.

STAND UP STRAIGHT. Poor posture can be a contributor to bursitis or tendinitis in the shoulders, says Dr. DiFiori. Pay attention to your posture and be sure to incorporate your abdominals and upper back into your flexibility and strength-training program. A physical therapist or trainer can be very helpful in providing specific posture-training programs.

How Not to Get Injured Again

"One of the best predictors of bursitis or tendinitis at a specific site is a previous injury at that site," says Dr. DiFiori. But how do you prevent an encore of pain? The best way is to make sure that any incident of bursitis or tendinitis is rehabilitated right the first time—that is, healed in such a way that there is never a repeat performance. Here's how.

MASSAGE WITH ICE. In the early stages of an injury—immediately after the injury and for the next few days—Dr. DiFiori says to treat the problem with ice. "We use a technique called ice massage.

"Purchase paper cups, fill them with water, and put them in the freezer. When the water freezes, the top of the ice will be higher than the rim of the cup. Three or four times a day, for 10 to 20 minutes each time, take one of the cups and rub the ice in a circular motion over the area of the bursitis or tendinitis. (If you experience a lot of irritation or stinging when applying the ice, place a thin cloth between your skin and the ice to avoid injuring your skin.)

As the ice melts, you can tear the cup to expose more ice to the skin. This reduces pain and inflammation in the area and allows it to heal more quickly," says Dr. DiFiori.

REST THE RIGHT AMOUNT. It seems obvious that if you have bursitis or tendinitis, you should give your sore limb some time out. But when can you stop resting: after a day, a week, a month? Dr. DiFiori and his colleagues at the University of California, Los Angeles, use a system that incorporates "relative rest" in treating these injuries. First, they rate the severity of an injury by *when* it hurts. Then they provide a safe level of activity—how many times a week, for how long, at what intensity—for every rating. "The idea of relative rest," says Dr. DiFiori, "is reducing the amount of activity based on the level of pain so that you are not aggravating the injury." Dr. DiFiori uses a five-level grading system to rate injuries and the extent to which activities should be decreased. Here is his system.

Grade One. If you only experience pain after you are finished with the activity or if you have pain at the onset of an activity but it doesn't persist during the activity, you have a Grade One injury. In other words, you may have pain only as you begin walking or playing tennis, or you may notice pain later that night or the next day. You should decrease the frequency, length of time, and intensity of the activity by approximately 25 percent.

While you are cutting back on that activity, substitute an alternative activity that doesn't put stress on the injured area. For example, if you are a runner who runs 20 miles a week and has a Grade One injury in the legs or feet, reduce your mileage to 15 miles per week and add bicycling or swimming to supplement your training.

Grade Two. If the pain occurs during the latter part of the activity but doesn't affect your ability to perform the activity, you have developed a Grade Two injury. You know the pain is there, but you are able to do what you want to do. Decrease the frequency, length of time, and intensity of the activity by 25 to 50 percent. Supplement with alternative activities.

Grade Three. If the pain starts soon after the onset of an activity but does not affect your ability to do the activity, you have a Grade Three injury. You should decrease the frequency, length of time, and intensity of the activity by 50 to 75 percent, remembering to supplement with alternative activities.

Grade Four. If you have symptoms that limit the quality or quantity of the activity, your injury is more severe and would be classified as a Grade Four injury. Reduce that activity by at least 75 percent, adding other activities that don't place stress on the injured area.

Grade Five. If you are experiencing symptoms that prevent you from doing the activity, stop it altogether and switch to an alternative activity. As your injury begins to heal, you can slowly ease back into your primary activity. But you should be working with a doctor or therapist as you strengthen the injured area and begin to restore flexibility, Dr. DiFiori advises.

Before you resume the activity that caused the problem, make sure that you figure out what contributed to the injury, Dr. DiFiori cautions. Was it trying to do too much too soon, not getting enough rest, or using poor equipment? If you have a racquet that is not the right size or a bike that doesn't fit you right, you risk repeating the injury if you don't correct the problem, notes Dr. DiFiori. "That's true even if you do all the strength and flexibility training, icing, relative rest, and alternative activities," he says.

CANKER SORES
Managing Mouth Ouch

Preventing canker sores—or by its fancy name, recurrent aphthous stomatitis (RAS)—is a little like preventing the tide from rolling in. "Canker sores are recurrent by definition," says Stephen Sonis, D.M.D., professor of oral medicine at the Harvard School of Dental Medicine. Lurking around the lips, gums, or even around the tongue, they are painful little ulcers that go ballistic when nudged by sour or salty foods.

For most people, recurrence means a sore two or three times a year. No big deal. But for some, recurrence means a nonstop parade of pain—sore after sore. When you have one, talking as well as eating makes the pain kick in. And if they are really bad, even sleep is haunted by their constant sting.

Although experts don't know what causes these little demons to pop up inside your mouth, they have identified many associated factors, sometimes indicating serious diseases that need to be ruled out by your doctor before you begin self-treatment for chronic canker sores, says Dr. So-nis. Eliminating those factors can help prevent the sores. "If you get canker sores all the time, you should be very aggressive in discovering and dealing with the factors that trigger them for you," he says.

If those pesky sores only appear now and then, however, a number of practical tactics can help prevent them. Here are the approaches that can help fend them off.

DON'T HURT YOURSELF. If you cut, scrape, or injure the soft tissue inside your mouth, that could lead to canker sores, according to William H. Binnie, D.D.S., professor and chairman of diagnostic sciences at Baylor College of Dentistry in Dallas. Here are some ways to avoid hurting yourself.

- Watch out for hard food like chips and pretzels. Eating too fast can also be risky, says Jonathan Ship, D.M.D., associate professor and vice chairman in the department of oral medicine, pathology, and surgery at the University of Michigan School of Dentistry and director of hospital dentistry at the University of Michigan Medical Center, both in Ann Arbor.
- Tell your dentist to take it easy. Some people experience canker sores after dental work, says Dr. Ship.
- Wear a mouth guard at night. Your dentist can easily construct a simple mouth guard to help keep you from biting your lips or cheeks while you sleep.

RINSE THEM AWAY. As a first line of treatment, Dr. Binnie suggests daily use of a prescription antiseptic mouthwash called Peridex. "Some patients get good control of canker sores by this one method," he says. But he adds that people with canker sores should avoid most mouthwashes because they contain too much alcohol and because they sting.

Is Stress Starting Your Sores?

If you are frequently getting canker sores, the most important factor to deal with may be yourself, says William H. Binnie, D.D.S., professor and chairman of diagnostic sciences at Baylor College of Dentistry in Dallas.

"The type of person who gets canker sores tends to be an anxious, high-strung, and perfectionist person," says Dr. Binnie. "People who are really cool and laid back and don't have many cares rarely have the problem."

But even uptight folks don't get canker sores all the time, Dr. Binnie says. They usually get them when they are about to undergo a specific stress, like a job interview, an exam, or a speech. In fact, Dr. Binnie's research shows that 54 percent of canker sore patients said that a stressful incident was the most common factor associated with an onslaught of canker sores.

"One way to prevent canker sores is to learn to live with the stress in your life," says Jonathan Ship, D.M.D., associate professor and vice chairman in the department of oral medicine, pathology, and surgery at the University of Michigan School of Dentistry and director of hospital dentistry at the University of Michigan Medical Center, both in Ann Arbor.

Meditation, yoga, or regular exercise are just some of the methods that may help you deal with stress.

SPOT YOUR SENSITIVITIES. Many experts think that a small percentage of people with the problem are hypersensitive to various foods, which trigger the ulcers. "For example, my wife gets canker sores if she eats strawberries or walnuts," says Dr. Ship.

Other common triggering foods include tomatoes, chocolate, cereals, cheese, cow's milk, and citrus fruit, says Dr. Binnie.

"If you see a repeating pattern where you eat a certain food and canker sores occur, stop eating that food for a while and see how you do," says Dr. Sonis.

USE A DAB TO DETER IT. To prevent a painful sore from getting a mouth-hold, ask your dentist about using Lidex, a prescription corticosteroid gel. "As soon as you feel a prickling or tingling sensation, put a thin smear of gel on that area," Dr. Binnie advises patients who use the gel. And you can use it a dozen times a day if you need to, he adds. "You can usually stop the ulcer from developing." Even if the gel doesn't stop the canker sore, it can reduce or prevent pain, he says.

CATARACTS
Vitamins May Help You See into the Future

When skin ages, it wrinkles. When hair ages, it turns gray. When eyes age, they often develop a condition called cataract. When someone's eyes are afflicted with this condition, they're said to have cataracts.

"The eye has a lens just like a camera has a lens," explains Robert Sperduto, M.D., chief of epidemiology in the division of biometry and epidemiology of the National Eye Institute at the National Institutes of Health. That lens focuses light onto the retina, the light-sensitive tissue at the back of the eye. When we are young, the lens is very clear, and the light has no problem getting through it. "But as we age, the lens becomes clouded, and the light can't get through it as effectively," he says. When that clouding is severe, that is called a cataract.

You can't prevent cataracts any more than you can prevent aging, explains Dr. Sperduto. But does that mean that cataracts can't be *delayed*?

"You can slow the onset of cataracts by taking some

extra precautions to save your eyesight," says Shambu D. Varma, Ph.D., professor and director of ophthalmology research in the department of ophthalmology at the University of Maryland School of Medicine in Baltimore. And one of those precautions, he says, is to make sure that you have a healthy level of antioxidant nutrients in your diet: vitamin C, bioflavonoids, and vitamin E.

Free Your Eyes from Free Radicals

To understand why certain vitamins may help battle cataracts, step into the laboratories of Dr. Varma and his colleagues. There, he works with animals, learning the exact chemical processes that create this eye disease. Dr. Varma has discovered that a major cause of cataracts are free radicals. The so-called radicals are destructive molecules formed when light hits the lens, or they are produced by the biochemical activity in and around the eye. "Free radicals are important contributors to the creation of cataracts," he says. And antioxidant nutrients are like a bomb squad that defuses these free radicals before they can do any harm to your eyes.

Fortunately, nutrients that take care of free radicals are easy to find. Just take a stroll in the produce department.

Munch on more fruits and vegetables. "Research has found that people who consume 3 1/2 servings combined of fruits and vegetables a day have a fivefold lower risk of developing cataracts compared to people who don't get the 3 1/2 servings," says Paul Jacques, D.Sc., an epidemiologist and associate professor of nutrition at Tufts University in Boston. "The antioxidant constituents of fruits and vegetables—particularly vitamin C and the bioflavonoids—may help prevent destruction of tissue in the lens of the eyes."

Take C for sight. In a scientific study of 247 Boston women, those who took vitamin C supplements for more than 10 years showed an impressive 80 percent reduction in cataract risk. But in order to get any protection, you need to take the vitamin C supplement on a long-term basis, notes Dr. Jacques. By that, he means a minimum of 5 years.

How much vitamin C is protective? When it comes to fending off cataracts, 150 to 250 milligrams a day is sufficient to saturate the eye tissue, according to Dr. Jacques.

EASE YOUR EYESIGHT. Vitamin E supplements may also protect you from cataracts. Multiple researchers have seen more than a 50 percent lower risk of cataract formation among people who take vitamin E supplements, compared to those who do not. How much vitamin E is protective? Again, no one knows for sure. But Dr. Varma says that a person could try taking 200 IU (international units) of vitamin E per day. If you are considering taking amounts above 200 IU, discuss this with your doctor first. One study using low-dose vitamin E supplements showed an increased risk of hemorrhagic stroke.

MULTIPLY YOUR PROTECTION. Nutrients other than the antioxidants may play a role in keeping your eyes healthy and preventing cataracts. One scientific study of male physicians showed that those who took multivitamin supplements had a decreased risk of cataract formation. Some of the B vitamins in the multivitamin may be what protect the eyes from the disease, says Dr. Varma. The B vitamins thiamin and riboflavin are necessary for the overall well-being of the eyes—a must for a healthy lens.

SAY AYE TO WEIGHT LOSS. If your eyes are bigger than your stomach at the average meal, your eating habits could be harming your eyes. Being overweight is a big risk for diabetes, and diabetes is a risk for cataract development, explains George Bunce, Ph.D., professor emeritus of biochemistry and nutrition at Virginia Polytechnic Institute in Blacksburg. "Diabetics have a three- to fivefold greater incidence of cataract. Therefore, controlling one's weight brings down the risk for cataract," he says.

Beware Corticosteroids

Corticosteroids are a group of powerful anti-inflammatory drugs used to treat many different conditions, including asthma, arthritis, and inflammatory bowel disease. Unfortunately, one of their side effects is that they can cause cataracts, says Robert Sperduto, M.D., chief of epidemiology in the division of biometry and epidemiology of the National Eye Institute at the National Institutes of Health.

If you do take this type of drug, your doctor should carefully monitor the condition of your lenses and consider other treatment options if there is an indication that a cataract is developing, cautions Dr. Sperduto.

DECLINE THE WINE. "Our studies have found that people who imbibe more than a couple of drinks a day increase their risk for cataract," says Johanna M. Seddon, M.D., associate professor of ophthalmology at Harvard Medical School and director of the epidemiology unit at the Massachusetts Eye and Ear Infirmary, both in Boston.

GO HOLLYWOOD. Ultraviolet radiation from the sun may damage the lens of the eye and increase the risk that you might get cataracts. A good precaution is to shade your eyes with some sunglasses or a hat, says Dr. Sperduto. In a study of 838 Chesapeake Bay fishermen who had spent years working on the water, researchers found that those who wore sunglasses or a brimmed hat were only one-third as likely to develop cataracts as those who did not wear sun protection.

That type of protection is particularly important if you live in higher altitudes, where ultraviolet light is less-filtered by the atmosphere. Look for sunglasses with a manufacturer's label that states, "blocks 99 percent of ultraviolet rays," says the American Academy of Ophthalmology. A hat with a brim that shades your eyes will decrease sun exposure to your eyes by 50 percent, says Dr. Sperduto.

PUT BUTTS OUT. Scientists have also found that another kind of light is bad for your eyes—lighting up a cigarette. Smoking is one of the most confirmed risk factors for cataract, explains Dr. Seddon. One reason is that smokers have more stress on their metabolisms and have lower levels of antioxidants. "The greater the number of cigarettes smoked per day, the higher the risk of developing cataract," she warns.

CAVITIES
Stop Decay with Food Fighters and Cleaning Tips

You weren't born with any *Streptococcus mutans* bacteria in your mouth. But around the time you got your baby teeth, you also got a smooch from one of your parents and some of their cavity-causing germs took up residence on your teeth. They have been living hungrily ever since, generating a potent acid that dissolves your tooth enamel. That's why you have all those fillings, says David Kennedy, D.D.S., a dentist and the president of the Preventive Dental Health Association in San Diego.

But there is no reason to ever get another cavity. You can prevent tooth decay, starting today. In fact, starting with your very next meal.

Choose a Dandy Dental Diet

Experts have identified foods that can help prevent tooth decay. "In fact, selecting more nutritious foods is probably as important as staying away from cavity-causing foods like sugar and other sticky foods," says Dominick DePaola, D.D.S., Ph.D., president of Forsyth Dental Center in Boston. Here are the best foods for keeping bacteria at bay.

TRY A CHEESE CHASER. Within the first five minutes of a sugar snack, nibble on an ounce of low-fat or nonfat cheese, advises Dr. DePaola. Eating a bit of aged cheese like Cheddar or Monterey Jack stimulates the flow of saliva, which contains buffers to neutralize cavity-causing acids. Also, some specific components in cheese may keep enamel from dissolving.

MUNCH AN APPLE. Any raw, crunchy fruits and vegetables can help delay decay. "Because they contain a lot of fiber and are crunchy, they scrape away some of the bacteria and plaque, so you get a cleansing benefit just from eating them," says Heidi K. Hausauer, D.D.S., assistant clinical professor in the department of operative dentistry at the University of the Pacific School of Dentistry in San Francisco.

SPICE UP YOUR SMILE. Try a lively salsa or toss some jalapeños on your next slice of low-fat pizza. You might not like the way chile peppers make your eyes water, but they make your mouth water, too—and that excess saliva helps neutralize corrosive acids and clean your teeth, says Dr. Hausauer.

GO FOR THE YOGURT. Nonfat plain yogurt is a great source of calcium, which not only helps build strong teeth when you are young but also fortifies the jawbone that supports your pearly whites. Skip the sugary, fruited yogurts and mix nonfat plain yogurt with fresh fruit. It is also a great baked-potato topper and a base for dips, says Dr. Hausauer.

WATCH OUT FOR STICKY SNACKS. Eating a nutritious banana or some raisins makes good sense for your body, but not necessarily for your teeth, says Sheila A. Mundorff-Shrestha, associate professor of dentistry with the Eastman department of dentistry in the School of Medicine and

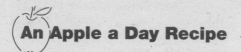

An Apple a Day Recipe

Pearly White Salsa

Spicy food may improve your smile by preventing cavities. Serve this spicy salsa with baked tortilla chips, over omelets, or on burgers. The recipe makes enough for a party or to freeze for future use. Reheat frozen salsa in the microwave or in a saucepan over low heat. For a spicier salsa, leave the seeds in the chile peppers as you mince them.

2 teaspoons olive oil
1 onion, finely chopped
1 rib celery, finely chopped
1 green, yellow, or red bell pepper, finely chopped
1 small jalapeño chile pepper, seeded and finely chopped (wear plastic gloves when handling)
1 clove garlic, minced
4 tomatoes, seeded and chopped
2 tablespoons fresh lime juice
1 teaspoon honey or sugar
½ teaspoon dried basil or oregano
½ teaspoon chili powder
¼ teaspoon ground cumin and/or coriander

Warm the oil in a large nonstick skillet over medium heat. Add the onion, celery, bell pepper, chile pepper, and garlic. Cook, stirring occasionally, for 5 minutes, or until the vegetables are soft. Stir in the tomatoes, lime juice, honey or sugar, basil or oregano, chili powder, and cumin and/or coriander. Bring to a boil. Reduce the heat to low, cover, and simmer for 20 minutes.

Makes 5 cups. Per ¼ cup: 13 calories, 1g. fat

Dentistry at the University of Rochester in New York. Mundorff-Shrestha and her research team found that these two healthy goodies did as much damage to tooth enamel as a cupcake and more damage than a chocolate bar.

Don't stop eating bananas or raisins and devour potato chips in their place. Just try to brush or rinse soon after eating sticky snacks and limit frequent, daily snacks, says Mundorff-Shrestha.

USE THE POWER OF GUM. Your teeth have their own favorite dessert—sugarless chewing gum. There is growing evidence that chewing a piece for 20 minutes after meals may reduce your risk of cavities. Bradley Beiswanger, D.D.S., professor of oral biology at Indiana University in Indianapolis did a study of 1,400 young people. The half who chewed sugarless gum two or three times a day after meals developed significantly fewer new cavities than their non-gum-chewing buddies. So stash sugar-free gum in your car, pocket, or purse. If you can't brush, chew.

Be a Clean Machine

From toothpicks to oral irrigators, there is an impressive array of low- and high-tech helpers to keep your teeth clean enough to prevent cavities. And here are some smart instructions on how to use them most effectively.

BRUSH UNDERNEATH THE "COLLAR." "If you look at a tooth from top to bottom, the top two-thirds of the chewing surfaces are relatively plaque-free from chewing," says Dr. Kennedy. But bacteria that live around the collar of the tooth—the part closest to the gum line—aren't removed by munching. To clean the collar during brushing, he recommends the following technique.

Aim the toothbrush so that the bristles are angled slightly downward into the gum for the lower teeth and slightly upward for the upper teeth. When the bristles

Sticky Situations

Tooth enamel is most vulnerable to foods high in sugar, starch, or stickiness. The following list from Sheila A. Mundorff-Shrestha, associate professor of dentistry with the Eastman department of dentistry in the School of Medicine and Dentistry at the University of Rochester in New York, ranks foods according to their cavity-causing ability. The higher the number, the worse the snack is for your teeth. If the number is over 0.5, it is a moderate to high likeliness that the food will cause cavities.

Corn chips	0.4	Graham crackers	0.8
Gelatin dessert	0.4	Milk chocolate	0.8
Peanuts	0.4	Bread	0.9
Yogurt	0.4	Granola cereal	1.0
Pretzels	0.5	Sugar	1.0
Dried fruit-and-nut mix	0.6	Bananas	1.1
Potato chips	0.6	French fries	1.1
Saltine crackers	0.6	Cupcakes	1.2
Doughnuts	0.7	Raisins	1.2

contact the tooth, they will deflect slightly into the gum. Then, instead of brushing, gently push and wiggle back and forth, working the bristles in between the teeth. "This will cleanse cavity-causing bacteria from the tooth around the gum line," says Dr. Kennedy. "It is also where the germs that cause gum disease are, so it is a brushing technique that will help protect you from that problem, too."

FLOSS TO PREVENT LOSS. To fully clean your teeth, you need to get in between them. For that, you need floss, says Dr. Kennedy. Here are his instructions on how to string up your germs.

Pull a two-foot length of floss from the dispenser—a shorter amount is too hard to grip. Wrap a lot of it around the middle finger of one hand and a little bit on the middle finger of the other (gently—you don't want to turn your fingers blue). Curl the middle fingers into the palms of your hands so that you have a "tightrope" between the two hands, and use your index fingers and thumbs to guide the floss as you clean. When the floss is in between the teeth, use your index finger and thumb to guide it so that it forms a semicircle around the tooth, and then slide it up and down and back and forth. "You're basically using it like you use a towel to dry your back—only you're scraping scum off the tooth," says Dr. Kennedy. And if you notice that the floss is shredding, unroll a little bit off one finger and roll it up on the other—like a ribbon moving across a typewriter.

DROWN THEM OUT. Use an oral irrigator after brushing and flossing, suggests Dr. Kennedy. "Once you've knocked all those germs loose from your teeth, send them on down the drain." He favors the brands with the rubber tip on the end because they will "reach down into the areas where the bacteria tend to accumulate, especially the part closest to the gum line, and flush them away." Check with your dentist to find out which type is best for you.

KEEP THAT MOUTH MOIST. Saliva is a natural cavity-fighter. Since some medications dry out your mouth, you should tell your dentist about any drugs you are taking. But if changing your prescription isn't an option, try to work harder on stimulating saliva and keeping your mouth super-clean. Suck on sugar-free candies or chew sugarless or Xylitol gum. Sip lots of water. Ask your dentist about anti-dry-mouth products like mouth rinse and artificial saliva, says Dr. Kennedy.

Toothpick: Small Size, Big Benefit

When it comes to preventing cavities, don't forget the toothpick, says David Kennedy, D.D.S., a dentist and the president of the Preventive Dental Health Association in San Diego. "Among the Native Americans in the East, when children reached the age that the elders taught them hygiene, they learned to select a prickly ash tree and use a sliver of that bark to clean their teeth. In this case, ancient and modern wisdom are the same. You can clean your teeth very easily and efficiently with a sliver of wood: a toothpick."

You can rub the enamel surfaces free of germs. To do that, make a circle around each tooth: First, using the point, place the toothpick in between the teeth and wipe up, away from the gums. Place the point of the toothpick against the front surface of the tooth and wipe around the neck, or collar, of the tooth to clean around the gum line. Then clean in between the teeth on the other side of that tooth.

Avoid the slivery, little flat toothpicks that have splinters all over them, Dr. Kennedy says. Look for toothpicks that are square in the middle and round on the ends.

CERVICAL DYSPLASIA AND CERVICAL CANCER
Planning Protection and Detection

Cancer of the cervix—the entryway to the uterus—used to kill more American women than most other cancers. Well, this former number one killer is now number nine, although rates are still disproportionately high among African-American and Hispanic women. The dramatic reduction in cervical cancer rates is mostly due to the success of a simple and almost painless medical test called the Pap test. A Pap test can detect the presence of precancerous or cancerous cells on the cervix. And, since the cure rate for cervical cancer is nearly 100 percent if it is detected in its early stages, this amazing test helps doctors save thousands of women's lives each year.

This is definitely great news, but it is still not enough. Far too many women fail to get a Pap test. Of the 15,000 women diagnosed with cervical cancer annually, 50 percent had never had a Pap test before diagnosis. "If we could reach all the women in this country who are not getting tested regularly, we could virtually eliminate deaths from this cancer," says Patricia Braly, M.D., professor and chief of gynecological cancer at the Stanley S. Scott Cancer Center of the Louisiana State University Medical Center in New Orleans and co-chairman of the National Institutes of Health Consensus Development Statement on cervical cancer.

Many of the women who are not getting Pap tests are postmenopausal, says Dr. Braly. When women are in their reproductive years, they are very conscientious about seeing a gynecologist and having an annual Pap test. But once they have gone through menopause, that may come to an end. Research shows that women start putting off their Pap tests at about age 45, and death rates from cervical cancer start to climb in this age group. "I don't think this point can be made strongly enough," Dr. Braly says. "There is no age at which a woman should stop having Pap tests."

Many women may also avoid the Pap test because they fear the results or find them confusing. "People need to understand that the vast majority of abnormal Pap tests are not telling us that the patient has cancer," says Yvonne Thornton, M.D., director of perinatal diagnostic testing at Morristown Memorial Hospital in New Jersey. When a Pap test finds abnormal cells, that may just mean that a woman has cervical dysplasia, a condition in which a few cells appear unhealthy or oddly shaped.

Dysplasia is a precancerous condition that may disappear altogether, with or without treatment, or it may develop into full-blown cervical cancer. There is no surefire way to predict its course. The bottom line, however, is this: Dysplasia is not cancer. And even if you have cervical dysplasia, there is a great deal that you can do to reduce your chances of getting cervical cancer.

Here are the steps to take to keep this cancer at bay.

A Pap Test Primer

Of course, a Pap test isn't the kind of diagnostic procedure that you can do on your own. You will need a doctor for the procedure and a lab to interpret the test. But even so, there are actions that you can take to assure that results are as reliable as possible. Here is what doctors advise.

HAVE ONE EVERY YEAR. "Every woman who is sexually active or older than age 18 should have an annual Pap test," says Dr. Braly. Sometimes Pap tests report false negative findings that say a woman does not have cervical dysplasia when, in fact, she does.

That is not a reason to worry. "Almost nobody is going to progress from a normal cervix to a cancer in one year," says Dr. Braly. But it is one of the main reasons that yearly Pap tests are a must. "If you have three annual Pap tests in a row that are normal, your risk of having precancerous cervical cells or cancer itself is about zero." But even then, you should continue to be tested throughout your life.

PREP FOR YOUR TEST. For the most accurate test results, don't have intercourse, douche, or use vaginal medications for 24 hours before your Pap test, says Dr. Braly. And have the test done mid-cycle so that menstrual blood doesn't interfere with the laboratory reading of the Pap test.

MAKE SURE YOUR DOC IS UP TO DATE. "A test called ThinPrep has made a great improvement on the standard Pap test technique," says Anne Carlon, M.D., an assistant attending obstetrician and gynecologist at New York/Cornell Medical Center in New York City. "For the improved method, the cervical sample is taken with a small brush, instead of a cotton swab, and it is then prepared in fluid, rather than on glass. As a result, there is less clumping in the cell sample," she explains. "A recent study of the method showed that it did a better job of picking up cervical dysplasia than did the standard test." If you decide to ask your doctor for ThinPrep, be aware that it is a little more

Put Down the Butts, Pick Up the Veggies

Cigarette smoking is a major risk factor for cervical cancer—second only to the human papillomavirus (HPV). In fact, women who smoke have a higher concentration of nicotine in the mucous membranes of their cervix than they do in their lungs.

"It is likely that nicotine or one of its breakdown products acts directly on the cervix as a toxin," says Joanna M. Cain, M.D., professor and chairman of the department of obstetrics and gynecology at Pennsylvania State University at the Milton S. Hershey Medical Center in Hershey.

Other research shows that the B vitamin folic acid that comes from supplements or the folate that is found in food may help decrease the risk of cervical cancer. But the best way to get your Bs is through food, not supplements.

Take these two steps to pump up your prevention plan.

- If you don't smoke, don't start. If you do smoke, here is how to get the help you need to quit. For information on smoking-cessation programs near you, you can contact the American Lung Association by writing to them at 1740 Broadway, New York City, NY 10019-4374.
- Fill your diet with lots of yellow and green leafy vegetables, citrus fruits, juices, brewer's yeast, and liver to get your 400 micrograms of folate a day.

expensive. But in Dr. Carlon's view, it is well worth its price since it provides superior early detection of precancerous cells.

READ YOUR OWN RESULTS. Don't assume that because you don't hear anything about your test results from the doctor, your Pap test was normal. "This is very important," says Dr. Braly, "because so many patients think that if they don't hear anything, they are fine." But your report may have been lost at the lab, mailed to someone else, or just plain lost at the doctor's office. Ask your physician for a copy of the report so that you are sure to see your results.

Protect Your Cervix from HPV

The human papillomavirus (HPV) is best known for its ability to cause ugly, itchy, and often painful genital warts. Scientists also know that this sexually transmitted disease can cause changes in the cells of the cervix, often leading to cervical cancer.

If you are sexually active and not monogamous, avoiding HPV isn't easy. The infection is very common, and there is no vaccine. Not everyone infected with the virus gets genital warts. In fact, many people never show any symptoms at all. But once you get HPV, you are stuck with it. Though the warts can be removed, there is no cure.

To avoid getting infected, any woman who has an active sex life needs to take this dangerous virus into account. Here is what experts advise.

ADOLESCENTS SHOULD ABSTAIN. Teenage girls have larger areas of squamous cells on their cervix—the type of cells that are easy targets for HPV. That is why the younger you are when you first begin having intercourse, the more at risk you are for developing cervical dysplasia and cervical cancer later in life. "I think that every young woman should strongly consider delaying the onset of intercourse until after the age of 18," says Dr. Braly.

MONOGAMY IS THE BEST POLICY. The more sexual partners you have, the more likely it is that you will be infected with HPV—and therefore, the more likely you will have cervical dysplasia and cervical cancer. "As best you can, ensure that you have a monogamous relationship," says Dr. Braly.

TAKE A "HIS-STORY" COURSE. The more partners someone has had, the more likely that they are infected with HPV. "Before you have sexual intercourse, you should know your potential partner's sexual history," says Dr. Braly. "Know the number of partners he has had. And know whether he has been exposed to sexually transmitted diseases." And then make up your mind about sexual intercourse.

COUNT ON CONDOMS. Unfortunately, condoms can't provide 100 percent protection against HPV because the virus can be transmitted through contact with the scrotum or anal area. But condoms should still reduce your chances of contracting HPV and other sexually transmitted diseases, such as herpes, that can increase your cervical cancer risk, says Dr. Braly.

Be sure to use latex or polyurethane condoms to be safe, says Joanna M. Cain, M.D., professor and chairman of the department of obstetrics and gynecology at Pennsylvania State University at the Milton S. Hershey Medical Center in Hershey. The natural ones, such as those made from lambskin, will not do the job.

MONITOR WHAT'S HAPPENING. "We test some women with HPV with Pap tests every three to four months," says Dr. Braly. So be sure that your gynecologist is aware if you have it and follow your doctor's advice on frequent tests.

CHAPPED LIPS
Seal Them with a Kiss of Moisture and Protection

They flake. They peel. They crack. They *hurt.* And they are about as kissable as sandpaper. Nobody wants chapped lips. But cold, dry, or windy conditions—or just some bad luck in the genes department—can dry out and roughen up that tender and sensitive section of your face. Here's how to stop the chapping from happening.

CALL IN THE BALM SQUAD. Using lip balm regularly is the best way to keep lips moist and prevent chapped lips, says Sylvia Brice, M.D., a dermatologist at the University of Colorado Health Sciences Center in Denver. "All lip balms, no matter what their ingredients, are basically a way to replace or add to the normal, moisture-retaining barrier of the skin," she explains.

How often should you use lip balm to prevent your lips from chapping? It depends on where you live and the time of year. "I live in Denver," says Dr. Brice. "It's very dry, it's cold in the winter, and there is lots of sun. A person living here should use lip balm on a daily basis, applying it a couple of times a day." If your neck of the woods is less dry, less cold, or less sunny, you may be able to use lip balm less frequently.

CHOOSE A PRODUCT WITH SUNSCREEN. The lips take a solar beating just like other areas of the face that are exposed to sunlight, but they typically don't get protection from sunscreen, says Richard Odom, M.D., interim chairman of the dermatology department at the University of California, San Francisco. That is why he suggests using a lip balm with a sun-blocking ingredient.

But he adds this caution: Some people are sensitive to sunscreen, and their lips can become chapped *because* they are using it on their lips. If you notice any itching or redness, go back to a lip balm without the extra protection.

USE THE STICK, NOT THE LICK. Yes, licking your lips moisturizes them, but only for a few seconds. The new coating of water on your lips evaporates immediately, and that makes your pucker even more parched. Not only that, but your saliva has digestive enzymes in it, which irritate your lips. "Licking your lips causes chapped lips," says Dr. Brice. But for many people, trying to stop lip-licking is about as easy as trying to stop blinking. She suggests carrying lip balm with you wherever you go and using it every time you feel like licking your lips.

Lipstick can function just like a lip balm with sunscreen, Dr. Brice says. Lipstick is based in a fatty ingredient, so it provides a barrier to keep moisture in. "And since most lipsticks are opaque, they protect you from the sun," she says. "It is probably the only makeup that is good for your skin."

HUM WHILE YOU SLEEP. During the winter, dry indoor air can turn your lips into little Saharas. To help counter the problem, Dr. Brice says to use a humidifier in your bedroom. Keep it on while you sleep, she advises.

BE CAREFUL OF ORAL HYGIENE PRODUCTS. A skin sensitivity or allergy to products like mouthwash or toothpaste can cause chapped lips, says Dr. Odom. If you have recently switched brands and notice that your lips are itchy, swollen, or have a rash, stop using the new product.

CHOLESTEROL PROBLEMS
Helping the Good Prevail

Cholesterol is bad for you, right? Not so fast. The truth is just a little more complicated.

Cholesterol comes in two varieties: low-density lipoproteins (LDL) and high-density lipoproteins (HDL). The low-density kind is the bad news, a trigger for the dismal chain of events that leads to clogging of the arteries. Worst-case scenario: From LDL damage, you get a buildup of artery-blocking plaque that often leads to heart disease. More than 100 scientific studies show that the higher your LDL, the higher your risk of a heart attack.

But the high-density kind is another matter. It is actually good for your heart and vascular health. This variety latches onto the plaque-causing low-density kind and helps usher it out of the blood. The higher your HDL, the *lower* your risk of heart disease.

"It is by keeping your HDL high and your LDL low that you prevent heart disease," says Michael Miller, M.D., associate professor and director for preventive cardiology at the University of Maryland School of Medicine in Baltimore. There are many ways that you can do exactly that.

Making Good Dietary Decisions

Smart eating habits can help drop your LDL levels. Your goal is to minimize your intake of dietary cholesterol and saturated fat. Once in your bloodstream, saturated fat prevents low-density lipoproteins from properly breaking down in the liver. As a result, the LDL levels in the blood rise. So even if a food is low in dietary cholesterol—"cholesterol-free" as the package may proclaim—it is just as bad for you as cholesterol if it has a lot of saturated fat.

There are two big dietary no-nos: (1) animal products like meat and dairy foods that have cholesterol and (2) oils that have saturated fat, specifically coconut, palm kernel, and palm oil, which are used in processed foods.

The formula for controlling cholesterol? Limit your dietary cholesterol to no more than 300 milligrams a day. Lower your intake of fat to no more than 30 percent of your total calories. And make sure that no more than one-third of those calories are from saturated or animal fat, says Dr. Miller.

Eating foods that will give you the best cholesterol profile is a lot easier than you may think, says Margo Denke, M.D., associate professor of medicine in the Center of Human Nutrition at the University of Texas Southwestern Medical Center in Dallas. Here are some key things that you can do to balance cholesterol in your favor.

CHOOSE BEEF WITH CARE. Beef isn't bad, says Dr. Denke. "But choose lean cuts like flank steak, round steak, filet mignon, or a lean cut of tenderloin," she says. Stay away from fatty beef like ribs or brisket and always choose select grade, which is lower in fat than choice and prime grades, she advises. Also, look at the piece of meat you are buying. If you see a lot of fat, trim it off when you get home. When buying hamburger, pick ground round, which has the smallest amount of fat.

As for other meats, the leanest cuts of pork are tenderloin, sirloin, and top loin. (Processed pork products like bacon, salami, sausage, and hot dogs are very high in fat.) The leanest cuts of lamb are the leg shank and the foreshank.

DISH OUT SOME FISH. "To help prevent high LDL cholesterol levels, include a lot more fish in your diet," says Wahida Karmally, R.D., director of nutrition at the Irving Center for Clinical Research at Columbia-Presbyterian Medical Center in New York City. Fish is much lower in saturated fat and cholesterol than red meat or poultry. The fatty fish like salmon, mackerel, and herring contain omega-3 fatty acids, which studies show may help protect against heart disease.

Try for a minimum of two six-ounce servings of fish a week to lower your risk for heart disease and to help protect you from arrhythmias (abnormal heart rhythm), says Paul N. Hopkins, M.D., associate professor of internal medicine at the University of Utah Cardiovascular Genetics Research Center in Salt Lake City.

SAY "LOW-FAT CHEESE." Dairy products are loaded with saturated fat, says Karmally. Always use nonfat or low-fat dairy products, like skim or 1% milk instead of whole milk. Look for cheeses with "fat-free," "reduced-fat," "low-fat," or "light" on their labels. One ounce of cheese should contain no more than three grams of fat, she says.

OIL YOUR HEALTH. Butter is loaded with saturated fat, and the fact is that you rarely need to use it in cooking. Instead, cook with small amounts of liquid oils. Corn, safflower, sesame, soybean, and sunflower oils have polyunsaturated fats, which won't bump up your LDL levels in the way that saturated fats will. And two oils, canola and olive, are high in cholesterol-lowering monounsaturated

Mini-Meals: The Perfect Eating Style to Prevent High Cholesterol

When you eat smaller meals throughout the day—five or six mini-meals rather than two or three big meals—your body may be more capable of clearing the cholesterol and fat from your blood, says Cheryl Rock, R.D., Ph.D., associate professor in the department of family and preventive medicine at the University of California, San Diego. She says that one mini-meal strategy for a typical 2,000-calorie day is to have a 400-calorie lunch and a 400-calorie dinner, eating the rest of the 1,200 calories in breakfast and three snacks. Here is a typical day of cholesterol-controlling mini-meals.

- Breakfast: A bagel with low-fat cream cheese and a glass of orange juice
- Midmorning snack: A slice of bread spread with a teaspoon of peanut butter and one banana
- Lunch: A bowl of soup and a pita pocket filled with low-fat cheese or turkey and lettuce, tomato, and sprouts
- Midafternoon snack: Some carrot sticks and a dozen whole-grain crackers with low-fat dip
- Dinner: Three ounces of chicken or fish, cooked broccoli, a small serving of spaghetti with tomato sauce, and a salad
- Evening snack: One cup of low-fat yogurt and one or two pieces of fresh fruit

fats. But don't overuse any oils. Remember that your goal is to reduce fat to no more than 30 percent of your calories.

BAN THE TRANS. Margarine is a source of trans fatty acids, which are created when a liquid oil is hardened during processing. They not only raise your LDL levels but also lower your HDL levels. They are very common in baked goods. To identify a product that has trans fatty acids, check the packaging label for the words "hydrogenated fat" or "hydrogenated oil."

If you must use margarine, Karmally suggests choosing a brand made with canola oil. Or select a low-fat liquid or soft (tub) variety, which has more unhydrogenated, unsaturated oils than stick margarine, she says.

EDIT OUT THE EGG YOLKS. Each egg yolk delivers a whopping 213 milligrams of cholesterol, about the same as nine ounces of beef. "To help prevent high LDL levels, I recommend limiting egg yolks to two to four per week," says Karmally.

Egg whites are fine. They don't have cholesterol. In recipes that call for one egg, try using two egg whites instead, suggests Karmally.

Toss in Cholesterol Combat

True, many foods can raise LDL levels, and you want to avoid them. But that also means that you need to favor foods that are low in fat and low in cholesterol—as well as foods that have cholesterol-cutting power. Here are recommendations from cholesterol-combat experts.

BE FULL OF BEANS. In 17 scientific studies, people who added beans to their daily diets lowered their total cholesterol by an average of 10 percent, says James Anderson, M.D., professor of medicine and clinical nutrition at the University of Kentucky and chief of endocrinology at the Veterans Administration Medical Center in Lexington.

Beans are both low in fat and rich in soluble fiber, which has a digestive by-product that reduces cholesterol production in the liver.

Both fresh and canned beans will help control cholesterol, says Dr. Anderson. And any variety of bean is effective, including chickpeas and navy, red, and kidney beans. The trick is to include about a half-cup of beans in your diet every day, he says. Add kidney beans to lasagna. Try mashed chickpeas (hummus) as a sandwich spread. Add black beans to soups.

To reduce discomfort from gas, introduce beans into your diet slowly, says Dr. Anderson. If they are not a regular part of your diet, eat them just once or twice a week. Then, add an additional day of bean-eating per week until you are having a serving of beans nearly every day. It usually takes about three weeks for your intestinal tract to adjust to the extra fiber, he cautions.

UP THE ANTI. Antioxidants, that is. Scientists theorize that LDL cholesterol damages your arteries when it becomes oxidized by the runaway molecules that also cause the deterioration of cells. Antioxidants can prevent this from occurring. The best dietary sources of antioxidants are fruits and vegetables. Dr. Hopkins recommends eating five or six servings a day of fruit and vegetables.

Emphasize tomatoes and tomato-containing foods like spaghetti sauce, he suggests. They contain lycopene, which has been shown to be particularly effective at stopping low-density lipoproteins from oxidizing, Dr. Hopkins says.

GO NUTS. "Eating nuts can lower high LDL cholesterol, and if you have normal cholesterol, eating nuts can *keep* it normal," says Gene Spiller, D.Sc., Ph.D., director of the Health Research and Studies Center in Los Altos, California, and author of *Eat Your Way to Better Health*.

In a study conducted by Dr. Spiller, people who added almonds and almond oil to their diets had a 14 percent drop in LDL cholesterol after three weeks. The fiber and the monounsaturated fats in the almonds may be the factors that control cholesterol, says Dr. Spiller. Those same factors are also found in filberts (hazelnuts), pistachio nuts, and pine nuts.

Eat these nuts as a snack—about a handful or one to two ounces per day. This is enough to trigger their anti-cholesterol action, according to Dr. Spiller. While they are high in fat, you are not likely to eat very many because they are so filling. "People in my study were afraid that they would gain weight from eating nuts," says Dr. Spiller. "But they found that a handful of nuts in the middle of the afternoon often satisfied their appetites for some time."

SCARE AWAY VAMPIRES—AND CHOLESTEROL. "Garlic can help prevent heart disease by lowering total cholesterol," says Stephen Warshafsky, M.D., assistant professor of medicine at New York Medical College in Valhalla. No one knows the exact mechanism by which garlic cuts cholesterol, but it may work by reducing the levels of enzymes that manufacture cholesterol in the liver.

One-half clove to one clove of garlic a day should help keep cholesterol under control, Dr. Warshafsky says. You can get that amount by including garlic in your diet or by taking a daily garlic supplement, following the dosage recommendations on the label. (Dr. Warshafsky says that only two brands of garlic supplements, Kwai and Kyolic, have been scientifically proven to lower cholesterol in people.)

Better yet, include your garlic in meals. "I put garlic in my pasta and salads," says Dr. Warshafsky. "It's nice to know that you can do a simple thing like adding garlic to your diet that will help keep cholesterol under control and prevent heart disease."

PACK IN THE PECTIN. Pectin is a type of soluble fiber found in citrus fruits and apples. Researchers at the University of Florida College of Medicine in Gainesville, led by professor of medicine James J. Cerda, M.D., have found that the pectin in grapefruit can lower total cholesterol and LDL cholesterol. High-pectin foods help lower the "bad"

An Apple a Day Recipe

Cholesterol-Lowering Skillet Dinner

Beans have the amazing ability to help lower your blood cholesterol. That's because they are high in soluble fiber, which helps reduce your body's internal cholesterol production. This spicy bean skillet dinner is ready in minutes, loaded with fiber, and full of rich flavors.

2 cans (15 ounces each) hot chili beans, drained

1 can (14½ ounces) stewed tomatoes

2 cups frozen mixed vegetables

¾ cup quick-cooking rice

1 tablespoon chili powder

½ teaspoon dried thyme

1 cup water

1 can (14¾ ounces) low-sodium tomato sauce

½ cup shredded reduced-fat Cheddar cheese

In a large skillet, combine the beans, tomatoes, vegetables, rice, chili powder, thyme, and water. Bring to a boil. Reduce the heat to low, cover, and simmer for 12 to 14 minutes, or until the rice is tender. Stir in the tomato sauce and cook for 5 minutes. Top with the Cheddar.

Makes 4 servings. Per serving: 371 calories, 4 g. fat, 11 g. dietary fiber cholesterol as much as any cholesterol-lowering medication available today, according to Dr. Cerda.

There is one problem, though. To get the amount of pectin necessary to stop or reverse cholesterol buildup, you would have to eat four grapefruit a day, including the white fiber between sections, where most of the pectin is contained. That's an unreasonable amount of grapefruit, but you can also take a pectin supplement, a powdered combination of pectin and protein that dissolves in liquids, according to Dr. Cerda.

Take one to three tablespoons a day of a pectin supplement in eight ounces of water or juice, recommends Dr. Cerda. Pectin supplements are available in most supermarkets and health food stores.

BUMP UP YOUR CHROMIUM. "When people take supplements of the trace mineral chromium, it keeps their levels of total cholesterol and LDL cholesterol lower and boosts their levels of HDL cholesterol," says Richard Anderson, Ph.D., lead scientist at the U.S. Department of Agriculture Human Nutrition Research Center in Beltsville, Maryland. Dr. Anderson theorizes that chromium is a powerful cholesterol beater because it improves the efficiency of insulin, the hormone that helps the body metabolize blood sugar. Many studies show that when blood levels of insulin are normal, so is the blood level of cholesterol. He recommends taking a daily "balanced nutritional supplement" and a daily chromium supplement of 200 micrograms to prevent cholesterol problems. Broccoli and turkey ham are good sources of chromium, and it is also found in grapefruit and fortified breakfast cereals.

The Cholesterol-Prevention Food Pyramid

A few years back, the U.S. Department of Agriculture introduced the Food Pyramid, a guideline to healthy eating that made recommendations for how much we should eat of each food group every day. If you are especially concerned about high cholesterol, consider this Cholesterol Prevention Food Pyramid, offered by Paul N. Hopkins, M.D., associate professor of internal medicine at the University of Utah Cardiovascular Genetics Research Center in Salt Lake City. Included in the lineup are many low-fat foods, beans, and nuts that have cholesterol-controlling qualities.

Grains, potatoes, and legumes. Six or more daily servings. Try to get many whole grains, including whole-grain breads and cereal, pasta, brown rice, tortillas, potatoes, sweet potatoes, beans, peas, and lentils.

Fruits and vegetables. Five or more daily servings. Shoot for a variety of leafy greens, red and yellow vegetables, and citrus fruits.

Low-fat and no-fat dairy products. Two to three daily servings. Use mostly the fat-free variety.

Fish, lean meat, poultry, and eggs. Two daily servings or fewer. Have at least two servings of fish every week. Choose the leanest cuts of meat. Eat all chicken and turkey without the skin. Limit egg yolks to no more than two per week.

Nuts and oils. One serving of nuts a day, four or five times a week. Cooking oils and salad dressings should be used sparingly. Use canola oil and extra-virgin olive oil, which are rich in cholesterol-lowering monounsaturated fat.

Angling for Cholesterol Control

A number of lifestyle factors have an effect on your cholesterol levels. Your weight and your exercise habits can make a difference. And your cholesterol levels are also influenced to a surprising degree by whether—and how much—you smoke and drink.

STAY LEAN. Putting on pounds can raise your LDL cholesterol and triglyceride levels and lower your HDL cholesterol level. "If you want to prevent cholesterol problems, do not become overweight," says Karmally.

GET YOUR BLOOD FLOWING. "Get your heart rate up and keep it up through brisk walking or any other type of aerobic exercise like bicycling or jogging," says Dr. Miller. "It will raise HDL cholesterol levels anywhere from 5 to 30 percent." Exercise works to boost HDL by improving your body's efficiency at breaking down blood fats or triglycerides, which are the building blocks of HDL. Dr. Miller recommends exercising three or more times a week for 20 to 30 minutes a session.

IF YOU DRINK—STOP AT ONE OR TWO. There is evidence that approximately one ounce of alcohol a day can help increase HDL cholesterol, says Dr. Miller. (One ounce of alcohol translates into two 4-ounce glasses of wine, two 12-ounce glasses of beer; or two 1 1/2-ounce shots of spirits.) It can also raise triglyceride levels if your genes lean this way.

But don't start drinking as a health move. "A cardiologist who tells nondrinkers to start drinking to control their cholesterol is not making a credible recommendation," Dr. Miller says.

One in every five people who starts drinking becomes a problem drinker, Dr. Miller notes. And the health risks from excessive drinking are serious. Having more than two drinks a day puts you at extra risk for stroke, high blood pressure, and various types of cancer.

Healthy by the Numbers

How often should you have your cholesterol levels checked? What are the numbers that you need to know?

Start with a baseline cholesterol/triglyceride/high-density lipoprotein (HDL) level check in your early twenties, says Paul N. Hopkins, M.D., associate professor of internal medicine at the University of Utah Cardiovascular Genetics Research Center in Salt Lake City. If there is no problem, you don't need to check again until you pass 40. If the 40th-year check is normal, then have the levels checked every five years.

As long as the readings continue to be normal, there is no need to check more frequently, says Dr. Hopkins. But you should know your levels of low-density lipoprotein (LDL) cholesterol, the "bad" kind that causes heart disease; triglycerides, which also contribute to heart disease; HDL cholesterol, the "good" kind that rids the blood of LDL; and total cholesterol, the combination of LDL and HDL. Here are the numbers you are shooting for.

Note: If you have already had a heart attack or have diabetes, your LDL should be at 100 or lower, says Dr. Hopkins.

LDL cholesterol: 130 or lower
HDL cholesterol: 35 or higher
Total cholesterol: 200 or lower
Triglycerides: Under 200

If your numbers move out of the desirable range, ask your doctor how often you should have your levels checked, suggests Dr. Hopkins.

SAY SAYONARA TO SMOKES. Cigarette smoke oxidizes LDL cholesterol, making it more likely to form artery-clogging plaque. "If you stop smoking, within two years your risk of a heart attack decreases to that of someone who has never smoked," says Dr. Hopkins. So if you are a smoker, have a head-to-heart talk with yourself and decide to quit.

COLDS
Blow Them Away

The nose wasn't designed to stop a cold virus. That's the conclusion of Jack Gwaltney, M.D., professor of medicine and head of the division of epidemiology and virology in the department of internal medicine at the University of Virginia in Charlottesville and one of the world's leading experts on colds. He has spent the last 20 years dropping cold viruses into thousands of people's noses, trying to figure out exactly how a cold virus works and how it can be stopped.

The good news for science is that he and his colleagues deciphered how cold viruses carry out their invasion. The bad news for cold sufferers—and that's just about everybody—is that a cold virus is just about unstoppable.

"If a cold virus gets in your nose—either directly or through the tear ducts, which lead to the nose—it's going to get you," says Dr. Gwaltney. "Your nose was designed to stop bacteria, dust, and other intruders by capturing them in the mucous membranes and sweeping them to the back of your throat for disposal." But the very part of your throat that blocks larger particles holds a warm reception for cold viruses. The virus actually attaches to back-of-the-throat receptors and infects your cells, which then produce lots of new viruses. To fight them, your body starts generating lots of virus-killing chemicals, and those powerful chemicals generate the unpleasant symptoms that you call a cold.

So what is the *best* way to prevent a cold? "Be a hermit," says Dr. Gwaltney. "You only get cold viruses from other human beings." But if a hermit's life isn't exactly your cup of tea, here are more practical avenues to prevention.

DON'T HANG OUT WITH THE NEWLY INFECTED. People are most infectious during the first three days that they have a cold, so avoid them during that time, says Dr. Gwaltney.

WATCH OUT FOR KID STUFF. Children are the major reservoirs of cold viruses because a child's immature immune system can't repel them as easily. Grandparents with chronic diseases should be especially wary, says Dr. Gwaltney, because a problem like chronic obstructive lung disease or heart disease could be complicated by the cold virus. Grandparents should steer clear of grandkids when they have a new cold, he says.

WASH AWAY THAT VIRUS. Most cold viruses come to you in the form of a "handout." When someone with a cold lifts his hands to his nose or eyes, he snags the virus. After that, the virus can rub off anywhere—on a doorknob, towel, pencil, or faucet. Just touch that object and then touch your nose or eyes, and you risk "inoculating" yourself with the virus. That is why Dr. Gwaltney says to wash your hands after any contact with somebody who has a cold or with something that they have touched. Both before and after you wash, try not to touch your eyes or nose with your hands, he adds.

DON'T COUGH WHEN YOU ARE CLOSE. Although most cold viruses are spread through touch, some are spread

---

Preventive Measures That Are Something to Sneeze At

Many of the ways commonly suggested to prevent a cold simply don't work, says Jack Gwaltney, M.D., professor of medicine and head of the division of epidemiology and virology in the department of internal medicine at the University of Virginia in Charlottesville and one of the world's leading experts on colds. Here is his list of time- and money-wasters.

USE DISINFECTANTS ON SURFACES IN THE HOME. The possibility of cleaning off the cold viruses from every contaminated area is very low, notes Dr. Gwaltney. "I don't think there's much practical value in that."

TURN ON THE HUMIDIFIER. Scientific research has shown that the nose works perfectly fine even when humidity is low, says Dr. Gwaltney. But even if humidity did help the mucous membrane of the nose, that membrane doesn't protect you from cold viruses. "The idea that low humidity can cause colds doesn't have any basis in fact," he says.

TAKE EXTRA VITAMIN C. Vitamin C can't prevent a cold, but it can shorten the length of a cold and reduce the severity of its symptoms, says Dr. Gwaltney. But, he says, in reality, these effects are pretty trivial.

---

through the air via a sneeze or cough. To prevent giving a cold to your family, friends, or co-workers, move away or turn your head before you cough, sneeze, or blow your nose. And afterward, wash your hands.

STOP A SUMMER COLD WITH CHLORINE. Most summer colds come from backyard swimming pools that don't have sufficient chlorine in them, says Dr. Gwaltney. "In the summertime, people get infected with the adenovirus, which causes a more severe cold than the rhinovirus, the

Relationships That Build Resistance

Dozens of scientific studies show that people with more diverse social networks—that is, a spectrum of interactions with spouse, family, friends, neighbors, co-workers, and others—are more resistant to heart disease and live longer. Now an experiment shows that having a wide variety of relationships may also prevent colds.

The team of scientists who made this surprising discovery was led by Sheldon Cohen, Ph.D., professor of psychology at Carnegie Mellon University in Pittsburgh. Dr. Cohen and his colleagues enlisted 276 participants for the study and asked them whether they had 1 or more of 12 varieties of social interaction ranging from their own spouses and other close family members to friends, neighbors, and workmates. Having determined varying degrees of social interaction, researchers gave nasal drops with cold-causing rhinoviruses to all the participants and waited to see whether or not they came down with colds.

According to Dr. Cohen, people with only a few types of relationships had four times the risk of developing a cold as those with six or more types of relationships.

The ongoing scientific research on social interactions and health is about five years away from providing specific advice, from telling people exactly what types and quantities of social interactions will produce the greatest health, says Dr. Cohen. But at least you have some heartwarming knowledge for the next cold-causing winter: If you have lots of different types of people in your life, you may have a lot more protection against colds.

type of virus that causes most winter colds. And people usually get an adenovirus from water in a swimming pool that doesn't have enough chlorine in it."

To prevent the problem, make sure that your own pool is sufficiently chlorinated before you jump in. And if you are swimming in a neighbor's, community, or club pool, ask when the water was last tested *before* you take a plunge.

COLD SORES
Let a Sleeping Virus Lie

This is one condition where what doctors call primary prevention—never getting the disease in the first place—is next to impossible. An estimated 80 to 90 percent of Americans are already infected with herpes simplex type 1, the virus that causes cold sores, those embarrassing eruptions around your lips.

The infection usually takes place during childhood. In many cases, the person doing the infecting doesn't have an active cold sore, and the person being infected doesn't get one. There is just an uneventful virus transfer during a kiss from Aunt Wendy or a sip from a friend's glass. In fact, in many people, the virus never produces an outbreak but simply hibernates in the nerves close to the lips. In approximately one-third of those who carry the virus, it crawls out of its cave 2 to 12 times a year and makes an unsightly, painful lip sore.

The outbreak lasts about 10 days. First, there is tingling and itching at the site of the sore-to-be. Next, the skin there swells slightly. That is followed by a herd of tiny blisters under the skin, which then erupt, forming a painful, visible ulcer. After a day or so, the ulcer scabs. After a couple of days, the scab falls off.

Various factors can trigger an outbreak. Sickness is a common cause, tagging the condition with its two non-medical names: cold sore and fever blister. Stress is often to blame, which is why cold sores have an uncanny ability to pop up exactly when you don't want them, like before an important date or job interview. Too much sunlight can often spark a sore. And so can direct trauma—for example, a shot of novocaine into nearby nerves.

Medical researchers have discovered numerous ways to help you stop cold sores, particularly if you get a lot of outbreaks. Here are some tactics to stop them cold.

FAVOR LYSINE, FORSAKE ARGININE. Lysine is an essential amino acid, a component of protein that is one of the body's nutritional necessities. But it is also on a biochemical seesaw with another amino acid, arginine, which helps viruses replicate. The higher the level of lysine in your cells, the lower the level of arginine. So it seems reasonable to suppose that you can help prevent cold sores by tipping the seesaw in favor of lysine.

To prevent cold sores, take lysine supplements, favor a diet high in lysine, and avoid foods that are rich in arginine, says Susan Zunt, D.D.S., associate professor of oral pathology at the Indiana University School of Dentistry in Indianapolis.

"Taking 500 to 1,000 milligrams of lysine a day can be very helpful in preventing cold sores," she says. "And if a patient gets a recurrence, he can minimize its severity by taking 3,000 milligrams—in three 1,000-milligram doses—for the duration of the outbreak." For some people, cold sores occur less frequently as they get older. If you don't want to take lysine for the rest of your life, says Dr. Zunt, you can stop after one year and wait to see if you still have frequent outbreaks.

A Med for Prevention

If you know that you are prone to cold sores in some situations, your doctor might be able to help prevent that predictable outbreak. "I prescribe acyclovir (Zovirax) to skiers who routinely get cold sores when they are in the mountains where the sun is more intense," says Sylvia Brice, M.D., a dermatologist at the University of Colorado Health Sciences Center in Denver. "They can start taking the medication the day *before* they begin their ski trip, and it is very effective."

Acyclovir works by traveling directly to cells infected with the herpes virus and ordering the virus to calm down, to stop generating so many copies of itself. You can take the drug before events that you know typically trigger a sore: a day at the beach, a trip to the dentist, or a major stress. Or, says Dr. Brice, you can take the drug immediately at the first sign of a cold sore—the tingling, itching sensation that is all too familiar to those who have frequent outbreaks. In either case, you don't have to make an appointment every time you want to prevent an impending sore. Your doctor can write you a prescription for a supply that is sufficient for self-treatment.

At the same time, you can also increase the amount of lysine in your diet by eating foods like chicken, fish, cheese, cottage cheese, eggs, milk, soybeans, and mung beans.

"When I counsel people about preventing or treating recurrences, I also point out that eating foods high in argi-nine can sabotage their dietary supplements of lysine," says Dr. Zunt. Foods to avoid that contain arginine include peanuts and peanut butter, walnuts, almonds, pistachio nuts, sesame seeds, sunflower seeds, coconut, cocoa powder, chickpeas, brown rice, and whole wheat.

BLOCK THAT SUN. "People who get sun-induced cold

sores need to be religious about using sunscreen lip balm," says Sylvia Brice, M.D., a dermatologist at the University of Colorado Health Sciences Center in Denver. "They can't just put it on once in the morning. They have to reapply it continually. But it can be very helpful in preventing cold sores, and I recommend it to every patient who has this problem."

FEND OFF KISSING AND SHARING. Unfortunately, you can transmit herpes simplex type 1 even if you don't have a cold sore. But when you do have one, be extra careful: No kissing, and no sharing glasses or utensils, says Dr. Brice.

DON'T INFECT ANOTHER PART OF YOUR BODY. In a very few cases, people with a cold-sore outbreak inadvertently infect another part of their bodies—the tip of a finger, the lining of a nostril, the eyes. To prevent this, be careful not to touch your sore, particularly before a scab forms, which is when it is maximally infectious.

COLON CANCER
Diet Makes a Big Difference

Of all cancers, lung cancer kills the most Americans. But the kind of cancer that occurs in the colon and rectum is the second biggest threat, stealing the lives of approximately 55,000 Americans per year.

In case you are wondering, the colon, or large intestine, is designed to collect the waste products of digestion and shuttle them out of your body via the rectum. Evidence suggests that exposing this organ to large amounts of certain harmful chemicals or digestive by-products can trigger either benign precancerous growths or outright malignant tumors in an otherwise-healthy colon.

A Colon-Friendly Diet

It is not surprising that what you consume (or don't consume) plays a big part in preventing colon cancer. In fact, scientists who have studied colon cancer say that up to 80 percent of all cases are preventable. And prevention starts with food.

EAT MORE WHEAT BRAN. The lower your intake of dietary fiber, the higher your risk of colon cancer. That fact has been proven in study after study, says Dr. Alberts. And the most powerful colon cancer–preventing fiber may be wheat bran, he says. His research shows that wheat bran helps to protect the body from some of the digestive byproducts that pass through the colon and may trigger cell mutations that lead to cancer. "To help prevent colon cancer, consider adding a bowl of cereal fiber to your five servings of fruits and vegetables each day," he advises.

FILL YOUR GROCERY CART WITH PRODUCE. More than 20 scientific studies have shown that eating more fruits and vegetables reduces the risk of colon cancer. "The evidence that a sufficient intake of fruits and vegetables helps protect against colon cancer is stronger than the evidence for any other possible protective factor," says Emily White, Ph.D., associate professor in the division of public health sciences at the Fred Hutchinson Cancer Research Center and in the department of epidemiology at the University of Washington, both in Seattle.

How much do you have to eat to lower your risk? Increase your intake of fruits and vegetables until you are eating the equivalent of five full servings a day, says David Alberts, M.D., professor of medicine in the cancer prevention and control program at the Arizona Cancer Center, a division of the College of Medicine at the University of Arizona in Tucson. (Any time you eat a fruit or vegetable—a banana sliced on your breakfast cereal, an apple for a snack, a salad at lunch, a baked potato with dinner—that's about a serving.) And don't worry if you love pears and red peppers but can't stand oranges and eggplant. Scientists have found that it is *fruits and vegetables,* not any particular food from the produce aisle and not any particular micronutrient in that food, that can help shield you against this disease.

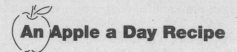

An Apple a Day Recipe

Fiber-Power Muffins

Wheat bran is a powerhouse for preventing colon cancer. Try it in these refreshing orange bran muffins. You can freeze the muffins and reheat them for a quick breakfast.

2 cups shredded all-bran cereal
¾ cup hot water
¼ cup canola oil
¾ cup buttermilk
1 egg
¼ cup honey
1 tablespoon grated orange peel
¼ cup orange juice

1 cup raisins
1¼ cups whole-wheat pastry flour or all-purpose flour
2 teaspoons baking soda
½ teaspoon salt
¼ cup chopped toasted walnuts (optional)

Preheat the oven to 400°F. Coat a 12-cup muffin pan with nonstick spray.

In a medium bowl, stir together the cereal, water, and oil until the cereal is soft.

In a small bowl, whisk together the buttermilk, egg, honey, orange peel, and orange juice. Add to the cereal mixture with the raisins, stir until well-blended.

In a large bowl, combine the flour, baking soda, and salt. Mix well. Add the cereal mixture and stir until just blended.

Divide the batter among the muffin cups, filling them about two-thirds full. Sprinkle with the walnuts (if using). Bake for 15 to 18 minutes, or until a toothpick inserted into the center of a muffin comes out clean. Cool on a rack for 5 minutes.

Makes 12 muffins. Per muffin: 184 calories, 5 g. fat, 8 g. dietary fiber

SLICE SOME MEAT FROM YOUR DIET. In one study, women who ate red meat (beef, lamb, or pork) five days in the week had a three- to four-times higher risk of developing colon cancer than women who didn't eat any. Fried or broiled meats may be particularly risky because they may increase levels of mutagens, substances that can trigger tumors, says Bandaru Reddy, Ph.D., associate director for research and chief of the division of nutritional carcinogenesis at the American Health Foundation in Valhalla, New York.

ENJOY SOY. In a study of nearly 1,000 Californians, the people who ate soybeans in some form at least once a week had half the risk of developing polyps (growths in the colon that are precursors to colon cancer) as compared to people who didn't eat soybeans.

GET PLENTY OF CALCIUM. "Calcium appears to be a significant agent in the reduction of risk for colon cancer," says Dr. Alberts. In his research, calcium worked in the same way as fiber, reducing the level of possible cancer-promoting bile acids in the colon.

Dr. Reddy recommends an intake of 1,500 milligrams of calcium per day, which can come from both dietary sources and supplements. Good sources of calcium in the diet include dairy products such as skim milk and nonfat yogurt and cheeses; green vegetables such as collard greens, mustard greens, kale, and broccoli; fish such as canned salmon with bones and sardines with bones; and calcium-fortified orange juice.

SEEK OUT SELENIUM. "The mineral selenium may

A Test That Prevents Colon Cancer

Alfred Neugut, M.D., Ph.D., is a very frustrated man. He knows that there is a screening test that can not just detect but also prevent a remarkable 80 percent of all cancers of the rectum and lower end of the colon. He also knows that very few Americans will get that test. And he doesn't know why.

"Screening for colon cancer is simple, easy, and effective—and it is sensational in preventing the disease," says Dr. Neugut, associate professor of medicine and public health at the Columbia University College of Physicians and Surgeons and director of the university's program in cancer prevention and control at its Herbert Irving Comprehensive Cancer Center, both in New York City.

To perform the test, called a sigmoidoscopy, the doctor inserts a flexible, fiber-optic lighted tube (a sigmoidoscope) in the rectum and lower half of the colon. The doctor looks for early-stage cancers and for polyps, abnormal growths from which most colon cancers

help protect against cancer of the colon," says Dr. Reddy. In one study, researchers determined that people who consumed 200 micrograms of selenium a day had a 60 percent lower risk of colon cancer than those who did not. Many of the best dietary sources of selenium aren't foods that you are likely to eat every day. Lobsters, cooked oysters, clams, crabs, and brazil nuts are five of the richest sources. Some doctors who recommend selenium for the prevention of colon cancer may suggest taking more than the Daily Value (70 micrograms). But anyone taking doses above 200 micrograms must be under medical supervision because of the potential for toxicity.

develop. As soon as the polyps are found, they can be removed, and that simple operation prevents them from developing into colon cancer.

"People are dying needlessly because they don't get this test," says Dr. Neugut. He recommends that you get a sigmoidoscopy every three to five years, starting at age 50. He also says that you should get a fecal occult blood test every year, also starting at age 50. If either of these tests is positive—if the doctor finds blood in the stool or polyps—the next step is a colonoscopy.

During a colonoscopy, the doctor explores the entire length of the colon for polyps. It is somewhat more elaborate and expensive than a sigmoidoscopy, and you have to prepare for the test by fasting overnight. Since the colonoscopy is not routinely covered by insurance and since it poses a very slight risk of perforation of the colon, Dr. Neugut doesn't recommend it as a routine procedure for everyone. But if there is visible rectal bleeding or a family history of colon cancer, your physician may bypass the fecal occult blood test and the sigmoidoscopy and suggest a colonoscopy right away.

SAY HELLO TO H$_2$O. Researchers at the Fred Hutchinson Cancer Research Center in Seattle studied 400 middle-aged men and women with a history of colon cancer, comparing their diets to those of cancer-free counterparts. They found that among women who drank more than five glasses of plain water a day, there were fewer cases of colon cancer. In fact, their risk was about half of what it was for women who drank fewer than two glasses a day. (The researchers didn't find the same protective effect in men, a finding they say they can't explain without more study.)

TAKE A WALK—OFTEN. In a scientific study conducted by Dr. White, people who participated in a moderate- or high-intensity recreational exercise program at least twice a week had a 30 percent reduced risk of colon cancer. Dozens of other scientific studies also show the same kind of protective effect. "One of the most consistent findings in the research on the prevention of colon cancer is that exercise reduces the risk of developing the disease," she says. And you don't have to enter a marathon to run away from colon cancer. Even 30 minutes of aerobics, dancing, or using an exercise machine a couple of times a week can be protective, she says.

Exercise may protect the colon against cancer by speeding up bowel transit time, that is, the time it takes for stool to pass through the bowels. A faster transit time helps stop potentially cancer-causing chemicals from loitering in the colon.

TALK TO YOUR DOCTOR ABOUT ASPIRIN. Scientific studies show that people who take aspirin seem to have a 50 percent lower risk of colon cancer than those who don't, says Dr. Alberts. But taking aspirin every day for a couple of months probably won't do it. In most of the studies, the protective effect kicks in only after about two decades or more of consistently taking the medication.

It is important to ask your doctor if regular doses of aspirin are right for you since long-term use of aspirin can damage your stomach lining or cause other side effects. If you start taking aspirin regularly, it should only be with your doctor's okay and supervision, says Dr. Reddy.

CONJUNCTIVITIS
Preventing Pinkeye

The conjunctiva is the thin, protective mucous membrane that covers your eyeballs and the inner surface of your eyelids. Any inflammation of that sensitive shield caused by viruses, bacteria, or even an inadvertent sudsing in the shower is called conjunctivitis.

Of course, if you get some soap on your conjunctiva, you can rinse it off, and the conjunctivitis will go away in a couple of minutes. But if you get an infection of your conjunctiva (typically called pinkeye), the symptoms are a lot worse than a little stinging and last a lot longer.

Viral conjunctivitis brings with it red, grainy, teary eyes. Bacterial conjunctivitis reddens your eyes and loads them with pus. Like a cold, those types of conjunctivitis tend to clear up in about a week. But in the meantime, you can infect your family and friends if you are not careful. And they are not going to appreciate the downtime any more than you do since schools and offices discourage people from showing up when they have this highly contagious infection.

Infectious conjunctivitis isn't always as minor as a cold. The infection can travel to your cornea, the layer of the eyeball underneath the conjunctiva. An infection of the cornea can blur or cloud your vision for weeks or months—or even ruin the cornea, requiring a corneal transplant.

Convinced that you don't want to get (or give) conjunctivitis? There are ways to prevent getting it in the first place and other ways to prevent spreading it around if you have it. For tips about both, turn an eye below.

WASH YOUR HANDS OF THE PROBLEM. Since the virus or bacteria usually hitches a ride on an infected person's hand, anything he touches turns to a polluted zone. Touch anything in that zone—a utensil, a doorbell, or a telephone—and you may be taking the infectious agent for a little ride. And when it touches down in your eye, your conjunctiva will be in trouble. The best way to cancel that infectious itinerary? Wash your hands frequently, says Richard Koplin, M.D., professor of ophthalmology at the New York Medical College in Valhalla and director of the Eye Trauma Center, New York Eye and Ear Infirmary in Manhattan. "This is particularly true if you are shaking a lot of hands and turning a lot of doorknobs."

DON'T LIVE HAND-TO-EYE. "You should keep your hands away from your eyes so that you don't infect yourself with something on your hands," says Dr. Koplin. If you must rub your eyes, use a tissue rather than your bare fingers.

GEL THEM TO DEATH. Dr. Koplin recommends that you use an antibacterial hand gel to prevent picking up somebody else's conjunctivitis. Scientific research shows that the instant antibacterial gels such as Vaseline Antibacterial Hand Lotion, Suave Antibacterial Hand Lotion, or Bath and Body Works Protective Antibacterial Hand Lotion, available at drugstores and specialty stores, are fairly effective at killing bacteria and most viruses, says Dr. Koplin.

"Put a little dab of the gel in your palm, spread it

Drop the Drops to Stop the Pink

Overuse of eyedrops containing tetrahydrozoline hydrochloride, like Visine or Murine, can cause one form of conjunctivitis, says Richard Koplin, M.D., professor of ophthalmology at the New York Medical College in Valhalla and director of the Eye Trauma Center, New York Eye and Ear Infirmary in Manhattan.

These drugs are vasoconstrictors, he explains. They constrict the blood vessels in your eyes so that they appear less red. "But if you use a vasoconstrictor consistently, in four or five days the muscles around the blood vessel will no longer react to the standard dose—it needs more. So you end up using the drops five times a day instead of once or twice a day. And after a month, the vessels won't constrict at all. In fact, you get a reverse reaction where the vessels expand more so that the eye is even redder."

Dr. Koplin tells his patients who use these products to switch to an ocular lubricant, a product such as Refresh or Cellufresh that does not contain a vasoconstrictor and is intended to reduce eye irritability. "You won't get rid of the red, but it will give you more eye comfort," he says.

around your hands, and in a few seconds, it evaporates. The gel can be kept near your desk at work or on the kitchen counter at home so that you can use it throughout the day. I use it in the office—it is an easy way to maintain my hand hygiene and avoid giving myself or my patients anything that I may have picked up in the last examining room," says Dr. Koplin.

Declare a "Mini-Quarantine"

Infectious conjunctivitis is a condition that is all too easy to pass around. That is why in the first three to five days of an infection—the time when you are most infectious—you want to put yourself in a mini-quarantine, says Dr. Koplin. "You have to be very unselfish and not pass the disease to somebody else." To prevent that from happening, here is what he tells his patients with conjunctivitis to do.

USE ALCOHOL PADS. "Go to the drugstore and buy 50 to 100 alcohol pads, the type doctors use on your arm before giving you a shot. Put a dozen in your pocket, and throughout the day, every half-hour or so, tear one open and wipe your hands with it. You are helping to prevent the most common way of giving someone else the infection, which is through your hands," says Dr. Koplin.

WASH, WASH, WASH YOUR HANDS. "Do it each and every time you think about it—as many times during the day as possible." And make sure that no one else uses your towels or washcloths, he adds.

BAG THE TISSUES. When you wipe your eyes with a tissue, immediately put the tissue in a separate plastic bag. When it is time to throw out that bag, do it yourself or make sure that whoever does it is wearing gloves or washes their hands carefully afterward.

SEGREGATE THE PLATES. The person who has conjunctivitis should pick their dishes and utensils and wash them himself or place them in the dishwasher, if he has one. "Those objects shouldn't be handled by anybody else," says Dr. Koplin.

DON'T MAKE THE BED. Beds should not be made by people who have the infection. "They'll spread it all over the place," says Dr. Koplin.

How to Avoid Contact Conjunctivitis

Using contact lenses the wrong way can cause conjunctivitis and, much scarier for the health of your eyes, keratitis, an infection of the cornea. Fortunately, tears contain a natural anti-infectious agent. But after you are 40 years old, the tear film is not as powerful an infection-fighter as it was when you were younger, says Dr. Koplin. People who have been wearing contact lenses most of their lives can suddenly start to develop problems like conjunctivitis.

The solution is just that—contact lens solution. Combined with other hygienic measures, you should be able to put in or take out your lenses without risking pinkeye problems.

BE HYGIENICALLY CORRECT. Clean and sterilize your lenses according to the manufacturer's instructions, says Dr. Koplin. And be sure to wash your hands before you put in or take out your contact lenses. Never take out a lens, clean it with saliva, and then put it back in your eye, he warns.

DON'T OVERDO. Dr. Koplin says that overusing your contact lenses is one way to end up with conjunctivitis. When your lenses bother you, take them out and rest your eyes. And don't take naps in hard lenses, he says. The pressure of the lens could cause a small abrasion or tear, which is a perfect entrance for virus and bacteria.

If you have disposable lenses, be sure to throw them out on schedule. "Some people try to get more out of those lenses than they should," says Dr. Koplin. "Sleeping in them after they should be disposed of is particularly dangerous."

CONSTIPATION
Keeping Things Moving

If you are like most folks, you have had at least one bout of constipation. And maybe the constipation that you have experienced—either once, occasionally, or often—was preventable. But before you take steps to prevent a future confrontation with constipation, it is judicious to make sure that you have a working knowledge of regularity. In other words, what *regular* really means.

"Many people think that they are constipated if they don't have a bowel movement once a day, every day," says gastroenterologist Marvin M. Schuster, M.D., professor of medicine and psychiatry at the Johns Hopkins University School of Medicine and director of the Marvin M. Schuster Center for Digestive and Motility Disorders at the Johns Hopkins Bayview Medical Center, both in Baltimore. But a normal, unconstipated rate of bowel movements can be anywhere from three times a day to three times a week, he says.

Staying Regular on the Road

Travel is a common cause of constipation because you disrupt the normal rhythm of your eating habits, says gastroenterologist Marvin M. Schuster, M.D., professor of medicine and psychiatry at the Johns Hopkins University School of Medicine and director of the Marvin M. Schuster Center for Digestive and Motility Disorders at the Johns Hopkins Bayview Medical Center, both in Baltimore. But it is easy to reduce your risk. Here's how.

LEARN TO LOVE THE LOCAL FIBER. You may not be able to get your favorite brand of cereal on the road, but take advantage of high-fiber foods in the local diet. If you are in Europe, for example, eat muesli, a high-fiber breakfast cereal, suggests Dr. Schuster. If you are concerned about possible poor sanitation and want to avoid the local fruits and vegetables, be sure to take along a bulk agent. Some brands, such as Metamucil, are available in individual packets or in wafer form.

DON'T FORGET TO DRINK. When you travel, it is easy to not get enough water, especially if you are avoiding the local tap water. Be sure to keep plenty of bottled water on hand or in your backpack and drink eight eight-ounce glasses every day.

SNACK ON A NATURAL LAXATIVE. Toss a few dried prunes or figs into your bag to munch on during the day.

STAY ON THE MOVE. Don't become a hotel-room couch potato. "Walk around and see the city you are in on foot," says Dr. Schuster. Or get some other form of exercise.

People age 65 and older shouldn't think that they are constipated if they begin to have some difficulty passing stool that is down near the opening, Dr. Schuster adds. "The muscles and nerves of the digestive system may degenerate somewhat by age 65, creating a slight difficulty. That does not mean that the individual has constipation."

But if your stools are usually small and hard, if you find yourself having to strain, or if three or more days pass between your bowel movements, then you genuinely have a problem. You may have to consult a doctor if the problem continues, and that's a good idea since constipation can be one sign of conditions like diverticular disease and colon cancer. It can lead to hemorrhoids as well. But usually, you can prevent constipation in the first place if you just pay closer attention to what you eat.

First, Fill Up on Fiber

Fiber is the wall, or cellulose portion, of every plant cell—including grains, beans, fruits, and vegetables. It is not digestible. Instead, it travels through the digestive tract into the large intestine, or colon. Once the fiber reaches the intestine, it combines with the water in your digestive track to create softer stools.

In people who eat high-fiber diets, the transit time of food is twice as fast as that of people who regularly consume low-fiber meals. Eat lots of fiber, and you will halve the time it takes for food to make its way through your whole digestive system. "Fiber is very good for preventing constipation," says Dr. Schuster. Here is how to get your share.

BREAKFAST WITH BRAN. Bran, the high-fiber portion of grains, is a constipation-prevention all-star. Study after study has shown that it is the most effective fiber you can eat to keep your body regular. "If you are really serious about preventing constipation, eat a cereal every day that is 100 percent bran," says Harris R. Clearfield, M.D., professor of medicine and section chief of the division of gastroenterology at the Allegheny University of the Health Sciences, Hahnemann Division, in Philadelphia. But go slowly, he suggests. Start by topping your regular cereal with a small amount of bran cereal and then gradually change the ratio of the cereals until you have a full serving of the bran.

FLAVOR YOUR HEALTH WITH FRUIT. Add a topping of sliced fruit to your bran cereal, Dr. Clearfield suggests.

"People have more frequent bowel movements during the summer simply because they are eating more fruit," says Dr. Schuster. Most fruits will help to some degree, but the best is famous for what it does: Prunes have a renowned laxative effect on the digestive system.

SIP THE RHUBARB REMEDY. For a tastier way to get your fiber, cook up one of the favorite recipes of James A. Duke, Ph.D., master herbalist and retired ethnobotanist and toxicology specialist at the U.S. Department of Agriculture and author of *The Green Pharmacy*. Cook three stalks of rhubarb without the leaves. Puree with one cup of apple juice, a quarter of a peeled lemon, and one tablespoon of honey, then drink up. Try this remedy three times for one day. The rhubarb not only provides fiber but also contains a natural laxative. But don't overdo it, he warns. The drink has powerful laxative properties.

ADD WATER. Fiber needs the assistance of water to soften the stool. Drink eight eight-ounce glasses of water a day, which will assist the fiber in your diet to help prevent constipation.

ADJUST AS YOU NEED TO. Adding fiber to your diet can sometimes create some intestinal activity that you didn't count on. "Adding fiber to the diet does produce more gas in some people," Dr. Schuster says. But, he adds, that gas problem usually goes away in about three weeks as your body adjusts to the dietary change.

Stick with your high-fiber diet for at least three weeks, Dr. Schuster suggests. If you still have a lot of gas, you may be one of the 15 percent of people who will always have excess flatulence on a high-fiber diet. Gradually cut back on your fiber intake until you find a level that is comfortable.

TRY A SUPPLEMENT INSTEAD. For those people who want a simple, reliable daily dose of fiber, Dr. Schuster recommends a supplement (also called a bulk agent), such as Metamucil, Konsyl, FiberCon, or Citrucel. Mix the supplement in a glass of water or juice to help it work more effectively and take it *with* a meal.

When you begin taking a fiber supplement, start with one dose and increase to three times a day as needed. The supplement forms larger, softer stools by combining with food. If you take it right before bedtime—as you would an over-the-counter laxative—it won't work nearly as well.

Check with your doctor about any medications you are taking that the supplement might block from being absorbed, Dr. Schuster says. If that is the case, take the medication about an hour before you take the supplement.

Try These Tips, Too

Bulking up your diet is the quickest route to regularity, but other little lifestyle changes may also help prevent constipation.

START THE DAY PIPING-HOT. Can't go to the bathroom in the morning without having a cup of coffee first? Join the unconstipated crowd. "A hot drink in the morning—tea, coffee, or even hot water—stimulates what is called the gastro-colic reflex, which often causes a bowel movement," says Dr. Clearfield. He recommends drinking a hot beverage when you get up or having it with breakfast.

GET UP AND GO. "Exercise definitely gets things moving—no doubt about it," says Dr. Schuster. "It is an im-

Where to Find Your Fiber

Bran is the best source of fiber for preventing constipation, say digestive experts, but it is not the only source. Here is a list of some non-bran foods that are good sources of fiber.

- Grains: bulgur, pearled barley, whole-wheat spaghetti
- Beans: chickpeas, kidney beans, lima beans, black beans, lentils
- Dried fruits: pears, apricots, peaches, figs, prunes
- Fruits: raspberries, blackberries, avocados

portant part of preventing constipation." Any type of aerobic exercise—walking, bike riding, or jogging—will do the job.

DON'T DELAY. When your body tells you it is time to go, do so. "If you habitually delay bowel movements, you can develop constipation because your body will lose the capacity to generate the reflex that tells you when it is time to defecate," says Dr. Schuster.

CHECK YOUR MEDICATIONS. There are many drugs that can produce constipation as a side effect. Painkillers, antidepressants, and antispasmodics are the biggest offenders. Ask your doctor whether constipation is a possible complication of the drug you are taking. If it is, check with your doctor about taking a daily fiber supplement.

PICK THE "M" ANTACID. If you take antacids and you are a person who is prone to constipation, Dr. Schuster says to choose an antacid with a name that starts with the letter M, like Maalox or Mylanta, rather than an A, like Aludrox or Amphojel. The "M" antacids usually have magnesium in them, which produces looser stools. The "A" antacids usually contain aluminum, which tends to be constipating.

JUST SAY NO TO LAXATIVES. Regular use of stimulant laxatives (not bulk agents) can actually *destroy* the reflex mechanism in the colon that stimulates defecation, says Dr. Schuster, leaving you permanently constipated and dependent on ever-increasing dosages of the drug. "Avoid using a stimulant laxative for more than a few days at a time if you possibly can," he cautions.

CORNS AND CALLUSES
Don't Give Them a Foothold

Feet are probably the body part that we use the most and think about the least. Day after day, mile after mile, we expect our sorely overused soles to keep us moving from place to place without a hitch.

Corns and calluses are little pads of dead skin that build up after all those miles of fancy footwork. Painful and protuberant, these islands of dead skin are a signal from our feet that they have had enough. Excess pressure or friction causes them. Corns develop on the toes only, while calluses show up on the heels or on the bottoms of the feet.

At the first sign, it is worth taking steps to stop them in their tracks. If the pressure isn't eventually corrected, it can affect not only the skin but also the bones and joints underneath. And any foot pain can cause you to change your gait, which can, in turn, throw your posture out of whack and lead to a bad back. Fortunately for most of us, preventing corns and calluses is just a matter of finding shoes that fit.

Pamper and Pumice for Prevention

Since corns and calluses are really nothing more than mounds of dead skin, doctors say it helps to keep your feet free of buildup. You can give yourself an excellent pedicure at home by following these steps from Douglas Hale, D.P.M., a podiatrist at the Foot and Ankle Center of Washington in Seattle.

- First, you will need a water basin, footbath powder (available at any drugstore), a towel, moisturizing cream, a pumice stone, toenail clippers, and a nail file.
- Add the footbath powder to the basin and run warm, not hot, water into it. Soak your feet for 10 minutes.
- Towel your feet dry. Gently clean away any dirt underneath your toenails.
- Rub the moisturizer on and give yourself a foot massage.
- With a pumice stone (never use a knife or sharp object to cut dead skin), gently rub dead skin away.
- Finish up by cutting your toenails straight across with clippers and filing away any rough edges.

Buy It Right

Let's face it, in the pursuit of fashion many women and more than a few men are likely to cram their feet into shoes or boots that are corn- and callus-creators. Narrow-toed shoes, boots, and high heels put plenty of pressure where the foot meets the footwear. Here is how to give your feet a little relief.

HEAVE THE HEELS. If you are a woman who is accustomed to high heels, it may be high time for a flatter-heel shopping spree. When you wear heels that are higher than two inches, you are putting too much pressure on the metatarsals, the bones directly beneath your toes. "You want to get the force off that area," says Lawrence Z. Huppin, D.P.M., a podiatrist at the Foot and Ankle Center of Washington in Seattle. Flat shoes are a much better bet.

ARCH YOUR FOOT. Another way to ease the pressure on your metatarsals is to buy over-the-counter arch supports, available at drugstores and discount department stores. "They shift the weight off the ball of the foot and onto the arch," says Dr. Huppin. But your heels need to go lower before the supports can be effective.

DON'T GET THE POINT. Many women's shoes and some boots for men and women are designed as if our feet were as pointed as Nixon's nose. Instead, look for a rounded toebox in shoes. In general, try to exercise good judgment by selecting shoes that best fit the shape of your feet, says William H. Rutherford, D.P.M., a clinical instructor in the podiatry section at Howard University School of Medicine in Washington, D.C.

REACH FOR THE RUNNING SHOES. Even if you are not a runner, many experts say that running shoes are the best all-around shoe for foot support because the heel is very thick and stable. "It is better than any other kind of athletic shoe," says Bruce Lebowitz, D.P.M., director of the podiatric clinic of the Johns Hopkins Bayview Medical Center in Baltimore. If you can't wear them on the job, you can still wear them to and from work, at home, and at play. Your feet will thank you for it.

LACE IT UP. A corn is caused by your shoe rubbing against a toe, and the rubbing is far less abusive if you wear shoes with laces, says Douglas Hale, D.P.M., a podiatrist at the Foot and Ankle Center of Washington. Because the laces make the shoe hug the foot, you feel less pressure on your toes than you feel from slip-on shoes.

SIZE THEM UP. Once we reach adulthood, we often

forget all about shoe size and just assume it stays the same. Not so. "Many people wear shoes that are too narrow or too small," says Arnold Ravick, D.P.M., a podiatrist at Capital Podiatry Associates in Washington, D.C. "Most people don't have their feet measured after they stop growing and figure that they will be the same size all their lives," he says. "But as you age, your feet swell and spread, and the bones buckle." Feet can grow from one to three sizes during your lifetime, Dr. Ravick points out. And during pregnancy, feet may swell or expand by as much as a size by the last trimester. To make sure that your shoes fit, he suggests having your feet measured by a shoe salesclerk at a specialty shoe store. "You must get your feet accurately measured," he says, "because if you wear shoes that fit poorly, you may get corns and calluses."

RESPECT YOUR DIFFERENCES. Keep in mind that your left foot may not be precisely the same size as your right. Get both feet measured when you go to the shoe store. If there is a big difference in sizes, you may want to shop at a store that allows you to mix and match sizes, suggests Dr. Hale. If the difference is a size or less, buy shoes that fit the larger foot and then apply heel pads and tongue pads to keep the smaller foot from slipping around.

BE ANTI-PRONATION. If a shoe salesclerk or a podiatrist has told you that your feet pronate, that means they roll inward when you walk. This may make you callus-prone. To prevent pronation, tell the salesclerk at the shoe store that you want an anti-pronation, extra-sturdy shoe, says Dr. Huppin. These shoes have especially well-built heels and soles that don't bend easily.

DANDRUFF
Rake Up the Flakes and Prevent Their Return

The epidermis—the outermost layer of skin—constantly renews itself. It sheds dead cells from its surface, replacing them with brand-new cells from underneath. Generally, this process goes on at a nice orderly pace. But sometimes, the skin on your scalp gets hyper and starts to shed the old cells at super speeds. Shed so quickly that they don't even have time to separate from each other, the cells get sloughed off in clumps or, rather, flakes. In other words, you have dandruff decorating the shoulders of your nifty navy blue jacket.

Dandruff is a fashion disaster, but fear not. You can prevent your scalp skin from shifting into super-shed mode. Here is how to keep dandruff from ever getting out of control again.

SHAMPOO DAILY. "Preventing dandruff can be similar to taking care of your teeth," says Diana Bihova, M.D., a dermatologist in private practice in New York City. "Just as you need to brush and floss daily to prevent a buildup of

The Fungus That Foments Dandruff

Dermatologists have discovered an unusual cause of
some severe cases of dandruff: the fungus *pityrosporun
ovale*. This fungus takes up residence in the hair follicles,
causing a very oily scalp and the greasy scaling
of dandruff.

If you have severe dandruff and you have tried lots of
over-the-counter dandruff shampoos without success, see
your dermatologist to find out if you have this fungus, says
Fredric Brandt, M.D., clinical associate professor of
dermatology at the University of Miami School of Medicine
and a dermatologist in Miami. The dermatologist can
prescribe a special antifungal shampoo or an antifungal
cream or pill.

plaque, all you may have to do to prevent dandruff is to
shampoo daily, using any regular shampoo."

STEP UP TO SELENIUM. For some people, though, a
regular shampoo may not do the trick. They need a therapeutic shampoo. Many are available, usually labeled as
dandruff shampoos.

Dandruff shampoos have a range of active ingredients. But there are some things that you should know to
pick the brand that is right for you.

Start with a dandruff shampoo that contains selenium
sulfide, suggests Dr. Bihova. "This is one of the best shampoo ingredients to prevent dandruff because it slows down
the extra-fast rate at which the skin cells on your scalp mature, and that is the process that creates dandruff."

Don't use it every day, however. Dandruff shampoos
are powerful medicine for your scalp. They can also over-
power your hair, making it dry and brittle. To prevent hair
damage, Dr. Bihova says to use the dandruff shampoo only
once or twice a week, alternating it with a regular shampoo.

SHOP AROUND, DOUBLE UP. If you don't get results from a dandruff shampoo, don't assume that none of them will work for you. You may just need a shampoo with a different active ingredient. Unfortunately, selenium sulfide may not work for everyone. If you have been using it for two months and don't see results, Dr. Bihova says to try a shampoo with one of these active ingredients: pyrithione zinc, sulfur, salicylic acid, or coal tar. Keep trying, she says, since almost all people will find an over-the-counter shampoo that works for them.

CHECK WITH YOUR DOC. When none of the over-the-counter shampoos are high-powered enough to prevent dandruff, you may need a prescription-strength alternative. See a dermatologist for a prescription shampoo, Dr. Bihova suggests.

BEWARE THE SEQUEL. Some people find a dandruff shampoo that works for them, but only for a while. After a couple of months of being dandruff-free, it is a head horror story, *The Return of the Flakes*. "Your scalp gets accustomed to the active ingredient, and it no longer works," says Dr. Bihova. At that point, you will need to switch to a dandruff shampoo with another active ingredient.

DELAY THE RINSE. For maximum effectiveness, leave the dandruff shampoo on for at least three minutes, says Dr. Bihova.

WASH THE SCALP, NOT THE HAIR. "Some people get overzealous and try to shampoo the hair excessively," says Dr. Bihova. "Use a conditioner on your hair. The dandruff shampoo is for the *scalp*." Be sure to apply it vigorously.

DOFF YOUR CAP. Wearing a hat can stimulate the process that is responsible for dandruff, says Dr. Bihova. So go without one whenever you can.

DEPRESSION
Some New Light on the Old Blues

Right now, 20 million Americans are in the midst of an episode of depression.

Some have the incapacitating symptoms of what doctors call a major depression. These are symptoms that usually require professional attention because they are very severe and demoralizing. Feeling hopeless and worthless, a person with major depression may sleep and eat irregularly. In the throes of severe depression, it is hard to concentrate, make decisions, or find the energy to do much of anything. Thoughts of suicide are common.

If someone has a minor depression, however, the problem is more manageable. "They feel lousy about themselves and lousy about their lives, but they are managing to function at a fairly high level," says Michael Yapko, Ph.D., a clinical psychologist in Solana Beach, California, and author of *Breaking the Patterns of Depression*. In fact, some of the newfound ways of battling the blues are related to what you do as well as how you feel. Here are some ways that you can prepare your body to help prevent minor depression.

PUT SOME SPRING IN YOUR STEP. "Regular exercise may be the most powerful natural antidepressant available," says Michael T. Murray, N.D., a naturopathic doctor in Seattle and author of *Natural Alternatives to Prozac*. He suggests taking a brisk walk. Exercise helps generate the release of brain chemicals called endorphins. "When endorphin levels are low, depression occurs," he says. And exercise also oxygenates the brain, keeping it healthy.

How much should you exercise? "Thirty minutes, five or six days a week, at moderate intensity is a nice level to aim for to help prevent the brain imbalances that can make you vulnerable to depression," says Michael Norden, M.D., a psychiatrist and clinical associate professor at the University of Washington in Seattle and author of *Beyond Prozac*.

NOURISH YOUR BRAIN. "Virtually any nutrient deficiency can result in impaired mental function, including depression," says Dr. Murray. To help prevent depression, he recommends that you take a high-potency multivitamin/mineral supplement.

GET ENOUGH SLEEP. Getting less than eight hours of sleep night after night may lower levels of the brain chemical serotonin, which can make you more prone to depression, says Dr. Norden. To sleep well, he recommends going to bed and waking up at the same time every day, including weekends. Relax before bedtime, perhaps with a hot bath, he advises. And for the soundest sleep, keep your bedroom quiet and dark.

Oil Your Brain

Your car needs oil to run smoothly. And new research is showing that your brain may need it, too. But the best brain fluid is a different kind of oil: fish oil.

Fish oil is rich in a substance called omega-3 fatty acids. "These fatty acids are important to behavior because they make up a crucial component of brain tissue," says Joseph R. Hibbeln, M.D., chief of the outpatient clinic at the National Institute on Alcohol Abuse and Alcoholism, and a leading expert on the role of omega-3 fatty acids in depression. In fact, getting enough of these fatty acids might help you prevent a major or minor episode of the blues, according to Dr. Hibbeln.

There has been a 100-fold increase in the rate of depression in America and other Western countries over the past century, Dr. Hibbeln observes. This increase occurred at the same time as a drastic decrease in the consumption of omega-3 fatty acids, the kind found in fish oil. When Dr. Hibbeln compared the current rate of depression in America to that of other countries, he found 10 times less depression in countries like Japan, Taiwan, and Korea where people eat more fish. In countries other

Try a New Spin

After 20 years of treating people with depression, Dr. Yapko is convinced that this most common of psychological problems is largely caused by people's interpretations about life. "Depression is not caused by the inevitable frustrations, difficulties, and disasters of daily living, but by what you think and feel in response to them," he says. With some new ways of thinking, you may be able to help fend than the United States where people eat less fish, like Lebanon and France, depression rates were far higher.

A Japanese study of 265,000 people, conducted over a 17-year period, showed that people who ate fish every day had a 20 percent lower risk of suicide than people who ate fish less frequently. Since suicide is often linked to major depression, this, too, seemed a significant finding. And in research yet to be published, Dr. Hibbeln says that he has found that omega-3 fatty acids may increase levels of the brain chemical serotonin. Low levels of serotonin have been linked to depression.

The link between low levels of dietary omega-3 fatty acids and depression is not fully proven, Dr. Hibbeln emphasizes. But we do know that increasing your levels of omega-3 fatty acids can help prevent heart disease, so getting more fish oil in your diet certainly won't do any harm. All the better if it helps prevent depression as well.

Good dietary sources of omega-3 fatty acids include fatty fish such as mackerel, tuna, salmon, and herring. In addition to fish sources, these fatty acids are also found in canola oil and flaxseed oil. Omega-3 fatty acids are also available in nutritional supplements.

off the feelings of bleakness. Here are some ways to make your mind turn in some new directions.

CONSIDER SOME ALTERNATE EXPLANATIONS. Your emotions—positive or negative—are created not by situations themselves but by the way you interpret those situations, says Dr. Yapko. A very common situation can turn into a reason for hand-wringing unless you take mental steps to prevent it.

"Suppose a friend is going to pick you up so that the two of you can go someplace and do something fun

Is Your Medication a "Pro-Depressant"?

Everybody has heard of the antidepressant medications, such as Prozac. But a doctor in Canada thinks that many common medications used to treat a wide variety of health problems might be dragging you down instead of lifting you up. "Our scientific research shows that there are medications that are quite potent in creating physiological changes that can cause depression," says Scott Patten, M.D., Ph.D., assistant professor in the departments of community health sciences and psychiatry at the University of Calgary in Canada, and a psychiatrist with the Calgary Regional Health Authority. Here are the categories to watch out for, according to Dr. Patten.

- Corticosteroids, a class of drugs used to reduce inflammation
- Tranquilizers and sleeping pills

together," says Dr. Yapko. "Now, suppose that time passes, and your friend does not arrive to get you. Your feelings change, quite literally, from moment to moment. If at first you think of your friend as being insensitive and irresponsible, you will find yourself feeling angry at him. If you think that perhaps something bad has happened to him, you will naturally become concerned. If you think that this person doesn't care much about you and that's why he is late, you feel rejected, lonely, even depressed."

Although the event doesn't change—your friend is delayed—you can have a whole range of feelings depending on how you interpret that event. "Situations are almost always ambiguous, open to any interpretation," Dr. Yapko points out. So your interpretation helps create your feelings

- Medications for high blood pressure, high cholesterol, and heart failure

In addition, he warns that two categories of drugs might lead to depression if you have been using the medication regularly and then stop. Drugs that can lead to this withdrawal side effect are over-the-counter decongestants and over-the-counter weight-loss drugs with the ingredient phenylpropanolamine.

But don't expect your doctor to warn you about the possibility of drug-induced depression when he writes a prescription. "Doctors don't usually think about depression as a drug side effect," says Dr. Patten. So if you start taking a new medication and begin to notice a sad mood, changes in your appetite or sleeping habits, lack of interest in life, or fatigue, talk to your doctor about choosing a different medication for your problem. Any of these could be the early signs of depression, possibly related to medications you are taking. "There are often alternatives for whatever drug you are using," he says.

about the situation. Positive interpretations lead to good feelings and enjoyment; negative interpretations lead to bad feelings and depression. To stay on the positive side, try to look for the positive interpretation, he advises.

DON'T JUMP ON THE ASSUMPTION WAGON. Before you conclude that something is negative, gather facts to clear up any ambiguities, says Dr. Yapko. "Don't assume, for example, what someone meant. Ask. Say, 'I'm not sure how to interpret that. What exactly did you mean?' Asking for facts is one of the best ways to prevent negative interpretations."

WATCH OUT FOR SELF-DEMOTION. If someone doesn't get a promotion at work and concludes, "I'm a loser," he is demonstrating all-or-nothing thinking, says Dr. Yapko. That kind of thinking is almost certain to give rise to the strong negative emotions of depression, he adds. Any time you are criticizing yourself or others, reexamine the situation to see if you have fallen into the trap of an all-or-nothing explanation.

If you are passed over for a promotion, it doesn't mean that you are a failure. Many factors—from office politics to lack of experience—could have played their parts. And those are factors that you can't control. By being less extreme, you will judge others and yourself less harshly, says Dr. Yapko. "And when you make the critic living in your head lighten up a bit, you will see more of what you and others do as being perfectly all right."

TAKE PRAISE—AND GIVE THANKS. If you can accept compliments, you can open the door to a more positive self-image, which is a good way to safeguard yourself from the blues. To boost a negative self-image, learn to accept compliments as genuine statements of how others feel about you, says Dr. Yapko.

To teach yourself how to accept compliments, Dr. Yapko suggests that you ask people close to you to tell you something positive about yourself, something they like or respect. "Then, with a straight face, respond to the compliment by saying, 'I'm sorry, I can't permit you to feel that way.' " Try it just once, and you will hear how absurd that sounds. Yet that is exactly what you are doing if you can't accept compliments. Welcome the compliments, he advises, and you will begin thinking better of yourself without even trying.

TRY AN ERROR. Learning to tolerate your mistakes without being nasty to yourself is a must for preventing depression, says Dr. Yapko. "You will make mistakes for as long as you live. The issue is how to treat yourself fairly and respectfully when you do."

To learn how to handle your mistakes in a positive way, Dr. Yapko suggests an exercise of making intentional mistakes in harmless situations. "Each day this week, deliberately make three obvious errors: get off the wrong freeway exit, mismatch your socks, dial a wrong number, or do some other silly thing. When you make the mistakes, does the world end? Does anything change?" This exercise will help you accept mistakes in a good-natured way instead of abusing yourself with negativity, he says.

CHOOSE TO REMAIN BLAMELESS. When a negative event happens—for example, you meet a close friend for dinner and she seems distant and in a bad mood—do you always blame yourself? Dr. Yapko calls this way of thinking and feeling personalizing—taking impersonal things personally. He says it is a reliable path to becoming over-emotional and depressed. In the case of your friend, for example, realize that you are probably not responsible for her bad mood. If you find that you are constantly blaming yourself for other people's unhappiness, gather the facts. Ask the person if you have done anything that's upsetting her. But until then, says Dr. Yapko, feel free to be guilt-free.

BE COMPLETELY POSITIVE FOR A DAY. The positive is always there, says Dr. Yapko. But most of the time we just don't notice it. To help you get accustomed to perceiving the positive, focus on positive things for a whole day. If your first perception of a person or an event is negative, push yourself to find at least a couple of positive aspects. If someone leaves a mess around the coffeemaker, for instance, say to yourself, "At least he was trying to make coffee fast." If your spouse forgets to mail a letter for you, think, "Maybe a day's delay will turn out for the best." After a full day of that, you may find yourself being a lot more forgiving to yourself, too.

DERMATITIS AND ECZEMA
Nip the Itch in the Bud

It's the Itch from Hell. Not the kind a little scratching can solve, but a constant, unrelieved, infuriating irritation. First, the red, swollen, scaly rash appears on your skin, and after that, it can get worse. Some people end up with oozing, crusty blisters that continue to itch like crazy. With so much misery to avoid, why not take some precautions against this devilish rash?

Fortunately, doctors say that there are a lot of ways that you can work around it. But first, it helps to understand what kind you have and what might be causing it.

Dermatitis means any inflammation of the skin, and if that sounds like a broad category, well, it is. Inflammation can range from a mild discomfort to the really miserable skin bubbles that make you wonder whether you are about to boil over. And the causes are just as various, ranging from your own genetic makeup to food, air, sun, artificial products, natural substances, and just about everything else.

When dermatitis develops to the stage where you can

see cracking, crusting, and oozing, it is generally diagnosed as some kind of eczema. But no matter what you call it, itchy, inflamed skin is something that everyone would like to avoid.

Counting the Kinds

Some people start getting skin outbreaks in childhood, with flare-ups that may continue off and on throughout their lives. Called atopic eczema, this rash is probably inherited from Mom, Dad, or other forebears who passed along the genes. The outbreaks can occur anywhere on the body, but the most common points of affliction are joint areas like the inside of the elbows or backs of the knees.

Another type of rash, allergic contact dermatitis, shows up when you have touched something that causes the outbreak. A rash from poison ivy is the classic example of this variety.

A skin irritation also can be caused by something you have repeatedly come in contact with, such as metal, latex, or some other substance. This falls under the category of irritant contact dermatitis.

But whatever kind of eczema or dermatitis you have, there may be ways to prevent the flare-ups in the first place.

"Prevention in eczema is key," says David E. Cohen, M.D., clinical instructor of environmental sciences at the Columbia University School of Public Health and director of occupational and environmental dermatology at New York University Medical Center, both in New York City. "If a patch of eczema starts, you will invariably scratch, and the scratching damages the skin and makes the eczema worse, which causes more scratching. Once eczema is out of control like this, getting it under control is far more difficult and requires far more effort than if you had just prevented it to begin with."

Countering the Contacts

Approximately 65,000 different substances can cause contact irritant dermatitis, with the rash usually occurring after repeated exposures, says Dr. Cohen. But there is one category of irritants, called solvents, that cause most cases of this kind of dermatitis. Solvents include water, soapy solutions of any kind, plus alcohol, acetone, varnish, thinners, gasoline, and kerosene. Often, people are exposed to these solvents at work, and the rash shows up as a result of frequent daily contact. Here are some things that you can do.

FAVOR NITRILE GLOVES. Nitrile gloves with cotton liners (available at medical supply stores) provide far more protection against many solvents than latex or vinyl gloves, according to Dr. Cohen. If you are cleaning up with water and mild detergent, however, you can use everyday latex gloves with cotton liners. Avoid using plain latex gloves; rubber can be irritating to some people.

SALVE UP FOR THE FUTURE. If you work with solvents, you should also moisturize your hands very frequently, ideally after every contact. If you notice a rash starting, you can usually prevent it from getting any worse by using an over-the-counter hydrocortisone ointment, following the directions on the product label. "These ointments can be very useful in aborting a minor attack and preventing it from becoming a major ongoing episode of eczema," says Dr. Cohen.

WASH NOT, ITCH NOT. Eczema on your hands is a painful affliction, particularly if the skin is sore and cracking, because you need to use your hands for so many things. "The vast majority of cases of hand eczema are caused by repetitive hand washing," says Dr. Cohen. Soap and water are very drying to the hands, and it is that lack of moisture on the skin that triggers the rash of hand eczema. So avoid washing your hands more often than necessary.

MOISTURIZE DAY AND NIGHT. "You want to constantly

keep moisturizer on the skin," says Dr. Cohen. Rub it on your hands whenever they start to feel dry. Use a light, fragrance-free moisturizer during the day and use petroleum jelly before you go to bed at night, he advises.

The best time to apply a moisturizer is in the morning right after your shower, he says. After you have patted yourself dry, "quickly apply the moisturizer while your skin is still hydrated with water." Even better is to moisturize a second time right before you go to bed. "When you put on the moisturizer at bedtime, you are less likely to rub or sweat it off, and it can really help your skin."

DON'T GET INTO SCENTS. In moisturizers as well as soaps, fragrances can irritate sensitive skin and actually cause eczema, says Dr. Cohen. "Avoid moisturizers with fragrance, period," he says. Even if the label says "unscented," the product might have a masking fragrance. "The label should say 'fragrance-free,' " he says.

RESERVE THE PRESERVES. As long as you are reading moisturizer labels, you may also want to avoid moisturizers with preservatives, Dr. Cohen warns. "Many of the preservatives have formaldehyde as a component, which can cause allergic eczema in some people."

CHOOSE JELLY. "The blander the moisturizer, the better off you are," says Dr. Cohen. His favorite is petroleum jelly. "It is an excellent barrier moisturizer, it is inexpensive, and it has virtually no chance of causing eczema." To avoid the greasy feeling of petroleum jelly, wait five minutes after you apply it to your skin, then remove the excess with an old cotton T-shirt. "Your skin won't feel greasy, and you will have given the moisturizer time to soak in," he says.

RING OFF. Remove your rings before you wash your hands, Dr. Cohen says. Irritants, particularly soap, get trapped under the ring, and those irritants can stay on your finger for hours, triggering the eczema.

Block the Poison in Ivy

Blame it all on urishiol, the nasty sap in poison ivy and poison oak. Every year it causes millions of cases of the red, blister-ridden, itchy, unsightly rash called allergic contact dermatitis. Until recently, the only way to prevent the rash was by watching out for the telltale three leaves and staying out of their way while in the woods and fields.

Now there is an over-the-counter product that blocks the effects of urishiol. Called Ivy Block, it is the first preventative of this kind that has been tested and approved by the government's Food and Drug Administration.

"Ivy Block is a lotion that stops poison ivy and poison oak," says James Marks Jr., M.D., professor of medicine in the division of dermatology at the Pennsylvania State University College of Medicine in Hershey. Dr. Marks was one of the scientists who conducted an experiment on the active ingredient in Ivy Block and helped to prove its effectiveness.

Too Clothed for Comfort?

If something is causing a dermatitis on various parts of your body, your clothing might be conspiring to cause trouble. Fabric, detergent, softeners, even fragrances are likely suspects. Here is how to flush them out.

BUY WEAVES THAT BREATHE. Synthetic fabrics like polyester and permanent press fabrics have a formaldehyde-based substance in them to keep them wrinkle-free. "This is an allergen, and it can irritate eczema-prone skin," says Dr. Cohen. If your skin is reacting, try some other types of clothing. "Fabrics like non-permanent press cottons and silk are more breathable and tend to contain fewer chemicals," he says.

In his study, Dr. Marks and his colleagues put a lotion containing the active ingredient (called Q18B) on the forearms of 144 volunteers. An hour later, researchers applied urishiol on the same area and left it on for four hours before washing it off. The volunteers were examined two, four, and eight days later. Remarkably, 68 percent of the volunteers never developed the characteristic redness, itching, and blisters usually caused by poison ivy or poison oak. Among those who did have symptoms, the reactions were mild, with some redness, swelling, or itching.

Ivy Block is available at drugstores and supermarkets all over the United States, according to Dr. Marks. You should apply it 15 to 20 minutes before a possible exposure to poison ivy or poison oak. If you think that you will continue to be exposed to the poisonous plants, apply Ivy Block once every four hours until you are out of harm's way.

Be sure to shake the bottle thoroughly before putting on the lotion, Dr. Marks advises. The active ingredient is a claylike substance, which needs to be mixed into the lotion.

BEWARE BARBS IN SHEEP'S CLOTHING. "When you look at wool under a microscope, you see little fishhook-shaped barbs, which can irritate the skin of someone prone to eczema," says Dr. Cohen. When you scratch to relieve the irritation, you can end up with a new patch of eczema. If you want to wear wool clothes for warmth or fashion, have a tailor put in a silk lining or wear a silk shirt or camisole underneath your clothing, he says.

WASH OUT WHAT YOU BUY. Many manufacturers of clothing, bedding, towels, and other fabric items use a fabric finisher on their products that can cause allergic contact dermatitis, says Rhett Drugge, M.D., a dermatologist in Stamford, Connecticut, who is president and founder of the Internet Dermatology Society, and chief editor of the

Electronic Textbook of Dermatology. To remove the finisher, run new clothes through the washing machine before you put them on, he advises.

DON'T GO SOFT. "I'm emphatically opposed to fabric softeners or dryer sheets for people who are prone to eczema," says Dr. Cohen. "They add a tremendous amount of unnecessary fragrances and irritant chemicals to your clothes."

NEVER MIND THE SWEET SMELL OF SPRING. Fragrance-free laundry detergents are always preferable, says Dr. Cohen. "It's nice to have your clothes smell like a spring day, but when you sweat, those fragrances leach out onto your skin and can trigger eczema."

Watch How You Are Washing

Your skin performs what scientists call the barrier function, helping to retain moisture inside your body. Once skin starts cracking because of eczema, you begin to lose body moisture through the tiny cracks. But you can avoid the start of this water-loss cycle if you watch your bathing habits and take steps to keep your skin moist and intact, says Dr. Cohen. Here are some tips to hold the barrier in place.

SHOWER, FOR SURE. People who are prone to eczema shouldn't take baths, says Dr. Cohen. "You tend to relax in baths and sit in them a long time, and you get that crinkled, white skin. That's simply a sign that you have compromised your skin's barrier function by overhydrating. Your skin will actually be drier after you get out." Instead, take a brief, cool shower lasting three to five minutes. "That is the most moisturizing, protective way to bathe," he says.

PICK A SENSITIVE SOAP. The best soaps to help prevent eczema are mildly moisturizing rather than drying, says Dr. Cohen. He recommends soaps that are fragrance-free and for sensitive skin, like Dove, Purpose, Basis, and Aveeno. Glycerine-based soaps such as Neutrogena advertise themselves as "smell-good deodorant soaps," which means that they are very drying and full of fragrances, according to Dr. Cohen.

BATTLE BACTERIA. Some people with eczema may find that antibacterial soaps help control the problem. Dr. Cohen recommends Lever 2000 and Dial, which he says are nondrying antibacterial soap bars.

PAT AND MOISTURIZE. When you get out of the shower, pat rather than rub your skin with a towel. When you rub too hard, you may rub right down to the raw areas that are most likely to develop into patches of eczema. And after you have patted yourself dry, don't forget to apply moisturizer right away, says Dr. Cohen.

Air and Mood

For people who are prone to eczema, everything from the air they breathe to the mood they are in can sometimes affect the skin. Here are some tips that could help prevent outbreaks year-round.

SEEK SOME SUN. The ultraviolet light of the sun can help prevent or reduce the inflammation of eczema in about 90 percent of people who are prone to the problem. "Since a lot of eczema is on the arms and legs, wearing shorts and short-sleeved shirts in the summer can often help prevent or relieve flare-ups of eczema," says Dr. Cohen. But since too much sun will cause its own problems, make sure to use a sunscreen that has a sun protection factor of at least 15 and reapply often. (For about 10 percent of people, sunshine makes the rash worse, and they should cover up or stay out of the sun.)

VAPORIZE YOUR BEDROOM. Winter is not a wonderland for people with eczema because the cold, dry air outside and the warmed, dry air inside suck moisture right out of the skin. Dr. Cohen recommends that people prone to eczema use a steam vaporizer in their bedrooms at night during the winter. "This humidifies the air, and your skin will feel a lot better in the morning."

DON'T BE FURIOUS. Your skin and your emotions are closely related, says Ted Grossbart, Ph.D., an instructor in the department of psychiatry at Harvard Medical School, senior associate and clinical supervisor for the department of psychiatry at Beth Israel Hospital, a clinical psychologist in Boston, and author of *Skin Deep: A Mind/Body Program for Healthy Skin.* "Stressful emotions and how you deal with them can play a large role in whether eczema is triggered or not. With eczema, one typical emotional trigger is anger," he says.

One way to deal with that anger is to express it verbally rather than through your skin, Dr. Grossbart says. But if expressing your anger seems inappropriate, don't give up. "Simply admitting to yourself that you are angry can often prevent your eczema from getting worse."

SOOTHE YOURSELF. Stressful emotions can make you want to scratch, which will just make your eczema worse and cause future flare-ups. But, says Dr. Grossbart, you can turn your scratching hand into a soothing hand.

"First, you need to be clear about what kind of stressful events push your buttons and make you scratch more. Then, instead of scratching at those times, rest your hand lightly over your skin or on your skin. Over time, this light, loving, soothing touch actually will soothe; you will feel much less itchy." These techniques are most effective when used as part of an ongoing professionally guided program, Dr. Grossbart adds.

DIABETES
Taming Type II

Insulin is your friend. Produced by the pancreas, a hard-working and necessary digestive organ, the hormone insulin is a royal escort service for blood sugar, or glucose. And that is a vital role because glucose is constantly pouring into your system. Some glucose is contributed by the obvious sugary food sources like candy bars and chocolates, but there is plenty that comes from less-obvious sources like spaghetti, potatoes, and your morning bagel.

It is the food-derived fuel that powers every cell. Normally, glucose is ushered out of the bloodstream and into the cells by insulin. But in people who have diabetes, the cells become insulin-resistant and won't accept all the blood sugar, or the pancreas wears out and generates too little insulin to do the job properly. The result is a flood of glucose in the bloodstream, which can damage almost every part of the body.

For the 15.7 million people with Type II diabetes in

the United States, the underlying culprit is often insulin resistance. But 1 million other people with diabetes have Type I, also known as immune-mediated diabetes, which means that their pancreases fail to produce any or enough insulin. Type I is an autoimmune disease that usually sets in suddenly during adolescence, and all people with Type I diabetes require synthetic insulin to manage their glucose levels.

Scientists aren't sure what causes either type of diabetes, but they know that genetics plays some role. Although people can be predisposed to Type II diabetes, it is actually a slowly developing metabolic disorder that is tremendously affected by lifestyle.

Diabetes is on the rise. The number of people diagnosed with diabetes every year increased by 48 percent between 1980 and 1994. Nearly all the new cases are Type II, or adult-onset, the kind that moves in around middle age. Symptoms of Type II diabetes include increased thirst, appetite, and need to urinate; feeling tired, edgy, or sick to the stomach; blurred vision; tingling or loss of feeling in hands or feet; and dry, itchy skin. People with Type II may also find that they have repeated infections that are hard to heal, especially infections of the skin, gums, vagina, or bladder.

The American Diabetes Association estimates that half of all Americans with diabetes don't even know they have it. So if you have these symptoms, by all means see your doctor. Even Type II diabetes can lead to serious complications such as blindness, kidney disease, nerve disease, heart disease, and stroke.

Fortunately, lifestyle factors can prevent or slow diabetes, or at least improve the quality of life of everyone who has the disease. "At least 75 percent of new cases of Type II diabetes can be prevented," says JoAnn Manson, M.D., associate professor of medicine at Harvard Medical School and Harvard School of Public Health and an endocrinologist in the division of preventive medicine at Brigham and

Women's Hospital, all in Boston. The exact cause of diabetes is not fully understood, according to the American Diabetes Association. But experts agree that Type II diabetes is affected by a combination of two lifestyle factors that are completely within your control: how much you weigh and how much you exercise. Here is some expert advice to help with a prevention campaign.

DO SOME D. When researchers in Sweden measured levels of vitamin D in 34 men, they saw that the more vitamin D in the blood, the better the insulin was at delivering glucose to the muscles. So vitamin D—an important nutrient for many other reasons as well—may help your body derail diabetes.

Though vitamin D is produced when your skin is exposed to sunlight, a more reliable year-round source is milk. Four eight-ounce glasses of fat-free milk a day can get you to the Daily Value of 400 IU (international units). Alternatively, you can supplement your diet with 400 IU of vitamin D, says Robert E. C. Wildman, R.D., Ph.D., professor of human nutrition at the University of Delaware in Newark.

LOSE EVERY EXTRA POUND. "If you keep your weight normal and you are physically active, you will decrease your risk of developing diabetes," says David Williamson, Ph.D., senior biomedical research scientist in the diabetes division at the Centers for Disease Control and Prevention in Atlanta. In a study conducted by Dr. Williamson of more than 8,000 people, he found that for every extra pound of weight, a person's risk for developing diabetes increased by 9 percent. That means an extra 10 pounds above your normal weight almost doubles your likelihood of getting the disease. (For tips on how to manage your weight, see Overweight on page 593.)

MOVE TOWARD PREVENTION. "There is a strong scientific link between Type II diabetes and sedentary living," says Andrea Kriska, Ph.D., associate professor in the department

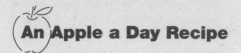

An Apple a Day Recipe

Vitamin D Chowder

Chunks of salmon turn this creamy corn chowder into something special. Plus, it is easy to make and is loaded with vitamin D, which may help prevent diabetes.

12 ounces boneless, skinless salmon fillet

2½ cups water

2 tablespoons lemon juice

¼ teaspoon hot-pepper sauce

1 large onion, chopped

2 ribs celery, chopped

1 large carrot, chopped

4 red new potatoes, scrubbed and chopped

2½ cups 1% milk

¾ cup fresh or frozen and thawed corn

2 tablespoons chopped fresh dill or 1 tablespoon dried

2 scallions, sliced

In a medium skillet, combine the salmon, water, lemon juice, and hot-pepper sauce. Bring to a boil over medium-high heat. Reduce the heat to medium-low and simmer for 5 to 8 minutes, or just until the salmon begins to flake easily. Remove the salmon, reserving the liquid. Cut the salmon into bite-size pieces.

Coat a large saucepan with nonstick spray and place over medium heat. Add the onion, celery, and carrot. Cook for 4 minutes, or until soft. Add the salmon liquid and bring to a boil over medium-high heat. Add the potatoes and cook for 6 to 8 minutes, or until soft. Add the milk, corn, dill, scallions, and salmon. Reduce the heat to medium-low. Cook for 2 to 3 minutes, or until hot. Do not boil.

Makes 4 servings. Per serving: 360 calories, 8 g. fat, 32% of Daily Value of vitamin D

of epidemiology in the School of Public Health at the University of Pittsburgh and an expert in diabetes and exercise. One study observed 577 residents of Daqing, China, who had impaired glucose tolerance, which made them susceptible to diabetes. They were separated into four study groups: those who exercised by doing 30-minute walks, those who modified their diets, those who both dieted and exercised, and those who didn't make any changes. The percentage that developed diabetes was significantly lower for the first three groups compared to those in the fourth group, who didn't diet or exercise, Dr. Kriska notes. "Physical activity combined with a modified diet appears to be the best combination in reducing the chances or effects of diabetes," she says.

"Frankly, we don't know exactly how much exercise is enough," says Dr. Kriska. But some sort of physical activity done most days of the week may be your best bet for regulating blood sugar levels and preventing Type II diabetes. "Try to get in $2^1/2$ to 3 hours of exercise a week, but be flexible with yourself about spacing it out. Even if you can walk for 15-minute sessions only, it will benefit you. I typically recommend walking because everyone can do it, it doesn't cost you anything, and you don't have to go to a gym."

PUT SOME E IN PROTECTION. In a study done at the Research Institute of Public Health in Finland, researchers found that men with the lowest blood levels of vitamin E were four times more likely to get diabetes than men with the highest levels. While no one knows how much vitamin E is needed to protect you from diabetes, the study noted

Snare Some Salmon

A scientific study hints that there may be even more that you can do to deter Type II diabetes than keeping your weight down and sticking with your exercise routine. It is possible that adding fish like salmon or sardines to your favorite-foods list may also help keep that illness upstream.

When scientists looked at the eating habits and blood tests of 666 people over age 40, they found that those who ate salmon every day had a 50 percent lower chance of having any glucose intolerance (a common signal of impending diabetes) than people who ate that fish less often. This preliminary evidence suggests that a daily dose of fatty fish may pack as much of a punch as exercise or losing weight does in staving off diabetes. No one should try to use fish alone to ward off the disease, however.

Researchers think that the fatty acids in the salmon may somehow grease the wheels of the "vehicles" that deliver glucose into cells, helping to prevent diabetes. If salmon doesn't sate your tastebuds, sardines, mackerel, and halibut are rich in fish oils, too.

good results in people taking 900 IU daily for four months straight. However, large doses can be toxic in some people, so discuss this with your doctor before taking any dose larger than 200 IU.

DIARRHEA
Don't Loosen Up

An entrée of shellfish. A new prescription. Aunt Sally's potato salad. A pack of sugarless gum. They all seem innocent enough. But any one of them—and dozens of other digestive devils in disguise—can infect or irritate your intestines and produce the watery, nonstop stools known as diarrhea. There is no foolproof plan to prevent a sudden run-in with the runs. But with a few dietary precautions, you may sidestep the problem.

Most cases of diarrhea are bad chain reactions. When any one of several common sugars combines with the bacteria that live in your intestines, the sugars ferment, creating by-products that draw extra water into the colon. Diarrhea is the disastrous result. To prevent loose stools, stay away from these sweeteners.

LOOK OUT FOR SORBITOL. This sweetener is used in lots of dietetic foods, especially in so-called sugar-free gum and diet candies. Sorbitol is also found in some wines and

---

Feel Fine with Wine

Researchers at Tripler Army Medical Center in Honolulu have found that both red and white wine are effective at killing the bacteria that cause many cases of traveler's diarrhea. In the Tripler study, both wines obliterated the most common perpetrators, including *E. coli*, shigella, and salmonella, within 20 minutes.

"You don't have to drink a bottle. A glass or two with dinner should do," says Martin E. Weisse, M.D., who conducted the study at Tripler and is now associate professor of pediatrics at West Virginia University in Morgantown.

But that doesn't mean that you should forgo other precautions, he says. While wine may help combat certain bacteria, it doesn't get them all, and it has no effect on viruses.

---

vinegars and in many fruits, including strawberries, cherries, plums, prunes, and peaches, according to Seymour Katz, M.D., clinical professor of medicine at New York University School of Medicine; attending gastroenterologist at North Shore University Hospital, Long Island Jewish Medical Center, and Saint Francis Hospital; and past president of the American College of Gastroenterology.

Our bodies just don't digest sorbitol well. If you are having trouble with diarrhea, make sure that you are not eating any sorbitol-rich foods. If you are, cut way back; it may help.

BEWARE THE SUGAR IN MILK. Lactose is the natural sugar in milk. Many people, including a large number of African-Americans, Asians, and people of Mediterranean descent, don't produce the enzyme lactase, which digests that particular sugar. The result can be what is called lactose intolerance, a bad case of indigestion that includes diarrhea.

If you have loose stools and don't know why, milk may be the culprit. Try avoiding dairy products for a while to see if your digestive problems go away. But boycotting dairy is easier said than done because it is not just a matter of shunning milk and cheese.

"Milk is hidden everywhere," says Dr. Katz. "It's in salad dressings, pancake mixes, lunchmeats, even powdered eggs." He says to examine labels carefully for not only the word *milk* but also the words *milk products, casein,* and *whey.*

HOLD THE FRUCTOSE, HONEY. The honey that you may pour into your tea to soothe a sore throat could give you diarrhea, according to one study.

"Some people don't have enough of the proper enzymes to digest fructose, the stuff that makes honey sweet," says gastroenterologist Marvin M. Schuster, M.D., professor of medicine and psychiatry at the Johns Hopkins University School of Medicine and director of the Marvin M. Schuster Center for Digestive and Motility Disorders at the Johns Hopkins Bayview Medical Center, both in Baltimore.

Honey is higher in fructose than any other foods (though fruit juices also have it). When the digestive enzymes are in short supply, fructose suffers the same fate as sorbitol. The bacteria in your intestines ferment the fructose, pulling excess water into your intestines, which brings on diarrhea. The solution? Use another sweetener in your tea.

Save Your Vacation: Avoiding Turista

Traveler's diarrhea, also called turista, is usually caused by the inadvertent ingestion of fecal bacteria. Vile as that sounds, the symptoms are even viler. And the victims are many: 30 to 40 percent of tourists who are from developed countries like the United States and who visit less-developed countries where sanitation isn't up to developed nation's standards are setting themselves up for turista. "The best way to avoid diarrhea is to avoid eating or drinking substances that are contaminated," says David R. Shlim, M.D., medical director of the CIWEC Clinic Travel Medicine Center in Kathmandu, Nepal. Here are some travel tips.

BOIL THE WATER. Avoid ice, locally bottled water, and water served at hotels and restaurants. The only safe water is boiled water. Since boiling kills bacteria, Dr. Katz suggests taking along an electric coil with an international adapter and boiling water in your hotel room. And be sure to use that boiled water when you brush your teeth.

KILL THE BUGGERS. Washing fruits and vegetables in an iodine-water solution is a very effective method for killing most diarrhea-causing organisms on food, says Dr. Shlim. You can purchase iodine tablets before your trip at most wilderness outfitters.

SIDLE UP TO SOME SOFT DRINKS. Carbonation makes soft drinks acidic, which kills the diarrhea bacteria. Beer is safe for the same reason. Don't add ice to your soda because the cubes are often made from untreated water. So to dodge diarrhea, stick to carbonated beverages or treated drinking water, says Dr. Shlim.

LIKE IT HOT. Food that is thoroughly cooked and served hot, which means that it hasn't been sitting around picking up nasty germs, is almost always safe. Do not eat raw food like steak tartare, sushi, or unpasteurized milk products.

DON'T EAT ON THE STREET. "Unless you are with a guide who knows the local scene, don't buy food from a street vendor," says Dr. Katz.

Always Check Your Meds

Some medications *can* cause diarrhea, says Christina M. Surawicz, M.D., professor of medicine and chief of gastroenterology at the Harborview Medical Center at the University of Washington in Seattle, and president-elect of the American College of Gastroenterology. So before you take a drug—whether it is a prescription or over-the-counter medication—read the label or accompanying brochure so that you know if diarrhea is a potential side effect. That way, if you do get diarrhea, you will realize that it is probably the drug, and you can talk with your physician about alternative medications.

One caution: If you are on antibiotics and develop diarrhea, a very common side effect, contact your doctor immediately, says Dr. Surawicz. If allowed to continue, this type of diarrhea can develop into colitis, a severe inflammation of the colon, or large intestine.

Managing Your Fridge

You may have the idea from the media that most cases of food poisoning happen at restaurants or by eating packaged foods. But that's not true, says Christina M. Surawicz, M.D., professor of medicine and chief of gastroenterology at the Harborview Medical Center at the University of Washington in Seattle, and president-elect of the American College of Gastroenterology.

"Commercially prepared food is unlikely to cause food poisoning," says Dr. Surawicz. Homemade food is the more likely source. To avoid picking up the virus or bacteria that cause diarrhea, follow these guidelines for safe handling.

KEEP IT COLD. An egg salad that sits for hours in the sun at the family picnic is a perfect incubator for bad germs.

This leads to a simple rule of thumb from the International Food Information Council Foundation for avoiding food poisoning: Don't eat anything that needs to be refrigerated but has been unrefrigerated for more than two hours.

PAY ATTENTION TO TIME. Even refrigerated food goes bad eventually, and foods with egg- or milk-based ingredients go bad faster. Different foods spoil in different time frames, but it is best to always check freshness dates on store-bought items.

Sniff for freshness if you have doubts and toss things that smell even slightly off. If you can't remember when you placed an item in the fridge, just toss it, says Dr. Surawicz.

DIVERTICULOSIS
Preventing Painful Pouches

It's been a long, strange trip—and what was once food has finally reached the colon, the last stretch of intestine before the rectum. There, muscular walls squeeze and relax, squeeze and relax, pushing the stool along. But if your stool is too small, the colon has to go into overdrive, squeezing extra hard to move it down the line. Sometimes, years of this high-pressure demand causes your colon to finally blow a gastrointestinal gasket: A portion of the colon wall pops outward through the muscle, forming a pouch. Doctors call these pouches diverticuli, and if you have them, you have diverticulosis.

About half of all Americans ages 60 to 80 have some of these pressure-caused pouches, and most of the time there aren't any symptoms. Our digestive systems work well enough to keep humming. But an unfortunate 10 to 25 percent of people with the condition suffer from bloating, abdominal cramps, and even internal bleeding. Indeed, in the

Soda: A Fiber Washout

Order a typical "large" soda these days, and you should probably order a reservoir to go—the amount of liquid you get is astounding. You also might get a huge load of calories, says Patricia Gregory, R.D., a dietitian at Shands Hospital at the University of Florida in Gainesville. And you don't get any fiber, the most important dietary factor in preventing diverticular disease. "One of the things I see with people who are on particularly low fiber diets is that they tend to get a lot of their total calories—sometimes 30 to 50 percent—from sodas, iced teas, and other sugary drinks." Her advice is to skip the 32-ounce soda and drink and eat more of the real thing: water and high-fiber foods.

worst cases, the pouches can become infected, a condition called *diverticulitis*.

But prevention is a piece of cake—well, maybe a piece of fruit after you have come in from your daily walk. "A high-fiber diet in combination with regular physical activity may be the most important preventive factors in reducing the risk of diverticular disease," says Walid H. Aldoori, M.D., Sc.D., a former research fellow in the department of nutrition and epidemiology at the Harvard School of Public Health. Dr. Aldoori was the chief investigator in three major scientific studies that looked at the dietary, exercise, and lifestyle habits of 47,678 American men ages 40 to 75 in an attempt to figure out why some of those men got diverticular disease and why some did not.

Here is what you can do to defend yourself against diverticulosis.

Put Faith in Fiber

"A healthy colon is a low-pressure colon," says Dr. Aldoori. "And to maintain this low pressure, you need a high-fiber diet."

Eating more dietary fiber—the indigestible portion of vegetables, fruits, grains, beans, and other plant foods—adds bulk to your stool, allowing the colon to exert a low, gentle pressure to move it along. In one of Dr. Aldoori's studies, the men who ate the most fiber (32 grams or more of fiber per day) had a 42 percent lower chance of getting diverticular disease than men who ate the least (13 grams).

FAVOR FIVE SERVINGS OF FRUITS AND VEGGIES. If it seems tough to track *grams* of fiber, just follow the government's current dietary recommendation to get three to five daily servings of fruits and vegetables. "That will get you close to 30 or more grams of fiber per day," says Dr. Aldoori. And that's good news because in Dr. Aldoori's study it was the fiber from fruits and vegetables that proved the most protective against diverticulosis. Apples, peaches, bananas, nectarines, and fresh vegetables are fiber-rich.

Five servings may be more than you are used to. Many people who think that they are eating lots of fruits and vegetables are surprised when they actually start to keep track, says Patricia Gregory, R.D., a dietitian at Shands Hospital at the University of Florida in Gainesville. "When we actually measure their fiber intake, it is often amazingly low." Gregory says that most of her patients get only 12 to 13 grams of fiber a day, the same amount as the folks in Dr. Aldoori's study who ended up with diverticulosis.

CHOOSE THE BEST BRAN. Wait a second, what happened to bran, the food that is practically synonymous with fiber?

It is true that bran, the outer husk of grains, can be an important component of a high-fiber, diverticulosis-preventing diet, says Dr. Aldoori. But he cautions that too many people eat grains and cereals that are highly refined or processed. "Foods like white bread, pancakes, and rolls are generally not as useful as whole-grain products in preserving the integrity of the colon," he says.

To get fiber from grains, says Gregory, choose a one-cup serving of a high-fiber cereal like raisin bran and then slice up a medium-size banana for a topping; the combo will net you 11 grams of fiber. And when you eat pasta, eat whole-wheat rather than the refined, white kind.

COUNT THE AMOUNT. To accurately measure your fiber intake, "go to a bookstore and purchase a book that helps you count your fiber intake," says Gregory. Her personal favorite is *Complete Book of Food Counts* by Corrine T. Netzer. It includes the fiber contents of both supermarket and restaurant foods. To keep accurate count, start a food diary, recording your daily intake of fiber until you get in the higher-fiber habit.

GET FIBROUS SLOWLY. To some people, eating more fiber to protect their intestines seems like a bad joke—with a punch line of flatulence, bloating, and abdominal cramps. But eating extra fiber doesn't have to mean digestive upset if you just increase your intake gradually. Up your average daily dose of fiber by 5 grams per week until—in about a month—you have reached 25 to 35 grams per day, suggests Gregory.

MODERATE THE MEAT. Dr. Aldoori's study also found that men who ate beef, pork, or lamb as a main dish more than two times a week had over three times the risk of diverticulosis compared to men who ate meat meals less than once a month. Nobody knows why meat may increase your risk for the disease, though Dr. Aldoori theorizes that it may trigger a type of bacterial activity in the intestines that weakens the walls of the colon. "You should reduce your meat intake," he says, "not only to help prevent diverticulosis but also to help prevent heart disease and many cancers."

Jog Your Colon

Regular physical activity may be an important factor in the prevention of symptomatic diverticular disease. In Dr. Aldoori's study on exercise, he concluded that men who exercised the least had the highest risk of developing the disease. (Those who had low levels of physical activity *and* low levels of fiber intake had the very highest risk of developing the disease—$2^1/2$ times higher than men who got plenty of exercise and fiber.)

How does exercise protect the colon from diverticula? No one knows for sure. But there are some theories. Exercise speeds transit time—the time it takes for the stool to move through the intestines—which means that the colon may have to generate less pressure. Exercise delivers more blood flow to the muscles of the colon, which may keep them stronger. Whatever the reason, your next step is to get more fit, says Dr. Aldoori. Check with your doctor before you take up any new fitness program, and then get started.

WALK. Increased physical activity—any kind of increased physical activity—can lower the risk of diverticular disease. And that includes walking briskly three to five times a week, depending on your current level of fitness and age, says Dr. Aldoori.

RUN. Dr. Aldoori's study also showed that those who participated in very vigorous exercise, like jogging or running, had the lowest risk of the disease. "The more you increase the level of physical exercise, the more benefits you will probably get," he says.

CHOOSE ANOTHER KIND OF EXERCISE FUN. The most important thing in regard to exercise and diverticular disease prevention is that you remain active, says Dr. Aldoori. Just moving about may get your digestion working and help prevent the disease. Stairclimbing, rowing, calisthenics, bicycling, and racquet sports all lower your risk of getting diverticulosis if they're performed regularly.

DIZZINESS
How to Keep a Level Head

For those of us who cruise confidently through life, it is easy to take our sense of balance for granted. But, in fact, balance requires a delicate coordination of many elements, including blood pressure, circulation, even conditions in our inner ears. If you have recurring problems with dizziness, you come to appreciate balance quite quickly.

Dizziness is a tricky problem. There are four distinct types, according to Terry Fife, M.D., professor of clinical neurology at the University of Arizona and director of the Balance Center at the Barrow Neurological Institute in Phoenix. The four types are: light-headedness, in which you feel faint when you stand up too quickly; imbalance, where you have trouble when you walk; spinning dizziness, which makes the world appear to be spinning around you; and physiological dizziness, which is a variation of motion sickness.

Each type of dizziness has many different possible causes. In fact, there are more than 100 different health problems that can produce dizziness as a symptom. That's why, if you're dizzy, you need to see your doctor and describe how often you have these symptoms, particularly if you ever faint or black out. Your doctor may recommend tests to determine the underlying cause. But if you experience dizziness now and then with no known cause, here are some measures that may prevent the different kinds of momentary spinning.

Light-Headedness: A Faint of the Heart

Feeling light-headed and dizzy is always caused by the brain not getting enough blood, says Dr. Fife. And the most common way for that to happen is a sudden glitch in the body's autonomic nervous system, which controls your blood pressure. The vasovagal reflex shunts blood away from the brain rather than toward it in times of stress. When someone faints at the sight of blood or after hearing bad news, it is the vasovagal reflex in action. Unfortunately, hundreds of thousands of Americans have a reflex that is triggered quite easily. If you are one of those folks who has this kind of triggered reaction, here is what Dr. Fife recommends to stop that light-headed feeling.

CHOW DOWN. Skipping meals and feeling very hungry can push the vasovagal reflex into action. Eat three meals a day.

DRINK UP. Getting dehydrated, particularly when it is hot outside, can also trigger the reflex. Drink eight eight-ounce glasses of water every day.

IF IT'S SWELTERING, SIT. Standing in the sun on a hot day is a setup for light-headedness. If you have to be outside when it is hot, find a place to sit. Be sure to wear a hat and lightweight clothing.

Ménière's Disease: Less Salt Equals Less Dizzy

In Ménière's disease, the inner ear has been damaged by an infection, a head injury, or some other problem. This causes excess fluid to accumulate in the inner ear, causing severe dizziness. "A person with Ménière's disease can get sudden, violent attacks of dizziness lasting anywhere from minutes to hours, and these attacks usually occur in groups," says Charles P. Kimmelman, M.D., professor of otolaryngology at Cornell Medical School and attending physician at Manhattan Eye, Ear, and Throat Hospital in New York City.

But there is a simple way to partially help the dizziness of Ménière's: Restrict the sodium, or salt, in your diet. "Salt has what is called an osmotic effect. It pulls water into any compartment," says Dr. Kimmelman. "By restricting the salt in the diet, less fluid might build up in the inner ear."

How low do you have to go? "I advise my Ménière's patients to get no more than 1,500 milligrams of salt a day," says Terry Fife, M.D., professor of clinical neurology at the University of Arizona and director of the Balance Center at the Barrow Neurological Institute in Phoenix.

WATCH TEMPERATURE TRANSITS. Walking from the hot outdoors into an air-conditioned building can set off the reflex. "As soon as you enter an air-conditioned building, sit down for a few moments until you are sure that you are not light-headed and dizzy," says Dr. Fife.

TAKE A DETOUR AROUND ODOR. Any noxious odor, such as the smell of vomit, can stimulate the reflex. If you can avoid a bad smell, do so, says Dr. Fife.

BE DECISIVE WHEN DIZZY. If you stand up and feel dizzy and light-headed, sit back down quickly, says Dr. Fife. "You don't want to faint and bang yourself up."

Slowing a Whirling World

There are dozens of health problems that can ruin your sense of balance or cause vertigo, the dizzying sensation that either you or the world is spinning around. The most common problem is damage to the balance organs of the inner ear, caused by infection or trauma, says Charles P. Kimmelman, M.D., professor of otolaryngology at Cornell Medical School and attending physician at Manhattan Eye, Ear, and Throat Hospital in New York City.

While the problem will most likely improve, it usually recurs. Fortunately, you can compensate for it. "You can train other parts of your balance system to help the inner ear," says Dr. Kimmelman.

Once your acute dizziness has subsided, Dr. Kimmelman says to do the following exercises twice a day, starting with 15-minute sessions and gradually increasing your time until you do two 30-minute workouts each day. It is better to stand, but let your own comfort guide you and sit, if necessary. Perform them slowly at first, then gradually increase to a comfortable speed.

LOOK DIZZINESS IN THE EYE. Without moving your head, swivel your gaze to look up, then down, at first slowly, then quickly. Repeat 20 times. Next, look from one side to the other, at first slowly, then quickly. Repeat 20 times. Then, focus on a finger at arm's length while moving one foot forward and backward. Repeat 20 times.

HEAD IN THE OTHER DIRECTION. With your eyes open, tip your head forward, then *slightly* backward. Do this slowly at first, then quickly. Repeat 20 times. Turn your head from side to side, first slowly, then quickly. Repeat 20 times. (As your dizziness improves, these head exercises should be done with your eyes closed.)

STAGE A SIT-DOWN STRIKE. While sitting, shrug your shoulders. Repeat 20 times. Now swivel in your seat so that you turn your shoulders to the left and then to the right.

Fight Dizziness with Nature's Medicines

Ginger may be an anti-dizziness option, according to James A. Duke, Ph.D., master herbalist and retired ethnobotanist and toxicology specialist at the U.S. Department of Agriculture and author of *The Green Pharmacy*. In one study of naval cadets, the sailors who took a half-teaspoon of powdered ginger before leaving the dock had fewer seasickness symptoms, including dizziness.

Other herbs may be antidotes for occasional dizziness, according to Dr. Duke. He suggests blending them all in this anti-woozy tea: Combine four teaspoons of ginger with dashes of ground pumpkin seeds, celery seeds, chamomile flowers, fennel, orange rind, peppermint, and spearmint. Add boiling water and steep for 15 minutes. These ingredients are available at most grocery and health food stores. If you have prolonged or recurrent bouts of dizziness, see a physician.

Repeat 20 times. Bend forward as if to pick up an object from the ground and then sit up. Repeat 20 times.

STAND UP AGAINST DIZZINESS. Sit down, then stand up and sit down again. Repeat 20 times.

GET ON A JUGGLING JAG. While standing, toss a small rubber ball from hand to hand above eye level. Do this for 30 seconds to one minute. Then lift one leg and toss the ball from hand to hand under the lifted knee. Do this for as long as you are comfortable, up to one minute.

WALK AWAY FROM IT ALL. Walk back and forth along a clutter-free hallway with your eyes open. Repeat 10 times. Now do the same exercise with your eyes closed. Repeat 10 times. If you don't feel at all dizzy after that, try walking up and down a slight slope—in your yard, for example—with your eyes open. Repeat 10 times, then try the same exercise another 10 times with your eyes closed.

The Dizziness of Motion Sickness

The most common kind of physiological dizziness is from motion sickness, says Dr. Fife. It is caused by a disparity in what you see—the objects whipping past the car window—while you are sitting or standing still. "There is a confusion between the brain and the inner ear, and that causes dizziness, nausea, and motion sickness." If you know that you are prone to motion sickness, here is what to do.

BE ILLITERATE. Motion sickness in a car, boat, or plane can easily make someone feel dizzy as well as queasy. If you are vulnerable, avoid reading while you are moving along, advises Dr. Fife. "Reading in a car is one of the worst things that you can do if you are prone to motion sickness," he says.

SIT CLOSE TO THE DRIVER. "In the front seat, you have a much better view of what is going on, so your vision and your inner ear are both reacting to the same environmental changes," says Dr. Fife. "This decreases the likelihood of motion sickness and dizziness."

ALL HEADS ON DECK. If you have to travel by boat, "you are better off up on deck and looking at the horizon than staying in the cabin below," says Dr. Fife.

DRY AND DAMAGED HAIR
Protecting Your Lustrous Locks

Everybody loves a thick, healthy head of hair. The problem is that lots of folks have a strange way of expressing that affection. The amazing array of styling, coloring, weaving, and waving techniques that people use today to achieve head-turning hair are actually very hard on tresses. When you add the drying effects of winter wind and summer sun, you have a prescription for disaster, which is why damaged hair is such a common condition, says Mickhael Cannon, of Seattle, a recipient of the Paul Mitchell World Medal of Honor in Hairdressing and artistic director at the Worldwide Beauty Store on the Internet.

But you can prevent (or at least dramatically reduce) hair damage by learning more about the fine art of hair care, says Cannon. Here is what dermatologists and cosmetologists recommend.

TURN OFF THE HOT WATER. "Hot water tends to dry out the hair," says Cannon. So turn down the temperature. Use warm water that is just a little hotter than body tem-

---

Brush Gently to Spare Your Hair

The wrong brush can rip your hair, causing breakage and contributing to split ends, says Mickhael Cannon, of Seattle, a recipient of the Paul Mitchell World Medal of Honor in Hairdressing and artistic director at the Worldwide Beauty Store on the Internet. To avoid breakage, he suggests using a natural-bristle brush rather than a plastic one. Plastic creates static, making the hair easier to break.

The right hair-brushing technique is also important for healthy hair, he says. Start brushing your hair at the ends, gently removing large tangles with your fingers. Then, gradually work your way up the length of the shaft until you reach the scalp. Finally, brush from the scalp to the ends with long, continuous strokes.

---

perature. Or even lather up with cool water—it can still get your hair squeaky clean, according to Cannon.

AVOID THE SHAMPOO OVERDO. Lots of people shampoo their hair too often. The best regimen for keeping hair healthy is to shampoo once a day using a pH-balanced product, says Rebecca Caserio, M.D., clinical associate professor of dermatology at the University of Pittsburgh.

"Your natural oils offer important protection to your hair shaft," she says. "If you strip too many of them by excessive shampooing, you create dryness, which eventually causes breakage."

RINSE IT CLEAN. Make sure that you rinse your hair thoroughly after shampooing. "Shampoo can leave a residue that can dry the hair," says Cannon.

CONDITION FROM THE ENDS IN. Conditioners help prevent dry hair, but there is a special way you need to apply them so that they will do the most good, according to Margie Ellis, of Highland Village, Texas, a hairstylist for 13 years and the creator of Hair Tips by Margie on the Internet. "A lot of people have the habit of putting the conditioner right on their heads, near the roots, which is the newest, healthiest part of the hair. But your hair is drier at the ends, so that is where you should apply the conditioner first." She suggests putting the conditioner in your palm, rubbing your palms together, and applying it first to the ends of your hair. Then work your way toward your scalp.

GET THERMAL PROTECTION. Use a conditioner that includes a component (sometimes called a thermal protector) that helps shield your hair from heat. Among the most common thermal protectors are cyclomethicone, dimethicone, and phenyl trimethicone. Read the label on the bottle to be sure that your conditioner has one. "Thermal protectors safeguard the hair against heat because they contain heat-absorbing ingredients," explains Cannon. Using them is one of the best things that you can do for your hair if you use a blow-dryer, a curling iron, or hot rollers, he says.

PAT, DON'T RUB. "A lot of people get out of the shower and rub the daylights out of their hair with a towel," says Ellis. Unfortunately, that habit can break the hair, especially if it is permed or naturally curly, leading to split ends. So instead of rubbing, pat or blot your hair with a towel or use it like a turban to wrap your hair.

BE COOL ABOUT HOT STYLING TOOLS. Styling devices that work their magic with heat—blow-dryers, curling irons, hot rollers, and the like—are hair destroyers, says Cannon. So you should limit your use of any high-heat styling method to once a day, suggests Fredric Brandt, M.D., clinical associate professor of dermatology at the University of Miami School of Medicine and a dermatologist in Miami.

CHOOSE DIFFUSION. If your hairstyle is curly, use a diffuser attachment on your blow-dryer, says Cannon. This causes less damage because it dissipates the heat and airflow. If your style doesn't lend itself to a diffuser, try using a lower heat setting on your dryer.

At-Home Herbal Hair-Care

Sometimes the best way to fend off dry, fragile hair is to get back to the basics. So toss your high-tech hair treatments aside and indulge in great-smelling herbs and essential oils. According to Kathi Keville, director of the American Herb Association, the herbs that do an excellent job of preventing dry hair are burdock, calendula, chamomile, rose geranium, lavender, rose, rosemary, cedarwood, and sandalwood.

You can make a strong tea with just one or a combination of a couple of herbs. This is done by using two tablespoons of the herbs you choose, covering them with 16 ounces of boiling water, and steeping for 20 minutes. Wait until this tea cools and then use it as a rinse.

Better yet, make your own warm-oil conditioner using ingredients that are available at most health food stores. Combine two ounces of aloe vera gel, two ounces of olive oil, six drops each of sandalwood and rosemary essential oils, and two drops of ginger essential oil (optional). Warm the oil mixture slightly. Comb and part your hair into different sections, then massage the oil into your scalp. Cover your head with a towel and leave the treatment on for one to two hours, then shampoo out.

CAST OUT THAT CURLING IRON. Try a heated styling brush instead of a curling iron. It is gentler on your hair, says Cannon.

SEEK SAFETY IN CERTAIN STYLES. Another way to prevent overdrying with styling tools is to wear your hair either very short or very long. Those types of cuts can dramatically shorten styling time, says Federico, owner and director of Federico Hair Salon in Manhattan. A short cut lets you just fluff with your fingers or blow-dry for a couple of minutes. Long hair can work well without a lot of styling because it can look great pulled up in a ponytail or back in a chignon.

WEAR A HAT. Too much exposure to the sun will dry and damage your hair, says Cannon. "For protecting your hair outdoors, you can't beat a hat," says Dr. Caserio. As for hair-care products with sunscreen, there doesn't seem to be any scientific research to show whether or not they really protect the hair.

JUMP FROM POOL TO SHOWER. Chlorine will dry out your hair. "Get chlorine off your hair as soon as possible after getting out of the pool," says Ellis. "If you can't give your hair a good rinse in the locker room, then do it as soon as you get home." Use one of the shampoos specially formulated to remove chlorine, since they can prevent the discoloring of your hair, says Ellis. Most drugstores and beauty supply stores carry these shampoos.

DRY EYES
Get Back Your Working Tears

Right now, as you are reading this, stop blinking. Keep your eyes completely open for the next 30 seconds or so, or at least until you feel that you have to blink.

How did your eyes feel? Probably a little irritated, with a slight burning sensation. Well, you have just experienced a case of dry eyes. In those 30 seconds, you normally would have blinked two or three times, restoring your tear film, a super-thin coating on the surface of your eyes that keeps them moist and comfortable. But when the tear film isn't replenished or is disturbed in any way, you experience the symptoms of dry eyes that can range from moderate itching and burning to light sensitivity and eye fatigue.

Sometimes dry eyes are a chronic problem because the tear film has been damaged by a disease, such as Sjögren's syndrome, in which the tear gland is inflamed and there are fewer tears to replenish the film. And many women experience dry eyes as a result of the hormonal changes that may occur during pregnancy or menopause. "The condition of the tear film may actually be related to a woman's hormonal status," says Mary Gilbert Lawrence, M.D., associate professor of ophthalmology at the University of Minnesota in Minneapolis.

But most people only experience dry eyes every now and then, in response to some environmental factor. Staring at a computer screen for too long can destabilize the tear film, says Dan Nelson, M.D., associate professor of ophthalmology at the University of Minnesota in Minneapolis and chairman of the department of ophthalmology at the Health Partners–Regions Hospital in St. Paul. Low humidity can dry your peepers, too. "It is much better to prevent dry eyes than to wait for problems to happen and *then* treat them," he says. "Once the eye gets irritated and sore, you get into a vicious circle, and the eye tends to keep getting worse." If you have had dry eyes in the past, here is how to keep your tear film intact.

GET THE DROP ON THE PROBLEM. Try bottled tears, better known as artificial tears, says Dr. Nelson. Don't use drops like Murine or Visine that are manufactured to reduce redness, but instead use artificial tears, drops designed to restore moisture to the eye. There are many different types of these drops: Some have preservatives, and some of the newer brands are more tearlike in their chemical composition. If you have dry eyes often, ask your doctor to recommend the right drops for you to help prevent the condition. If it is a problem every now and then, "any type of bottled tears, like Thera Tears or Bion Tears, will work well," he says.

DON'T OVERDO DAILY TEARS. If your eyes are normal, you shouldn't have to use more than an occasional eyedrop to help prevent dryness, no matter how many eye-drying situations you are in, says Dr. Nelson. If you find that you need to use eyedrops more than four times a day to keep your eyes moist, make an appointment with an ophthal-

mologist. You may have a medical problem more serious
than dry eyes that requires treatment.

GET PREPPED FOR DRY-EYE SITUATIONS. If you are
about to be in a situation where you know you usually get
dry eyes—when you are about to spend time in front of a
computer, for instance—put in a drop before the activity. Or
put in a drop at the first sign of discomfort.

READY YOURSELF FOR TAKEOFF. The air in airplanes is
uniquely drying and irritating, says Dr. Nelson. First, the
plane has probably just been cleaned, so the air is loaded
with chemicals. Second, the air in the plane is pressurized at
5,000 feet, which means *dry* air. Third, that air is recirculated for the entire flight. "Many flight attendants have
trouble with dry eyes," he says. Use eyedrops before you get
on the plane and while flying, he suggests.

KEEP YOUR EYES MOIST ON THE ROAD. "People often
experience dry eyes in cars," says Dr. Nelson. Make sure
that the vents aren't blowing in your eyes. Or sit in the back
seat if you are not driving.

BLOCK OUT WIND AND COLD. Being outdoors in cold,
dry, windy climates can steal moisture from your eyes, says
Dr. Nelson. The best way to protect your eyes is with a pair
of glasses. If regular sunglasses don't help, he says, try wraparound sunglasses with lenses that are close to your face.
If wraparound glasses don't help, try moisture-chamber
glasses. These have pieces of plastic film on the sides of
the frames that form an enclosure around your eyes. They
are available at your local optician, eyeglasses stores, and
some outdoor and wilderness outfitters. And if they don't
work, try wearing ski goggles, says Dr. Nelson. "The complete enclosure prevents evaporation and increases moisture. They keep the wind out, and they can be worn over
other glasses."

WATCH OUT FOR DRY INDOOR AIR. Being indoors in
winter can also take a toll on your eyes, since the heating

Meds That Leave You Dry-Eyed

People with chronic dry eyes may be suffering from a drug side effect, says Dan Nelson, M.D., associate professor of ophthalmology at the University of Minnesota in Minneapolis and chairman of the department of ophthalmology at the Health Partners–Regions Hospital in St. Paul. The drugs that cause dry eyes are called anti-cholinergic—they block the cholinergic nerves that control the secretion of mucus to the eyes.

Some medications that cause dry eyes can also dry out the mouth, nose, vagina, and all other areas where there are mucous membranes. If you think that a drug is causing dry eyes or other dryness problems, Dr. Nelson says to work with your doctor and pharmacist to pick an alternative drug that won't have this side effect.

Here are a few common drugs that can cause dry eyes.

- Antihistamines
- Cough medications with codeine
- Antidepressants (tricyclics and MAO inhibitors)
- Tranquilizers
- High blood pressure medications (beta-blockers and diuretics)
- Heart medications (beta-blockers)
- Parkinson's disease drugs

dries out the air. To prevent dry eyes, Dr. Nelson recommends using a vaporizer next to your bed while you are sleeping or in your office while you are working. "They tend to work better than humidifiers in really making the air wet."

MONITOR YOUR MAKEUP. Perhaps your makeup or eye cream should take the blame for early-morning dry eyes. If you have dry eyes and routinely apply makeup or creams to your eye area, stop using them for a few days and see if your symptoms go away, Dr. Nelson suggests. And be sure to take off all of your eye makeup at bedtime. "Leaving your makeup on just exposes your eyes to irritating or drying chemicals."

For Computer Users

Working long hours at a computer can cause dry eyes, says Dr. Nelson, and he suggests a few ways to prevent the problem.

CHECK YOUR GLASSES. "You want to make sure that your prescription allows you to see the screen clearly so that you are not struggling to focus," he says.

CUT THE GLARE. "There should be adequate light in the room, and the contrast on the screen should be good," says Dr. Nelson.

ADJUST SCREEN HEIGHT. "The screen should be positioned so that it is lower than your eyes and you have to look down slightly to read," he explains. "This will cause your eyelids to lower, so there will be less of the eye exposed and less evaporation."

DUCK THE DUCTS. "If your computer at work is right below a heating or air-conditioning duct, ask your supervisor if you could move," says Dr. Nelson. "If you can't switch locations, use artificial tears." Also, adjust your at-home workstation as necessary to help prevent dry eyes.

GIVE YOURSELF A BREAK. "Looking at the computer screen is strenuous work for your eyes," he says. "Take a break every now and then; get up and walk around."

DRY MOUTH
Mouthwatering Strategies

Saliva is one versatile fluid. Besides helping us talk, chew, kiss, and digest, it also helps us avoid many ailments, from infections to bad breath and tooth decay. A saliva shortage can be a big problem. "Having a dry mouth is a major negative factor in the quality of life," says Ronald Ettinger, D.D.Sc., professor at the Dows Institute for Dental Research at the College of Dentistry at the University of Iowa in Iowa City.

Dry mouth is also quite common, especially as we age. Approximately 40 percent of people over age 65 have it, says a study from the Eastman Dental Center in Rochester, New York. Some cases are caused by radiation treatments to the head and neck that destroy the salivary glands or by an autoimmune disease called Sjögren's syndrome. Other times, our mouths lose moisture because of a medicine. But most cases of xerostomia—that's the medical-school name for dry mouth—are preventable. Here are a few methods for keeping your whistle wet.

Saliva-Stimulating Herbs

Nature's pharmacy may well offer relief from dry mouth. Here are some herbal options for preventing that parched feeling.

TRY ECHINACEA. For short-term relief, take 10 to 15 drops of tincture in juice, once every hour as needed, says David Winston, founding member of the American Herbalist Guild and a clinical herbalist in Washington, New Jersey. It is a proven saliva producer. The reputable German government herbal advisory agency, Commission E, recommends limiting your use of echinacea to a duration of eight weeks at a time.

CONSIDER CAPSAICIN. This is the active ingredient in hot pepper. It can produce all kinds of moisture—sweat, tears, or saliva, according to James A. Duke, Ph.D., master herbalist and retired ethnobotanist and toxicology specialist at the U.S. Department of Agriculture and author of *The Green Pharmacy*. Add some red pepper to soups and stews, and put a shaker of it on the kitchen table.

QUESTION THE DRUGS THAT DRY OUT. There are more than 400 different medications that can cause dry mouth, says Dr. Ettinger. Some of the more commonly prescribed remedies that do are drugs used to treat heart disease, high blood pressure, depression, and anxiety. Decongestants and antihistamines used to treat colds and allergies can leave you with a parched pucker, too. Ask your physician if a drug could be the source of your problem. But don't be surprised if you don't get much of a response. Physicians are often not sensitized to all the personal problems caused by dry mouth, he says.

So what should you do? Dr. Ettinger suggests that you ask your dentist for guidance. Your dentist will understand just how serious dry mouth can be and work with your physician or pharmacist to figure out if a drug could be the source of your problem. "There are now many medications available that are much less drying than the older, more commonly prescribed drugs," he says.

Drink plenty of water. A dry body produces a dry mouth. To prevent dehydration, carry a water bottle around and sip from it regularly, says Dr. Ettinger.

Or suck on a few ice chips if you can stand the chill, says Donna Stach, a registered dental hygienist and associate professor of dental hygiene at the University of Colorado School of Dentistry in Denver.

Cut the java and the booze. Coffee and alcohol can leave your mouth feeling like the Sahara. Both are diuretics, so they tend to take fluids out of your body. Limit them, Stach suggests.

Make tobacco taboo. Add one more to the reasons to stop smoking. Most experts believe that it aggravates dry mouth, says Stach.

Watch your mouthwash. Whiskey and wine aren't the only sources of alcohol. Most mouthwashes on the market contain significant amounts of alcohol. Choose one made specifically for people who have dry mouth, advises Dr. Ettinger. These mouthwashes not only are alcohol-free but also contain mouth-moistening ingredients.

Go with the flow. Reach for an over-the-counter saliva substitute such as Salivart, says Dr. Ettinger.

"Treat" your mouth right. Sucking on candies and chewing gum stimulates the saliva glands, helping to prevent dry mouth, says Dr. Ettinger. But those goodies have to be sugarless; otherwise, you are inviting tooth decay.

Any kind of sugarless candy is fine, and the flavor you like best will stimulate the salivary glands the most, says Ibtisam Al-Hashimi, Ph.D., director of the Salivary Dysfunction Clinic in the department of periodontics of the Baylor College of Dentistry at Texas A&M University in Dallas.

Prevent Tooth Decay, Too

"People with dry mouth, or xerostomia, are at risk for massive amounts of tooth decay," says Donna Stach, a registered dental hygienist and associate professor of dental hygiene at the University of Colorado School of Dentistry in Denver. Saliva, she explains, contains protective agents that shield teeth from decay-causing bacteria. It also helps flush away the bacteria. Saliva also contains calcium that constantly remineralizes your teeth. If you have dry mouth, try these cavity-prevention tips.

CHAT WITH YOUR DENTIST. The more the dentist knows about your condition, the better he can help you prevent tooth decay. People's needs are different—talk with your dentist about setting the best cycle to see him regularly (some people need to go at least three times a year), says Robert Ettinger, D.D.Sc., professor at the Dows Institute for Dental Research at the College of Dentistry at the University of Iowa in Iowa City.

USE FLUORIDE. Fluoride also helps the teeth stay mineralized, preventing decay. Use a fluoride toothpaste and follow brushing with a fluoride rinse or gel, says Stach. For those with severe dry mouth, she recommends talking to your dentist about creating a customized "fluoride tray" (a mouth-guard-like device) for your mouth. You put a few drops of fluoride rinse in the tray and leave it in your mouth for five minutes or so a day.

PAY ATTENTION TO THE BASICS. Don't forget to brush and floss after every meal and avoid sticky, sugary foods, says Dr. Ettinger.

"I always encourage the use of fruit flavors, which are mild," Dr. Al-Hashimi says. And she cautions not to chew gum for more than 10 minutes without a break, or you may strain your jaw joints. If you prefer to steer clear of sweets altogether, munching on celery and carrots can also make your mouth water, she adds.

HUMIDIFY YOUR HOME. Winter heating and summer air-conditioning can suck the moisture out of the air—and out of your mouth. Using a humidifier (or vaporizer) at night in the bedroom is a good way to prevent the problem, says Dr. Ettinger.

DRY SKIN AND WINTER ITCH
How to Stay Supple and Moist

Nothing takes the moisture and softness out of skin faster than winter's dry indoor heating and icy, face-chapping winds. Even if you pamper and protect your skin all year long, it needs a little extra attention when the temperatures begin to fall. As the moisture level in the air drops, the dry air tries to rehydrate itself by borrowing moisture from your skin. When that happens, your body's natural protective barrier, made of water, oils, and a protein called keratin, can get dehydrated to the point where your skin gets taut, wrinkly, cracked, and itchy.

But winter doesn't have to turn your epidermis into a desert. Just use some lotions and precautions, and you'll keep your skin at its best.

Nature's Way of Soothing Winter Skin

If dry skin is your issue, Mother Nature is definitely part of the problem, but she can also be part of the solution. Tuck a few of these natural remedies into your medicine chest for those days when your moisturizer just isn't doing enough to prevent dry-skin discomfort, says expert herbalist James A. Duke, Ph.D., master herbalist and retired ethnobotanist and toxicology specialist at the U.S. Department of Agriculture and author of *The Green Pharmacy*.

Aloe vera. This skin soother has been a hot topic since the days of ancient Egypt when the pharaohs used it to help them look their best. The gel is excellent for treating all kinds of skin problems and keeps them from going from bad to worse. It can also speed the healing process for itchy, irritated skin. Pick up a bottle at just about any drug or health food store and just rub on the contents.

Avocado oil. Sure, avocados are great on a salad, but did you know that avocado oil has superior powers when it comes to slowing down attacks of dermatitis (a skin inflammation) and eczema, which can be aggravated by dry conditions? Apply it directly to any potentially itchy, red, or irritated areas. Avocado oil is available at health food stores.

Marsh mallow. No, not the sugary, white pillows that you drop into hot cocoa. This is an herb that contains a soothing, water-soluble fiber called mucilage. In Europe, it is a key ingredient in ointments used to prevent and treat chapped skin. Easy-to-use preparations are available at health food stores. Spread some on for protection the next time you are about to go out into the winter wind.

Master the Moisturizers

Buying a moisturizer used to be simple. Your choices were limited to a few oil and water emulsions that did an okay job of soothing your skin. They were basically the same, except for variations in scent, packaging, and price. Not anymore. Now we have lotions and potions that include everything from acid to megadoses of vitamin C. Here are some guidelines to skin-care products.

Assess the AHAs. Alpha hydroxy acids, or AHAs, are the stars of the new skin-care revolution. They help your skin to look and feel a little better by removing dead, dry surface cells.

All skin has a dense structure of vital living cells (the *stratum compactum*) and a top layer where cells are loose and dead cells accumulate *(stratum disjunctum)*, says Gary Grove, Ph.D., vice president of research and development for the Skin Study Center, an independent testing laboratory in Broomall, Pennsylvania. People with very dry skin tend to have more of that loose top layer.

In the "old" days (prior to the early 1980s), there was no way to get rid of those unsightly, old cells except to rub them off with a rough scrub or cloth. Now, the best way to get those troublesome layers out of the way is with AHAs.

AHAs actually help loosen the cells without abrading the skin and making it more vulnerable to dehydration. Although these acids are widely known for their ability to help preserve youthful-looking skin (they reduce the appearance of wrinkles and make some fine lines disappear), they first made their mark as a weapon against skin dryness.

Not all alpha hydroxy acid products are created equal. Some are stronger than others and may cause redness if used on fair-skinned complexions. Other formulas slough off dead skin but do not provide moisture, so you still need to top them off with a moisturizer.

The trick to finding the right AHA for you is to

discover a strength and mixture that agrees with your skin. You may have to test a few different brands before you have success. "Some of the over-the-counter products may work for you," says Alan B. Fleischer, M.D., associate professor of dermatology at Bowman Gray School of Medicine of Wake Forest University in Winston-Salem, North Carolina. "If not, your dermatologist can recommend prescription AHAs, such as Lac-Hydrin 12 percent."

A few words of caution: Overusing very strong alpha hydroxy acid preparations can actually increase dryness or irritate some people with sensitive skin. So, if you are using a product and you begin to have a problem, stop using it and call your doctor for advice.

SELECT A SIMPLE LOTION. Since many AHA formulas do not contain moisturizers, you will still need a good, basic moisturizer that you can use twice a day in addition to an AHA. To give your after-bath moisturizer a boost, leave a light film of water on your skin before you apply the cream or lotion. The oil in the moisturizer will help keep the water from evaporating quickly. Look for ingredients such as petrolatum, lanolin, or mineral oil in your moisturizer. "They tend to be most effective at sealing in moisture," says Dr. Fleischer.

SMOOTH ON A SUPPLEMENT. Antioxidant lotions, face creams, and even transdermal patches packed with vitamins—mostly A, C, and E—are the new wave in skin care. They are supposed to ease the effects of aging, but the jury is still out on whether or not they work. "There is some evidence that they can prevent some of the acute sun damage done to the skin," says Lorraine Kligman, Ph.D., research associate professor of dermatology at the University of Pennsylvania School of Medicine in Philadelphia. Sunburn causes cells in the epidermis to die, and some of these preparations may reduce the number of sunburned cells present. Their long-term benefits, however, are still unknown, she adds. They may be worth a try, though, because sun-damaged skin is dry skin.

Get Better at Basic Care

In addition to taking care of your skin with lotions, you can adopt some everyday strategies that help prevent dry skin. Here are a few simple tips that can help you win the battle.

LAY OFF THE LOOFAH. Tempted to try a loofah to slough the dry stuff off? Don't. Though gentle exfoliation is good, it is too easy to get carried away and remove healthy cells in the process. And too much exfoliation can actually encourage drying. Even a washcloth can be too harsh. For washing, your hands are the best equipment that you can use, says Dr. Fleischer.

STAY COOL. In the winter, hot air and water (as in bathtub, shower, and wash-basin water) are your skin's worst enemies. Indoor heat is especially bad because when dry air gets heated up, it becomes even drier. Set your thermostat to around 68°F (or lower if you like). You can save a bit of your skin's natural moisture and a bit of fuel while you are at it.

DAMPEN YOUR HOME—AND OFFICE. Buy a humidifier, especially if you can't face turning your thermostat down. Try putting it in your bedroom. After all, you spend a lot of time there. You can also put a pie pan filled with water on your radiator or near your heat ducts.

MAKE BATH TIME BRIEF. Ironically, you can't get water into your skin by dousing yourself with it. Quite the opposite. "There are valuable natural humectants (moisturizing factors) in your skin that are, unfortunately, water soluble," says Dr. Grove. For the first few minutes, these humectants help the water bind to your skin, so it puffs up a bit and looks good. But if you stay in the water longer, these humectants dissolve and are washed away. Five minutes is pretty much the maximum advisable time for winter showers and baths. And adding a little bath oil or moisturizing shower gel to your routine can help.

DIP IN THE EVENING. Doing your cleansing in the evening is best. That way, if you do strip off some of your natural moisturizers, your skin can replace them overnight. Showering in the morning and then going outdoors into the elements gives your skin a double whammy, says Dr. Grove.

CHOOSE SENSIBLE SUDS. The type of lather you work up when you are in the bath or shower can also help or hurt your cause. Avoid harsh soaps and restrict your scrubbing to the areas of your body that need it most. "Most deodorant bars are too drying," says Marcia Glenn, M.D., a dermatologist in private practice in Marina del Ray, California. She recommends mild emollient soaps or cleansers such as Cetaphil, Dove, Oil of Olay, Neutrogena, Basis, and Alpha-Keri.

EARACHES
For a More Sound Future

Lend us your ears—because to understand how to prevent the different kinds of earaches, you need to hear a little bit more about them.

The ear has three parts: outer, middle, and inner. The outer ear is the part that you can see as well as the ear canal. At the end of your ear canal is your eardrum, a thin membrane across the entrance of the middle ear. That is where you will find the eustachian tube, which is connected to your nose and throat. The tube allows for the drainage of bacteria- and virus-encouraging fluids from the middle ear. Go deeper, and there is the inner ear, which houses your hearing and balance centers.

Most earaches are caused by infection. And most outer-ear infections happen when the ear canal is too moist, allowing bacteria to grow. These infections temporarily reduce hearing, cause pain, and may produce an itch. Sometimes infections of the middle ear happen when the draining

How to Jettison Airplane-Ear Pain

The ear pain we get when we are climbing or descending from eight miles above the earth isn't caused by infection. Our ears often ache when we are aloft because of unequal pressure on the inside of the eardrum and the outside. The pressure pushes the eardrum inward and causes sharp pain. Try these airborne ear-savers.

CLEAR THE WAY BEFORE TAKEOFF. Taking a simple over-the-counter decongestant 30 minutes before your next flight leaves the ground can put an end to air-travel-related earaches, say researchers. In a study of 190 fliers with recurrent ear pain, only 32 percent of the people who received a decongestant containing pseudoephedrine before takeoff had ear pain. Sixty-two percent of those in the no-decongestant group felt some pain and popping.

The decongestants work by opening up the eustachian tube, which prevents pressure (the source of the pain and popping) from building up inside your ears. The medicines also help decrease secretions that might block the tube, says study co-author Jeffrey Jones, M.D., director of the department of emergency medicine at Butterworth Hospital in Grand Rapids, Michigan.

Be sure to take the decongestant *before* you fly, says Dr. Jones. It won't work as well if you take it after your earache gets started. Building on his earlier study, Dr. Jones also found that oral decongestants work better than nasal spray. One dose should last you all day, so you don't have to keep popping decongestants if your flight is delayed. The only side effect seen in the study was drowsiness.

eustachian tube is blocked so that bacteria and viruses can flourish in the middle ear. An untreated middle-ear or respiratory infection could lead to an inner-ear infection,

One caution: Avoid pseudoephedrine if you have thyroid disease, heart disease, high blood pressure, diabetes, or an enlarged prostate.

CONSIDER THE FRENZEL MANEUVER. If you don't want to take decongestants—or you can't for health reasons—try the Frenzel method of clearing your ears instead, says Dr. Jones. Pinch your nose closed and push your tongue firmly against the back part of the roof of your mouth. That works a little air through your eustachian tube. This method works best for preventing the problem rather than treating it, says Dr. Jones, so you will want to start doing it as soon as the plane begins its descent.

DON'T POP UNDER PRESSURE. Don't try to clear your ears by holding your nose, closing your mouth, and then trying to build the pressure inside your eardrum. "This routine tries to force air through a tube that may already be blocked, and it can actually injure your ears," says Dr. Jones.

GIVE BABY HIS BOTTLE. To prevent a baby from developing an earache during takeoff or landing, give him a bottle to suck on as the plane climbs or descends. The sucking action can help clear his ears. For extra insurance, make sure that the baby is sitting upright during his feeding, says Dr. Jones.

GIVE THE KIDS SOME SUCKERS. Older children can suck on candy or lozenges during the flight—or give them gum if they are old enough (try this tip yourself, too). The idea is to keep them swallowing so that their ears stay clear. If they have complained about ear pain before, Dr. Jones says, you may want to give them a decongestant recommended by your pediatrician.

which often causes nausea and vomiting because it induces vertigo (a feeling that your surroundings are spinning).

The premier preventive principle when it comes to

earaches caused by infection is to keep those ears nice and dry inside, says Anu Sheth, M.D., lead physician at the Egleston Children's Health Care Center in Dunwoody, Georgia. Try these tips to prevent another round of pain.

BLOW-DRY YOUR EARS. Swimmers get lots of ear infections. They spend almost as much time with water-clogged ears as they do with wet hair. "Swimmer's ear may be prevented by keeping the ear canal dry," Dr. Sheth says. "And blow-dryers make it a breeze." The warm air evaporates trapped moisture.

Just be careful not to toast your own or anybody else's ears. Use a warm—never hot—dryer setting on low speed and test the temperature on your wrist after the hair dryer has been running a bit. Hold the dryer as far as you can from your ear and slowly move it back and forth for a few minutes.

PULL AND TIP. After you get out of the pool or shower, remember this infection preventer. Pull your earlobe down and tilt your head. Then wiggle the earlobe to shake the water out of each ear, says Dr. Sheth. This motion helps straighten your ear canal and let trapped water escape.

PLAY DEFENSE WITH DROPS. You can also prevent ear infections by using homemade ear drops of equal parts rubbing alcohol and distilled white vinegar, says Dr. Sheth. Put three or four drops in each ear after swimming, she advises. This won't make your ears more moist. As the alcohol evaporates, it absorbs some water that has collected in the ear. And the vinegar helps to discourage the growth of bacteria and fungi in that warm-water medium.

FATIGUE
Holding On to High Energy

Call it fatigue, listlessness, tiredness, lethargy, or just plain feeling pooped, seven million Americans visit their doctors each year seeking an answer for why they are dragging. Well, you don't have to be one of them. Here are some ways to avoid the most common causes of fatigue.

GET STRESSED LESS. "Stress is the number one cause of fatigue in this country," says Reed Moskowitz, M.D., clinical assistant professor of psychiatry, founder and medical director of the stress disorders service at New York University Medical Center in New York City, and author of *Your Healing Mind*. Stress causes your body to go into fight-or-flight mode. When that occurs, you produce excess adrenaline and other hormones that make your heart beat faster and energize your body. As soon as that burst is over, however, you slump into fatigue.

"Being constantly stressed-out is like living with one foot on the brake and the other on the accelerator; you are eventually going to strip your gears," says Dr. Moskowitz.

Catching Some Afternoon Zzzs

Want to prevent the midafternoon slump? Try a short siesta. "You can wipe out the midafternoon blahs very quickly with a 20- to 30-minute nap," says Mary A. Carskadon, Ph.D., professor of psychiatry and human behavior at Brown University in Providence, Rhode Island. "I think napping is undervalued in American society." Timing is important, however. "To avoid insomnia at bedtime, don't nap too late in the day," she adds.

Peter Hauri, Ph.D., director of the insomnia program and co-director of the Mayo Clinic Sleep Disorders Clinic in Rochester, Minnesota, says that he often tells his patients who get the afternoon swoon to put the phone on voice mail, turn the ringer off, and steal a 20- to 30-minute snooze (if, of course, your office culture allows). "They almost always tell me how great they feel and how much more productive they are when they do this," he says.

The later in the day you nap, the more likely you will enter deep sleep, so nap in the early or midafternoon, says sleep researcher Michael Bonnet, Ph.D., professor of neurology at Wright State University School of Medicine in Dayton, Ohio. He also warns that you should limit naps to around 30 minutes. "The longer you sleep, the greater the chance you will enter deep sleep and wake up groggy and worse off than before."

Stress also triggers other physical responses that compound fatigue, including muscle tension.

The first step to minimizing stress, says Dr. Moskowitz, is to develop an awareness of when and how stress affects you. Observe your physical and emotional states. When someone or something upsets you, ask yourself: Do I get tension in my neck? Does my stomach get queasy or tight? Do I feel anxious? Once you have identified the things that

Watch the Meds

Staying energized means paying close attention to everything that goes into your mouth, medications included. Antihistamines, high blood pressure drugs, and cough suppressants can all make you tired. But plenty of other common medicines can also leave you feeling lethargic. Some anti-diarrheals, even over-the-counter (OTC) varieties, contain opiates and other agents that can be sedating. Similarly, some anti-nausea drugs, including those containing meclizine or dimenhydrinate, can cause sleepiness. Some nonsteroidal anti-inflammatory drugs such as ibuprofen and naproxen (Aleve), many of which are now available without a prescription, may be at the root of your lethargy as well. And look out for the load of OTC drugs, like pain relievers, that contain caffeine.

"Many people assume that their fatigue is coming from the headache, arthritis, or whatever and don't realize that it is really coming from the medications," says Mack T. Ruffin IV, M.D., associate professor of family medicine at the University of Michigan Medical Center in Ann Arbor. If you are taking medicine and often find yourself feeling groggy or low on energy, Dr. Ruffin advises talking to your doctor about the side effects of medications and asking for alternatives to drugs that may be sapping your energy.

bring on stress for you, the second step is to figure out how to calm down when a stress-inducing event occurs.

Take the time to learn a few relaxation techniques like meditation or deep breathing. Try them out the next time you are under pressure. If need be, consult a qualified mental-health professional who specializes in stress. Once you find something that helps you relieve excess tension, you are less likely to become tired.

BEAT DESK-JOCKEY SYNDROME. Believe it or not, just

sitting for long periods can actually wear you out. Also, intense mental activity is tiring. If you spend the whole day poring over the sales figures for the last quarter, you use up incredible amounts of energy.

The office solution? Instead of taking a coffee break at work, try an exercise break. No need to work up a major sweat, but it will help if you pep up your heart rate just a bit. "A brisk 10-minute walk will help you feel more energized and less fatigued for 30 to 90 minutes following the walk," says Robert Thayer, Ph.D., professor of psychology at California State University in Long Beach and author of *The Origin of Everyday Moods*. Or just get up from your desk and stretch for a few moments, being sure to work any tightness out of your neck, shoulders, and lower back.

EXERCISE FOR ENERGY. "Even though energy is used during exercise, it also creates more energy," points out William J. Evans, Ph.D., director of the nutrition, metabolism, and exercise program in the Donald W. Reynolds department of geriatrics at the University of Arkansas for Medical Sciences in Little Rock. "The muscles and cardiovascular system are like a car engine. Regular exercise increases the efficiency and the horsepower of the engine." He notes that people who are physically fit have an easier time with daily activities like climbing stairs, carrying things, and walking from the car into the shopping mall. "So the more fit you are, the more energetic you feel at the end of the day."

While health officials used to recommend that all Americans get 20 to 60 minutes of moderate- to high-intensity exercise three to four times per week, they now say that 30 minutes of moderate activity daily is enough to gain major health benefits. You can accumulate those 30 minutes in short bursts of activity that include walking up stairs, walking short distances quickly, gardening, and even dancing, says Dr. Evans.

BREAK OUT OF BOREDOM. Let's say that you get plenty of exercise in short bursts on Saturday when you clean the house. You run laundry up and down the steps or clean the gutters or mop and wax the kitchen floor. Why, then, are you dead-tired by midafternoon?

It may be that you are bored, which saps the energizing benefits from activity. "It is all about exercise that's refreshing versus exercise that isn't," says Gregory Heath, a doctor of health sciences and an epidemiologist and exercise physiologist at the Centers for Disease Control and Prevention.

That's why it is important to find some exercise that's enjoyable or challenging. "Taking regular breaks throughout the week to engage in some exercise or other physically demanding, but interesting, activities should help prevent fatigue," says Dr. Heath.

CLOSE THE SLEEP GAP. Frequently, fatigue has a simple cause—too little sleep. Even being an hour or so short on high-quality slumber can make you fade. "Many Americans force their bodies to run day after day on five to six hours of sleep, when they really need seven to eight," says sleep expert Mary A. Carskadon, Ph.D., professor of psychiatry and human behavior at Brown University in Providence, Rhode Island.

In her research, Dr. Carskadon monitored 66 Brown University students before and after extending their usual sleeping time for an hour or two each night. "They couldn't believe how much more energetic they felt after sleeping just a little more each night," says Dr. Carskadon, who also notes that many other studies have confirmed that adequate sleep improves energy levels. Shoot for a minimum of eight hours to feel your best.

LIGHTEN YOUR LOAD. Are you one of the countless Americans who has no downtime? Do you go from work to home to your volunteer position or children's activities, leaving no time for your pleasures? Then you may be on overload, says Dr. Moskowitz.

Overload is being active without ever attending

to your own human needs. "Absolutely everyone needs true downtime to relax and recover," says Dr. Moskowitz. By downtime, he means that time when you don't have to answer to anyone, when you have no responsibilities. It is that time when you garden, read a mystery novel, go for a walk, or lose yourself in gourmet-food preparation. He argues that to avoid becoming what he calls a human "doing" instead of a human being, you have to prioritize your activities. To avoid overload that leads to fatigue, cut activities that are a low priority and reclaim that time for yourself.

Fuel Up for Fatigue Fighting

Your body's fuel is a blend of water and nutrients, along with bulk—the substantial mass of food that carries them through your body. What you eat and drink today can help ward off tomorrow's fatigue. Here are some basics of fueling up right.

GET WATERED DOWN. Unwatered, your houseplants quickly droop. If your body isn't hydrated properly, it may respond by wilting, too. Many people walk around slightly dehydrated, according to E. Wayne Askew, Ph.D., professor and director of the division of foods and nutrition at the University of Utah in Salt Lake City. "Fatigue is a very likely consequence."

To stay ahead of dehydration, drink the equivalent of at least eight eight-ounce glasses of fluids a day (including water, juice, and soup, but not alcohol and coffee), advises Dr. Askew. That's enough to replace the fluid lost each day via exhaled breaths, body waste, and sweat.

FEED THE MACHINE. Often, even modest calorie restriction can lead to marginal vitamin levels. And if you are short on vitamins, you may feel tired as a result. "Consuming fewer than 1,800 calories per day is a risk factor for low-nutrient intake simply because nutrient intake is tied to calorie intake," says Jo Ann Hattner, R.D., a clinical dietitian at Stanford University Medical Center. She advises dieters who eat fewer than 1,800 calories per day to take a multivitamin/mineral supplement.

WATCH WHAT YOU EAT. Certain nutrients are superstars when it comes to building energy. B-complex vitamins are the ones that doctors recommend most when you are running low on stamina. To make the most of these energy boosters in your diet, make sure that you get plenty of servings of whole grains each day and get plenty of fruits and vegetables. Apples and bananas with whole-grain crackers, for example, are great afternoon pick-me-up snacks.

CUT THE CAFFEINE. As you know, coffee has eye-opening power—it's the caffeine in your cup. But scientists have discovered that coffee can also leave you dragging. Here's how. Caffeine actually locks onto receptors in the brain that usually mediate the effects of adenosine, a chemical that is meant to keep us calm and clearheaded. By blocking the natural adenosine action, caffeine allows the brain to function more quickly in the short term, but with more negative effects in the long term.

Even when you kick coffee, it kicks back. "Fatigue may be the first sign of caffeine withdrawal," says caffeine researcher Roland R. Griffiths, Ph.D., professor in the departments of psychiatry and neuroscience at the Johns Hopkins University School of Medicine in Baltimore. "Someone experiencing unexplained fatigue should take a hard look at his caffeine intake."

Take it slow, however, when you cut back to avoid withdrawal symptoms like nervousness and headache. The typical American who consumes about $2^1/2$ cups of coffee per day should gradually cut out coffee over a one- to two-week period to avoid withdrawal symptoms.

BANISH THE BOOZE. Alcohol is one of the quickest routes to a snooze that you can find. First of all, it is a sedative. And, to make matters worse, it forces your body to give B vitamins the boot. So skip the wine with dinner unless you want to take a nap before dessert, suggests Dr. Moskowitz.

FLATULENCE
Minimize Bloating and Rumbling

Each of us—man, woman, and child—emits our daily share of vapors like methane, hydrogen, carbon dioxide, and the most "aromatic," sulfur dioxide. Wondering if you are normal? The average is 14 episodes of flatus a day. But, aside from the risk of embarrassment, is intestinal gas really a problem?

"In Europe, if you would ask the question 'Is flatulence a problem?' they would look at you funny and say, 'No, it's a normal part of life. It's healthy,'" says Dennis Savaiano, Ph.D., professor of nutrition and dean of the school of consumer and family sciences at Purdue University in West Lafayette, Indiana. "And they would be right. A healthy colon produces gas."

The colon, or large intestine, is the final stretch of digestive tract before the anal canal. It is also "home smelly home" for more than 400 varieties of helpful bacteria. And they are not waiting for you to bring home the bacon; they are waiting for you to bring home the bread, the bananas, and the beans. Those bacteria live on a steady diet of the complex sugars known as carbohydrates, some of which are not digested until they reach the colon. When the bacteria feed, the sugars ferment. They give off sulfur dioxide and other gases. It is simple biology.

The problem, of course, is when there is so much gas that you feel uncomfortable—when your insides rumble like a bowling alley, and you feel as bloated as a balloon. Or maybe you feel fine, but you are way above the norm of 14 flatus emissions a day and wish that your colon was a bit more restrained. Or perhaps gas isn't a problem for you, and you definitely want to keep it that way.

Well, to outsmart gas, you just have to use the old bean—before you eat any.

Make Peace with Beans

The reason that beans have such a reputation for producing excess gas is that they contain the carbohydrate raffinose. Oddly enough, sometimes the body doesn't have enough enzymes in the small intestines to digest this carbohydrate. So it reaches the colon, and that's where, in some people, the musical fruit cranks up the volume. Other gas-producing foods like cabbage, brussels sprouts, broccoli, asparagus, and whole grains also contain raffinose but in smaller amounts.

Beans aren't all bad, however. They are packed with cholesterol-lowering fiber and bone-protecting calcium and can help protect you against heart disease, brittle bones, and even colon cancer. And they are a plentiful source of low-fat protein, making them a valuable part of a healthy diet. Here's how doctors suggest that you can make beans behave.

FIND A BEAN THAT SUITS YOU. All beans are not created equal, says Eugene Oliveri, D.O., professor of medicine at Michigan State University College of Osteopathic

Medicine in East Lansing and a gastroenterologist in Milford. The worst culprits are usually pinto beans, black beans, and great Northern beans. But a gas producer for you may be a gas reducer for somebody else. "I think that people's reactions to beans is an individual matter. Some people will produce a lot of gas with one bean and much less with others." He says to try different varieties to find the most benign bean for you.

CHANGE THE WATER. Except for lentils and split peas, dry beans need to be soaked overnight before they are cooked. But don't cook them in the same water in which they have soaked. Instead, pour off the water, give the beans a final rinse, and then cook them in fresh water. "This should help reduce any flatulence caused by the beans," says Dr. Oliveri.

GET OUT THE PRESSURE COOKER. Beans that are undercooked can also cause more flatulence, says Dr. Oliveri. Cook them thoroughly to help reduce their explosive effects. "I recommend pressure-cooking," he says. "It's fast. Otherwise, you would have to boil them for four hours or so. Pressure-cooking guarantees that beans are completely cooked." For best results, pressure-cook the beans for 30 minutes at 15 pounds per square inch.

RUN 'EM UNDER THE FAUCET. Canned beans are a great convenience. Before cooking canned beans, drain off the liquid and rinse the beans in water to remove the gas-causing carbohydrates that leached out of the beans' skin. "This reduces flatulence—no two ways about it," says Dr. Oliveri.

SPRINKLE ON SOME BEANO. If beans in any form are a problem for you, there is hope: Scientists have discovered a way to grow an enzyme that can digest raffinose, one of the troublesome complex carbohydrates in beans. The product, called Beano, is available as a liquid that you sprinkle on your beans before you eat them or as a tablet that you take before a meal. Just follow the dosage directions on the label.

"Using Beano makes a dramatic difference in reducing the discomfort in people who have had difficulty eating beans," says Dr. Oliveri. "Use it once, and you may have no gas at all after that particular meal." He also says that you could also try Beano if you have excessive discomfort from other gas-forming foods.

Help for the Dairy-Phobic

If milk gives you gas, relax—you are normal. We are all born with fair amounts of lactase, an intestinal enzyme that enables us to digest lactose, or milk sugar.

Approximately 75 percent of the world's population loses lactase between the ages of three and five. As for the other 25 percent, the theory is that thousands of years ago their ancestors lived where dairy foods had become a regular part of the diet—northern Europe, central Africa, the Middle East—and they developed a helpful genetic mutation that allowed them to keep the enzyme and digest milk.

For these few fortunate digesters, drinking and eating dairy foods is no problem, says Dr. Savaiano, one of the world's leading experts on lactose intolerance. For the rest of us "maldigesters," dairy foods can produce a lot of extra gas (and sometimes even diarrhea). But lactose intolerance is not a disease.

In fact, Dr. Savaiano's research has convinced him that lactose intolerance is easy to prevent, no matter how much of a problem you think you have. That is very good news for the typical American woman, many of whom don't get their Daily Value for osteoporosis-preventing calcium, a mineral that is readily available in dairy products.

DRINK MILK WITH A MEAL. "People have three times more symptoms of lactose intolerance if they drink a glass of milk alone than if they drink it with a meal," says Dr. Savaiano. One suggestion is to pour milk over your morning cereal. And make it skim. Whole milk generates less gas, but it is high in fat, so he doesn't recommend it.

TRAIN YOUR BODY TO DIGEST DAIRY. The intestinal bacteria in the colon that produce gas are incredibly adaptable, says Dr. Savaiano. "When we gradually feed people increasing amounts of milk, their colon bacteria change so that they more easily handle milk sugar. When people adapt to dairy in this way, they have very little gas when we give them lactose."

To study this adaptation process, Dr. Savaiano first "challenged" people who had trouble digesting lactose with high levels of the milk sugar, then measured their gas production. Not surprisingly, they produced excessive gas. Then he gave them the equivalent of one cup of milk three times a day with each meal. Over a period of 10 days, he gradually increased that amount to the equivalent of two cups of milk at each meal. After 10 days, he again challenged them with high levels of lactose. "They generated no extra gas," he says. "They produced the same amount of gas as they would have had they been living on a lactose-free diet. Essentially, we turned them into digesters."

Try the same experiment on yourself, suggests Dr. Savaiano. Once you have adapted, he says, you can dine freely on low-fat dairy products.

YOGURT: GO FOR IT. "The bacteria in yogurt naturally contain a very high level of the enzyme lactase (which digests lactose), so yogurt is very well tolerated by people who have trouble digesting lactose," says Dr. Savaiano. In fact, he has given people in studies up to 16 ounces of yogurt at a time—a whopping two cups—with no symptoms of excess flatulence. He says that any commercial brand with the words "live cultures" on its label or in its ingredient list will do the trick. Frozen yogurts don't qualify, however. "They are more like ice milk. Most have very little yogurt in them," he says.

USE ENZYME SUPPLEMENTS. If you can't digest lactose,

lactase supplements can also help. "Stirred into milk or taken before you eat dairy, enzyme supplements work to reduce flatulence," says Dr. Savaiano. You can find the supplements in most health food stores. Instructions are on the label.

LOOK FOR LACTASE-TREATED DAIRY PRODUCTS. For convenience, look for milk, cottage cheese, and other dairy products that have been pretreated with lactase. Most supermarkets sell at least one brand of lactase-treated products. Look for "lactase enzyme" in the ingredients.

CHOOSE "SAFER" DAIRY. Hard cheeses contain very small amounts of lactose. Chocolate milk is kind to those with lactose intolerance because the cocoa and sugars slow down the rate of digestion, allowing the small intestine more time to break down the lactase. You may also find that you can tolerate ice cream pretty well—the high levels of fat and sugar slow down digestion. But if you are watching your intake of fat and calories, you will want to keep portions small, cautions Dr. Savaiano.

More Fiber with Less Gas

If raffinose and lactose were the only carbohydrates that produce gas, preventing excess flatulence would be fairly simple. But all high-fiber foods are packed with potentially gas-producing carbohydrates. Given the benefits of a high-fiber diet—to prevent constipation, certain forms of cancer, and a number of other conditions—you don't want to avoid fiber. You want to eat more of it, 25 to 35 grams a day, according to experts. To get that much fiber, start the day with some bran cereal, eat up to five servings of fruits and vegetables a day, and maybe even take a fiber supplement, all of which can challenge your digestive system if you are not used to the fiber.

Here's how to put more health-giving fiber in your diet without violating the Clean Air Act.

STEP UP TO THE VEGETABLE PLATE—SLOWLY. "I tell anyone who is thinking of increasing the fiber content of their diet to go very slowly," says Dr. Oliveri. To increase your fiber, he suggests adding one additional serving of a fruit or vegetable to your diet per week, until you have reached your daily minimum of five servings per day.

GO EASY WITH BRAN. If you are thinking of adding extra fiber to your diet with bran, you will want to do it gradually, says Harris R. Clearfield, M.D., professor of medicine and section chief of the division of gastroenterology at the Allegheny University of the Health Sciences, Hahnemann Division, in Philadelphia. "People who are going to eat bran cereals should start with small amounts until their bowels adjust to it." He suggests adding two to three tablespoons of All-Bran or 100% Bran cereals to your regular cereal every day for a week. Then add another tablespoon or two for the next week. "Keep increasing the amount of bran cereal and decreasing the amount of regular cereal until you are eating nothing but bran cereal," he advises.

SCALE YOUR SUPPLEMENT INTAKE. Dr. Oliveri recommends a similar strategy if you want to get extra fiber from a fiber supplement like Metamucil or Citrucel. "Start off with one tablespoonful a day for the first week, then add one tablespoonful a week until you reach the dosage recommended on the label."

CHARCOAL TO THE RESCUE. People who have had no success with other methods of preventing gas may want to try charcoal capsules (such as CharcoCaps), available at health food stores. Taking two after each meal may provide some benefit by absorbing intestinal gas, says Dr. Clearfield. They are safe, he says, but will turn the stools dark or black.

FLU
An Annual Episode You Can Skip

Who would spend a week each year in bed with the flu if they didn't have to?

No one has to get the flu, but plenty of people do. Between 25 million and 50 million Americans get the flu each year. Worse, 500,000 are hospitalized and 20,000 die.

"Those numbers drive me nuts because flu is preventable," says Steven R. Mostow, M.D., professor of medicine at the University of Colorado, chairman of the American Thoracic Society's committee on the prevention of pneumonia and influenza, and chairman of medicine at the Rose Medical Center in Denver.

Commonsense measures like washing your hands frequently, especially during flu season, and trying to steer clear of people with obvious flu symptoms can minimize your exposure. But those measures are a little like gambling—you might avoid the flu, and you might not. If you get a shot of the flu vaccine, however, "your chances of getting and transmitting the flu virus are almost nil," says Dr. Mostow,

Can I Get Sick from the Flu Shot?

Some people experience side effects from a flu shot, but this is relatively uncommon, says Steven R. Mostow, M.D., professor of medicine at the University of Colorado, chairman of the American Thoracic Society's committee on the prevention of pneumonia and influenza, and chairman of medicine at the Rose Medical Center in Denver. "The chance of having a fever or feeling sick the next day is 1 percent or less," he says, which means that 99 out of 100 people won't get sick after the shot. About 20 percent of those who get the shot, however, will have "a very mild sore arm the next day, which will last for one to two days."

calling himself a zealot for the flu vaccine. Nearly all adults and most children should get the vaccine, he says. It is particularly important if you have a higher-than-normal risk of getting the flu—that is, you are over 65 or (at any age) you have heart disease, lung disease, kidney disease, or insulin-dependent diabetes. And anyone living with someone at high risk should also get the vaccine, he says.

Getting a flu shot is easy and inexpensive. You can get vaccinated at your doctor's office, at a public medical clinic, or even at supermarkets, drugstores, or other stores during special promotions. If you are under 65, expect to pay $8 to $10, says Dr. Mostow. For those 65 or older, the flu vaccine is paid for by Medicare. Either the physician charges you and you get reimbursed, or the shot is free and the physician is reimbursed.

Never Get the Flu Again—Ever

To make sure that you are not risking your health or even your life the next time flu season rolls around, just follow Dr. Mostow's flu-foiling advice.

GET A SHOT EVERY YEAR. The flu vaccine is different every year. That is because flu viruses are constantly mutating, or changing, as they travel around the world infecting different populations. To battle the current year's version of the flu, experts at the World Health Organization, the Centers for Disease Control and Prevention, and the Food and Drug Administration collect and analyze those mutations in laboratories in dozens of countries. They choose the three most likely viral suspects for the current year's vaccine and, almost invariably, their selection is accurate. Upon injection, your body reacts to their presence by creating specialized immune substances called antibodies. These antibodies will attack the live virus or viruses should they ever pay you a visit.

GET A SHOT IN OCTOBER. Doctors recommend that you get the flu shot anytime from October 1 to November 15. If that seems earlier than necessary, it is because experts think that the flu is arriving earlier in the United States. Increased jet travel may be the cause of earlier arrival, says Dr. Mostow.

If you miss getting the flu shot in October, get it later. The vaccine can protect you even during the middle of a flu outbreak, says Dr. Mostow. Here is the scenario: "Say you live in Madison, Wisconsin, and there is no flu in Madison, and it's Thanksgiving. You feel healthy, everybody else feels healthy, so you think it was okay that you didn't get a flu shot. Then around December 15, lots of people have started to get the flu, but you are not infected yet. The problem is that even if you get the shot today, it takes two weeks for the vaccine to provide full immunity." But, he says, it is still not too late to get the vaccine. "Your doctor should give you a flu shot and put you on a prescription medication called rimantadine hydrochloride (Flumadine), which is a drug you take once a day for two weeks until the immunity from the vaccination kicks in. If a person is religious about taking this medication, they cannot be infected. So that is the prevention strategy during an outbreak."

GET A SHOT IF YOU ARE FLYING OUT OF THE COUNTRY. There are a couple of reasons why this is a good idea, says Dr. Mostow. First, when it is summer in the United States, it is winter—and flu season—in the Southern Hemisphere. Second, if you are traveling to a developing country, medical care might not be up to par, so being hospitalized with a bad case of the flu is the last thing that you want. Third, air travel itself puts you at high risk for a rendezvous with a flu virus because lots of people are in close proximity on a plane, and the cabin's air is being continually recirculated. "If you are leaving the country by airplane, get a flu shot," he says.

DON'T GET A SHOT IF YOU ARE ALLERGIC TO EGGS. The viruses for the vaccine are grown in a chicken's egg, so anybody who is allergic to eggs will also be allergic to the flu vaccine and shouldn't take it.

DON'T GET A FLU SHOT FOR CHILDREN UNDER SIX MONTHS OF AGE. There is no scientific data showing whether the flu shot is safe or effective for this age group, says Dr. Mostow.

FOOD ALLERGIES
Discover the Culprits, Prevent the Symptoms

Think you have a food allergy? If so, you have lots of company. More than one-fourth of all adult Americans are convinced that some of the foods they bite into wind up biting them back with recurrent symptoms such as hives, skin rashes, diarrhea, and vomiting—the most common telltale signs. So they make drastic changes in their diets. Aside from the inconvenience of avoiding foods that everyone else seems to enjoy with impunity, staying away from an otherwise nourishing food, like milk or wheat, can deprive you of key vitamins or minerals.

If you have a bona fide food allergy, you must learn how to avoid the culprit, says Hugh Sampson, M.D., professor of pediatrics; chief of the pediatric, allergy, and immunology department; and director of the Jaffe Institute for Food Allergy at the Mount Sinai Medical Center in New York City. Detective work, not guesswork, is the key to sorting it out and staying well.

Allergic to Latex? Think "Bananas"

Not surprisingly, if you are allergic to one food, you may also be allergic to related foods. And sometimes, you are allergic to a *nonfood* relative.

How do two related substances cross-react? "Most likely, they share common allergens or allergens that closely resemble each other," says Dean D. Metcalfe, M.D., chief of the Laboratory of Allergic Diseases at the National Institute of Allergy and Infectious Diseases (a division of the National Institutes of Health). A good example is cantaloupe (a food) and ragweed (a nonfood). "People who have a cantaloupe allergy sometimes report that they only have trouble with it during ragweed season," he says. This is because the ragweed has already caused their allergic immune system to respond. So eating the cantaloupe makes matters worse.

So, if you know that you are allergic to certain foods or plants, you need to get acquainted with their relatives to avoid trouble. Common allergens are listed here with related foods or nonfoods that could trigger reactions.

Bananas: Latex (used in gloves)
Birch pollen: Carrots, apples, filberts (hazelnuts), potatoes
Celery: Mugwort (an herb)
Ragweed: Watermelon, cantaloupe, honeydew, bananas, chamomile tea, sunflower seeds

Allergy or Intolerance?

"True food allergies are quite rare, probably affecting less than 2 percent of the adult population," says Dr. Sampson.

"Some individuals who think that they have a food allergy actually have a food intolerance," says Wesley A.

Are You Allergic to Food?

If you experience bloating, cramping, gas, or diarrhea after eating, you may or may not have a food allergy. Answering the following questions provided by Dean D. Metcalfe, M.D., chief of the Laboratory of Allergic Diseases at the National Institute of Allergy and Infectious Diseases (a division of the National Institutes of Health), can help you determine if you have a food allergy and not merely a food intolerance or another problem.

If you got sick or felt unusual after a meal, was anyone else sick at the same time? If others who ate the same meal also felt sick, it is possible that you ate a contaminated food rather than an allergen.

Does your mouth itch after eating a suspect food? This is often the first symptom of an allergic reaction because the lips, tongue, palate, and throat are the first to come in contact with a food. When these areas react, this group of symptoms is sometimes called the oral allergy syndrome. Oral allergy syndrome is far more common in people with allergies, and the syndrome has been linked to specific foods, including watermelon, cantaloupe, honeydew, and bananas. So if you experience oral allergy syndrome in reaction to these or any other foods, it is likely that you are allergic.

Burks, M.D., an allergist-immunologist and professor of pediatrics at the University of Arkansas for Medical Sciences in Little Rock. Food intolerances—lactose intolerance is the most well-known example—can be quite nasty in their own right. "Food intolerances produce some of the same uncomfortable symptoms that food allergies create, including bloating, cramping, gas, and diarrhea," he says.

Of course, whether it is an allergy or an intolerance, you will want to prevent the host of symptoms that are ini-

Do you break out in a rash after eating certain foods? Hives or skin rashes are among the most common allergic reactions to food. Skin reactions, however, have a wide variety of causes beyond food allergies. And while food allergies frequently cause acute hives, they are rarely responsible for chronic hives.

Do you have difficulty breathing after eating certain foods? A food allergen can affect breathing by causing your windpipe to swell, and it can also affect the lungs. People with asthma are at special risk. There can be, however, multiple triggers for an asthmatic attack besides foods.

Does your discomfort begin within 45 minutes of eating? Most allergic reactions occur within 45 minutes. And some reactions may be immediate. If your reaction is delayed by hours, you are probably dealing with a food intolerance, not an allergy. The method of preventing symptoms is the same in either case: Avoid the food.

Do you have other, nonfood allergies? Food allergies are more common in people who have other kinds of allergies. If you are allergic to cats or ragweed, for example, you are at higher risk for developing a food allergy. Food allergies can also worsen asthma and skin conditions like eczema.

tiated by the particular food or food group. Initially, this hunt for a prevention regimen may turn you into a world-class detective. Once you know the culprit, prevention may not be easy, but at least you will know what you need to avoid.

In any case, knowing once and for all whether you have a food allergy is the first step toward prevention. This is especially important for those who actually do have a food allergy but suffer in silence, thinking that their symptoms are just a normal part of life.

An allergy is the body's abnormal reaction to a harmless substance. In fact, even the healthiest foods may trigger a reaction in susceptible people. Ironically, it is your body's immune system—designed to protect you from naughty invaders—that accounts for the symptoms. Histamine and other chemicals released from specialized cells, called mast cells, cause a wide range of allergic symptoms.

Although you might think that food allergies are a lifelong affliction, the symptoms of these allergies can appear for the first time in adulthood. "Why allergies strike when they do remains a mystery," says Dr. Burks.

Figuring out whether you actually have such an allergy and tracking down the culprit food is not easy. Just consider the sheer number of foods and ingredients you ingest at every meal. Even a simple breakfast menu can leave you asking, "Was it the cereal? The milk? Or the sliced banana on top?"

If all this sounds daunting, rest assured, there is a way to get answers and to prevent the symptoms. The first step is to do some detective work. Maybe you have always believed that you had a food allergy but never knew for sure. Or you have had symptoms such as the characteristic hives or rashes that very well could be food related, but you always blamed the symptoms on something else. It is likely that you will still need to consult your doctor. But if you follow the guidelines here, you will discover a lot of the information that you and your doctor need to arrive at a conclusive diagnosis.

Keep a Diet Diary

If you think you have a food allergy, consider keeping a diet diary for one to two weeks, says Dr. Sampson. That is, write down everything you eat, the time you eat it, the amount, and any symptoms that occur throughout the day. Then

---

The Food Allergy Network

Living with food allergies can make life complicated. The Food Allergy Network (FAN) is an organization that helps people with food allergies and their families cope so that they can lead normal, healthy lives.

FAN helps people find their way through the maze of ingredients found in supermarket aisles and overcome the difficulties inherent in ordering restaurant food. It keeps members up-to-date on changes in label laws and new food products and ingredients. And it publishes handy, wallet-size cards listing ingredients to watch out for if you are allergic to a certain kind of food. If you are trying to prevent food-allergy symptoms and you have done your detective work, these cards can be your ticket to relief.

To get a copy of FAN's booklet *Understanding Food Labels*, send $5 to Food Allergy Network, 10400 Eaton Place, Suite 107, Fairfax, VA 22030. For free information and a sample newsletter, send a self-addressed, stamped business envelope.

---

take the diary with you when you see your doctor. By examining your diet diary, you and your doctor may be able to spot unforeseen relationships between symptoms and the foods you have eaten.

Here is how to get the most useful clues from your diet diary, according to experts.

CARRY IT WITH YOU. Have it with you at all times. Don't wait until the end of the day to fill it in.

WRITE DOWN EVERYTHING. Yes, everything. That includes beverages, medicines, and even chewing gum. And be very specific. For example, don't write down "ham sandwich," instead list all the fixings: "smoked ham, white bread, brown mustard . . ."

SPECIFY SYMPTOMS. Indicate the symptoms, when they began, and how long they lasted.

ATTACH LABELS. Whenever possible, attach ingredient labels to your diet diary as a handy quick reference for your doctor. Labels are extremely helpful when considering food allergies.

TALLY THE AMOUNT. If you don't react to a food every time, that doesn't always mean that the food is innocent. Sometimes, it depends on how much of the food you ate.

"If you eat a little, you may not react. If you eat a lot, you may react," says Dean D. Metcalfe, M.D., chief of the Laboratory of Allergic Diseases at the National Institute of Allergy and Infectious Diseases (a division of the National Institutes of Health).

"Say that you ate lobster tail once and reacted, then ate some lobster salad and didn't react. That doesn't mean you are not allergic. The key may be in the amount consumed."

ACCOUNT FOR ALCOHOL. Drinking alcohol increases the absorption of food allergens. So if you take a drink, you are more susceptible to an allergic reaction. That means that you may react to some food only after you have had an alcoholic drink along with it.

RECORD EXERCISE, TOO. In susceptible people, exercise can cause an allergic reaction to a food just eaten.

90 Percent of the Problem

The following foods account for 90 percent of all food allergies, says Dr. Sampson. So if your diet diary indicates that you have consistently reacted to any of these foods, the odds are good that you have a true food allergy.

DON'T SHELL OUT FOR PEANUTS. As a legume, the peanut can be a healthy addition to most diets. But it is among the most allergenic of all foods. In people with se-

---

Allergic Emergencies: Be Prepared

Anyone who has ever experienced an allergic reaction to a food should carry a kit to self-administer epinephrine, a form of adrenaline. Check with your doctor to find out whether you might need one of these. Epinephrine kits must be prescribed by a physician.

"Allergies are potentially fatal when they cause an anaphylactic reaction," says Dean D. Metcalfe, M.D., chief of the Laboratory of Allergic Diseases at the National Institute of Allergy and Infectious Diseases (a division of the National Institutes of Health). Characterized by severe itching, hives, sweating, swelling of the throat, difficulty breathing, and a sudden and severe drop in blood pressure, anaphylaxis can lead to loss of consciousness. If not treated immediately, anaphylactic shock can be fatal. People with asthma appear to be at special risk.

Also, some people will have an anaphylactic reaction only after exercising. But prevention is simple: Before exercising, just don't eat any food that you suspect is causing you a problem, says Hugh Sampson, M.D., professor of pediatrics; chief of the pediatric, allergy, and immunology department; and director of the Jaffe Institute for Food Allergy at the Mount Sinai Medical Center in New York City.

---

vere allergies, just a fraction of a peanut kernel can be enough to set off a reaction.

LEAVE TREE NUTS ALONE. Walnuts and other tree nuts—Brazil nuts, almonds, cashews, pistachios, filberts (hazelnuts), pecans, hickory nuts, pine nuts—are among the most allergenic foods. If you are allergic to one true nut variety, there is a chance that you are allergic to others, but not necessarily to peanuts, which are legumes.

BE A CRAB ABOUT SHELLFISH. Although shrimp gets much attention as an allergen, a broad class of shellfish can cause an allergic reaction. This class includes other crustacea (lobsters, crabs, and prawns) and mollusks (snails, mussels, oysters, scallops, clams, squid, and octopus).

THROW BACK THE FINFISH. Compared with other major food allergens, the proteins in fish are more vulnerable to heat and other forms of preparation. So some people allergic to fresh cooked fish can eat the canned version without difficulty. You might be able to eat canned tuna, for instance, but have a problem with fresh grilled tuna—but don't count on it. In people with extremely severe fish allergies, even inhaling the vapors from cooking fish can set off a reaction.

Reactions to toxins in fish are sometimes mistaken for fish allergies. Scromboid poisoning from fish occurs when fish are contaminated with high levels of histamine, the primary irritant in classic allergic reactions. If you get an immediate reaction, try to save a portion of the fish serving so it can be tested for this histamine.

BYPASS MILK. Most adverse reactions to milk are not allergies but rather lactose intolerance. That is, insufficient amounts of the digestive enzyme lactase lead to cramping, bloating, and other abdominal symptoms. Most individuals with lactose intolerance can generally manage small amounts of milk. In people with a true milk allergy, any consumption of milk or milk-related proteins can be dangerous, says Dr. Sampson. Knowing the difference is critical.

REVIEW TOFU. Tofu is made from soy, a major allergen in children. Some adults react, too.

DON'T EAT WHEAT. If you notice that wheat products cause symptoms, it is quite possible that you are allergic to that grain. But be sure to see a doctor, too, says Dr. Sampson. Some people have celiac disease, a rare condition resulting from an intolerance to gluten, which is present not only in wheat but also in rye, barley, and oats.

Avoiding a Run-In with Your Allergen

Once you have completed your diet diary and perhaps isolated a food or foods that you think may be causing your allergic symptoms, you can start preventing the uncomfortable symptoms just by avoiding that food, says Dr. Sampson. Improvement in symptoms, however, doesn't always mean that you are allergic. But you may need the help of an allergist to do the definitive test for a food allergy. The doctor might outline a diet in which you cut out highly suspect allergens for a few weeks. He may be able to help you determine your allergies with the help of a skin-prick test. Or the allergist might run a specific kind of blood test, called a Radioallergosorbent (RAST) test, that determines the allergens that are in your system.

According to experts, here are the best ways to avoid a run-in with your allergen.

AVOID IT FOR LIFE. In a few cases of adult food allergies, reactions to the allergen disappear within one to two years following complete avoidance. The development of tolerance depends on the food, however. Major allergens, especially peanuts, are likely to be lifelong enemies. So before attempting to reintroduce any food that you have had an allergic reaction to in the past, it is best to check with your allergist beforehand, says Robert Plancey, M.D., assistant clinical professor of medicine at the University of Southern California in Los Angeles and an internist and allergist in Arcadia. Ultimately your best prevention will always be avoidance.

"In adults, it is simply not reliable to stop eating a food and hope that your allergy will not come back," says Dr. Metcalfe. "I think once you are allergic to a food, it is safest to assume that you are allergic to that food for the rest of your life."

BE LABEL-SAVVY. The toughest part of living with a food allergy is knowing what to look out for. For example, nondairy products routinely contain casein, a protein derived from milk. And sometimes the same food can be disguised under different names. For example, *lactalbumin* is another name for milk protein. Even when you think that you know what's in a product, the ingredients change. "So you must always check, even when you think you know," says Anne Munoz-Furlong, founder and president of the Food Allergy Network in Fairfax, Virginia.

QUESTION THE MANAGER. Cafeterias and restaurants can be precarious. Since there are no labels to read, you have to count on the reliability of the chef to let you know the full ingredients in any menu selection. Munoz-Furlong has this advice: "Speak with the restaurant manager rather than relying on your waiter or waitress. And don't ever be afraid to ask questions." Among the best: What other foods have been prepared on the same grill? If an allergy-causing food has been cooked earlier, small amounts of cross-contamination could infiltrate your meal.

"I tell people to go to smaller restaurants that are more responsive to their individual needs," says Dr. Plancey. "Explain to the owners or the chef what your sensitivities are, get a meal you can eat, and go back to that restaurant again."

FOOD POISONING
Do's and Don'ts for Wholesome Eats

We've all done it: Opened a container of leftovers or a half-used jar of spaghetti sauce, long forgotten in the back of the fridge, and reeled at the sight and smell of fuzzy mold. Food that is obviously spoiled gets pitched. But what about stuff that looks and smells okay, but has been around awhile? Do you play it safe and pitch it? Or throw it into the microwave and take your chances?

"We can't rely on our eyes, nose, or tastebuds to tell us whether or not a food is safe," says Don Schaffner, Ph.D., an extension specialist in food science at Rutgers University Cooperative Extension in New Brunswick, New Jersey.

Disease-causing microorganisms that creep into food sure can make you sick, sometimes for as long as several weeks. For the very young, the very old, the pregnant, and people with illnesses like cancer and AIDS, food poisoning can be even more serious. In fact, people can even die from a severe case of food poisoning. So it pays to have a little extra information on your side. The trick is knowing which food to get rid of before it can hurt you, says Dr. Schaffner. With the right prevention tactics, you never need to second-guess your toss-or-keep policies.

Six Golden Rules

To steer clear of food poisoning, start by following six simple, germ-savvy rules, says Dr. Schaffner.

1. Keep cold foods cold (34° to 40°F, 1° to 4°C).
2. Keep hot foods hot (140° to 165°F, 60° to 74°C).
3. Keep food storage and preparation areas clean (that includes shelves and counters as well as your refrigerator).
4. Before starting food preparation, wash your hands with hot soapy water for at least 20 seconds.
5. Refrigerate leftovers quickly.
6. When in doubt, throw it out.

Sounds easy enough. But there are always murky areas, such as food that is kept too long or raw foods that carry troublesome bacteria. Follow the tips outlined here, and you will prevent food-borne disease from sneaking into your kitchen.

Stanch the Spread of Salmonella

The sneaky salmonella bacteria are probably the most common cause of food poisoning. Infected food usually tastes fine, but you won't feel fine. Within 12 to 20 hours after eating, you may develop nausea, abdominal pain, diarrhea, headache, and sometimes fever.

While salmonella rarely lasts more than three days,

these symptoms can last two weeks or longer. The main hosts of salmonella are raw eggs, poultry, fish, and other meat. Lettuce and other produce can also be contaminated. Here is how to prevent salmonella poisoning, according to Manfred Kroger, Ph.D., professor of food science at Pennsylvania State University in University Park.

DON'T EAT RAW EGGS. Be wary of uncooked foods that contain eggs, like eggnog or steak tartare. Don't buy cracked eggs, and if you crack one at home, cook it within a few hours or give it an immediate burial. And always keep eggs refrigerated in the carton, preferably on a shelf, not the door, which can be 1° to 2°F warmer.

STAY COOL. When shopping, put refrigerated items like meat, chicken, and dairy products in your cart last, and pack them in an iced cooler if you are not heading straight home. Use poultry and ground meat within two days of purchase or freeze it.

DON'T THAW AT ROOM TEMPERATURE. Thaw foods only in the refrigerator, microwave, or in cold water. Marinate only in the refrigerator—and never reuse the marinade.

USE A FOOD THERMOMETER. Don't guess if your goose is cooked. Cook meats until the center reaches 165°F (74°C). The only way to tell is with a thermometer that goes all the way into the center of the bird or roast.

WASH FRESH PRODUCE THOROUGHLY. Cool to warm plain running water and a vegetable brush are all you need to wash produce. Throw away the outer leaves on produce like lettuce, cabbage, and brussels sprouts.

X Out *E. Coli*

Some strains of the bacterium *Escherichia coli* can cause a life-threatening inflammation of the colon. While the potentially deadly strain of *E. coli* is sometimes found in raw or undercooked ground meat, it can also be carried in

Play It Safe with Take-Home Chow

No longer called doggie bags, take-home containers are a routine part of many restaurant meals. With dinner portions approaching gargantuan scale, it makes sense. Why waste half your Nantucket Seafood Grill when you can enjoy it again tomorrow? Still, food is food, and some cautions are in order. To help you avoid a potential case of food poisoning, here are helpful steps as provided by Don Schaffner, Ph.D., an extension specialist in food science at Rutgers University Cooperative Extension in New Brunswick, New Jersey.

EAT TAKE-HOME FOOD WITHIN 48 HOURS. Remember that the food already has an extra load of bacteria from your fork, and it sat unchilled while you chatted. Refrigerate it within two hours of the food being served, within one hour during the summer, then reheat it to 165°F (74°C) or higher within two days. And if you left your chicken cacciatore in the car for more than an hour, sorry. Even doggie should bag it.

EAT OR CHILL TAKEOUT WITHIN ONE HOUR. Your chow mein may have waited on a counter for 25 minutes and then spent another 20 riding home in your car. Put it in your fridge, microwave, or tummy within one hour of leaving the restaurant.

produce and unpasteurized apple juice. If you are a victim, within eight hours you will likely be doubled over with diarrhea, abdominal pain, nausea, vomiting, and sometimes fever. The misery lingers for a week. This infection can be deadly, especially for young children. Here is how to avoid it, says Dr. Schaffner.

COOK MEAT THOROUGHLY. Never eat burgers with pink centers and make sure that all your cooked, ground-meat juices run clear. Although whole cuts of meat are

Pitch Those Moldy Oldies

All sorts of fungi just love to grow into many-celled, filamentous colonies, especially on bread and in spaghetti-sauce jars. Some molds just destroy taste, but others make people extremely sick. If you are lucky, you'll vomit quickly. If not, this toxin might linger in your system, potentially leading to liver disease or worse.

Mold usually forms on dairy products, bread, and acidic foods like tomato sauce or jelly that are stored in moist, dark areas in airtight containers, according to Manfred Kroger, Ph.D., professor of food science at Pennsylvania State University in University Park.

If food is covered with mold or it is moldy throughout, toss it, advises Dr. Kroger. Small spots of mold on hard cheese and firm fruits and vegetables, however, can be cut away, he says. To be safe, remove a half-inch margin of nonmoldy area around and below the spot. You can also scoop out tiny spots of mold from jelly and jam. First remove the mold itself, then, with a clean spoon, the half-inch area around it. Though experts don't all agree, most advise discarding other foods with mold, including bread and cottage cheese.

not as dangerous as ground meat, prime rib that runs red (or other cuts ordered rare) can spell trouble and should be avoided.

WASH FRESH PRODUCE THOROUGHLY. The same procedure you use to prevent salmonella poisoning will also banish *E. coli*. Plain running cool or warm tap water and a vegetable brush are all you need. If you are washing a vegetable that tends to wilt, use cool water instead of warm and remember to discard the outer leaves of the lettuce and greens that you wash.

Beat Back Botulism

Though it happens rarely, a toxin made by spores of *Clostridium botulinum* can cause botulism. This is an often-fatal illness, even if treated. These spores are found in improperly canned or preserved foods. Commercially canned foods have an excellent safety record. Home canning and preserving can be riskier when approved methods aren't followed. If you eat tainted food, within 12 to 36 hours you could experience fatigue, double vision, nausea, vomiting, or difficulty speaking. Respiratory and muscular paralysis soon follow. Obviously, this is very serious stuff. According to experts, here is how to avoid trouble.

EXAMINE CANS AND JARS. Never, ever use cans of food that are bulging, rusting, leaking, dented, or smell foul when opened, says Dr. Kroger. The same goes for cracked glass jars or those with loose or bulging lids.

And if the liquid surrounding the food is cloudy when it is supposed to be clear, that is a danger sign as well, warns Dr. Schaffner.

TOSS IT IF IT BLOWS. Growing bacteria can inflate a container. So if food oozes or squirts when opened, don't eat it, advises Dr. Kroger.

COOK IT JUST RIGHT. Even if none of these warning signs are present, Dr. Schaffner suggests that you bring all canned foods to a full boil. "The boiling process destroys any butulinum toxin if it is present," he says.

FOOT ODOR
Keep Your Feet Sweet

Feet are faithful, if not entirely problem-free, servants. While happily performing their tasks, they may work up quite a sweat. And that can be a problem for another part of the human anatomy, the nose.

"There are a tremendous number of sweat glands on the feet, and sometimes the combination of sweating and bacteria can cause an obnoxious odor," says Marc A. Brenner, D.P.M., a podiatrist at the Institute for Diabetic Foot Research in Glendale, New York.

Fortunately, say doctors, there are plenty of ways to banish sweat and bacteria and keep your feet odor-free in the bargain. Here is how to prevent the malodorous march.

CLEANSE YOUR SOLES. The best way to deodorize smelly feet is to wash them with regular soap and water. "That may sound simple," says Glenn Gastwirth, D.P.M., executive director of the American Podiatric Medical Association, "but a lot of people quickly step in and out of the shower, forgetting to bend over and scrub the tops and bottoms of their feet, which washes away much of the bacteria."

DRY THEM WELL, TOES AND ALL. Once your feet are clean, be sure to dry them well, even taking care to get between the toes. This removes the moist environment where smell-producing bacteria thrive, explains Douglas Hale, D.P.M., a podiatrist at the Foot and Ankle Center of Washington in Seattle.

SMOOTH AWAY ODOR CATCHERS. Rough, scaly skin can provide an excellent breeding ground for stinky bacteria. "It is a good idea to get rid of any calluses and excess skin, especially around the heels," says Dr. Brenner. Try rubbing the scaly skin with a pumice stone while in the tub.

DUST THEM OFF. Once you have smoothed the skin, top it off with an antifungal foot powder. Just make sure to apply powder to very dry feet: Any moisture will make the powder cake, defeating the purpose, says Lawrence Z. Huppin, D.P.M., a podiatrist at the Foot and Ankle Center of Washington in Seattle.

STOCK UP ON SOCKS. The best odor-fighting socks are made of special moisture-wicking synthetic fibers like orlon, polypropylene, or CoolMax. If foot odor is especially problematic for you, it is best to change your socks frequently, even two or three times a day, suggests Dr. Hale.

DEODORIZE. If you wear panty hose, changing footwear during the day may not be practical. In that case, try a couple of swipes along the bottom of the foot with an antiperspirant roll-on that contains an aluminum-based active ingredient, says Dr. Huppin. In fact, anyone can do this before getting dressed in the morning, whether or not the person wears panty hose. But the antiperspirant has to contain that aluminum compound in order to be effective—so read labels.

LAVILIN UP. To keep your feet sweet-smelling day in and day out, Dr. Brenner recommends a natural product called *Lavilin Long Life Deodorant,* made especially for the feet. It is available in many health food stores. "Rubbed on the feet once or twice a week, this cream is like a miracle," he says.

GIVE 'EM A DAY OFF. Try wearing a given pair of shoes only every other day to allow them to air out. On their day off, keep them fresh with a cedar shoe tree.

While women tend to switch shoes to fit their outfits, some men get in the habit of wearing the same pair every day. If you are wedded to one style, buy two pairs of that style of shoe and alternate them day to day, says Dr. Huppin.

LAUNDER YOUR SHOES. When you buy athletic shoes, ask the salesclerk if they are washable—and if they are, put those shoes in the washer about once a month, says Dr. Hale. This will reduce colonies of odor-producing bacteria in the shoes, he says.

GALLSTONES
Exit the Stones Zone

The gallbladder is nothing more than a small sack attached to your liver, but it does a terrific clean-up job. Think of the gallbladder as a washing machine.

Bile is a digestive fluid manufactured by the liver and stored in the gallbladder. Think of bile as a detergent.

Cholesterol is a soft, waxy substance found in food and in your body. Think of cholesterol as the dirty laundry.

Now think of a gallstone as a stain that just won't come out.

Though we are accustomed to hearing about cholesterol in terms of heart disease, 80 percent of gallstones are *cholesterol* stones. Scientists aren't sure how cholesterol stones form. One theory suggests that they form when there is too much cholesterol in the gallbladder for the bile to "wash." Others suggest that the bile itself isn't an effective-enough detergent, or the gallbladder's wash cycle has been set way too slow. And, strangely enough, most of the cholesterol in that stone doesn't come from your diet. Rather, it is choles-

Take Your Gallbladder for a Walk

In analyzing who gets gallstones and who doesn't, researchers noticed that people who didn't get much exercise did get more than their share of gallstones. Right now, the link is more of a hunch than a proven cause and effect.

But researcher Alan Utter, Ph.D., assistant professor of health and exercise science at Appalachian State University in Boone, North Carolina, is trying to find out why exercise might work to help prevent cholesterol stones. One possibility is that exercise may speed up how much bile the gallbladder releases, and how quickly. If the gallbladder empties more slowly and less completely than normal, it leaves a small pool of bile behind. The bile puddle that remains is a perfect breeding ground for a cholesterol stone.

When Dr. Utter tested the theory on real people, he found that after one aerobic exercise session, slightly more bile was emptied from the gallbladder when compared to the gallbladder following no exercise session.

Another theory is that regular exercise protects against gallstone disease by helping you prevent weight gain, since being overweight is a potent risk factor for gallstones (along with health problems like heart disease, high blood pressure, and diabetes, to cite just a few examples).

In other words, preventing gallstones is yet another good reason to exercise. Walk briskly, bicycle, or swim for a minimum of 30 minutes, three or four times a week, suggests Dr. Utter.

terol manufactured by the liver for many crucial bodily functions, including the production of bile.

Gallstones themselves can be as small as a grain of sand or as big as a golf ball. You may have one stone or thousands. And every year, one million Americans—the majority of them women over age 40—will be told by their doctors that they have gallstone disease. For most people, gallstones are no big deal. Usually detected during a medical checkup or exam, they are called silent stones because there are no symptoms to speak of and no treatment is necessary.

But for hundreds of thousands of people, the stones are attention-getters. The worst symptom of an attack is severe pain in the upper abdomen, sometimes accompanied by a pain between the shoulder blades or in the right shoulder. And once you have had one attack, future assaults are more likely. When the stones hold repeat performances, they are more difficult to tolerate. So 600,000 people undergo gallbladder surgery to remove the organ. No more gallbladder, no more gallstones. It is reasonably simple, but it is still surgery.

Make the Fish Connection

Even though gallstones are common, there are ways that you can avoid getting them in the first place.

And if you already have them, you can avoid repeat attacks. As you might guess, avoidance strategies involve diet. Here are the keys to a stone-stopping food plan.

ORDER TUNA SALAD. "Scientists have discovered that Eskimo populations in Alaska who consume diets rich in marine fish oils have almost no gallstone disease," says Thomas H. Magnuson, M.D., assistant professor of surgery at the Johns Hopkins University School of Medicine in Baltimore and an expert in gallstone disease. He says that plenty of additional scientific evidence indicates that a diet rich in fish oils, either from fish or from fish-oil supplements, may help prevent cholesterol gallstones.

One study, for example, looked at several tribes of Es-

kimos, including traditional people living near the ocean
and eating a diet high in fish and people that had moved in-
land and were eating a "modern" diet low in fish.

Those who worked on the medical problems of the
Eskimos for many years reported rarely seeing a case of
gallbladder disease until a few years ago. But at one hospital serving the more modernized group, operations for
gallbladder disease outnumbered any other kind of operation. Not only do the urban Eskimos eat less fish than their
traditional kin, but they also get less exercise and eat a lot
more sugar.

Studies on animals (prairie dogs, to be exact) conducted by Dr. Magnuson and his team suggest that omega-3
fatty acids—the active ingredient of fish oils—seem to account for the protective effect of fish. Research suggests
that these omega-3's replace the types of fatty acids that are
normally in bile and keep the cholesterol soluble, in a liquid
rather than a solid form.

CONSIDER FISH-OIL SUPPLEMENTS. Could a diet rich
in omega-3's prevent cholesterol stones in people? "Some
studies show a dramatic effect, so it is a reasonable assumption," says Dr. Magnuson.

To benefit from omega-3's, you don't have to live
on tuna-noodle casserole and canned mackerel for the rest
of your life (unless you want to). Dr. Magnuson says that
daily supplements of omega-3 fatty acids can provide the
same amount of omega-3's eaten by Eskimo populations.
Most health food stores stock a variety of fish-oil supplements. He suggests following the dosages recommended on
the label.

Put Your Stones on a Diet

There is more to gallstone prevention than tuna sandwiches and fish-oil supplements. No one knows why, says

Dr. Magnuson, but being overweight can load you down with gallstones. One theory is that overweight people secrete excess cholesterol into their bile. The greater amount of cholesterol in the bile obviously means a higher risk for cholesterol stones. Whatever the reason, studies show that the heavier a person is, the greater the risk for gallstones.

To calculate the risk, scientists use a mathematical formula called the body mass index (BMI). Research shows that women with a BMI of 30 or higher have at least double the risk of developing gallstones compared to women with a BMI of less than 25. To calculate your BMI, grab a calculator and divide your weight (in pounds) by your height (in inches) squared, then multiply the resulting number by 705. If you are 130 pounds and 5 feet 3 inches (63 inches) tall, that's 130 divided by 3969 (63 × 63), which is 0.032. Multiply the number you get by 705 (0.032 × 704.50 = 23). The number you get is your BMI. If your BMI is over 25, it may be a good idea to lose weight if you want to take a giant step toward preventing gallstones, says Mitchell Shiffman, M.D., chief of the hepatology section of the Medical College of Virginia at Virginia Commonwealth University in Richmond.

SHED TWO POUNDS AT A TIME—NO MORE. Crash-dieting may peel away a few extra pounds in a matter of days, but if that happens, your risk for developing gallstones will go up, not down. That's because when you shed pounds, you mobilize fat stores, including stored cholesterol. To get rid of that cholesterol, your body sends it through the liver into the bile, where it will be squirted out into the intestines and excreted. But, as you already know, too much cholesterol in the bile translates into cholesterol stones. Sounds like a lose-lose situation, right?

The secret is to limit your weight loss to less than two pounds a week, says Dr. Shiffman.

EAT JUST ENOUGH CALORIES A DAY. If you eat a sensible number of calories—not too many, not too few—you will lose weight at the slow and steady rate of about $1^1/2$ pounds per week, says Judith S. Stern, R.D., D.Sc., professor of nutrition and internal medicine at the University of California, Davis.

GASTRITIS
Protecting Your Tummy

Your stomach is a miraculous sack. It produces a powerful acid to digest the food you send its way. And it has a lining of gellike mucus to stop the acid from making the stomach itself part of the meal. But even though your stomach lining is pretty tough, sometimes it gets inflamed. The result is tummy pain, a condition called gastritis.

Gastritis can be tough to pin down. To begin with, the pain of gastritis presents itself in varying ways. For some people, it is a painful burning or gnawing sensation in the upper abdomen, right below the breastbone. (Often, this kind of gastritis is mistaken for heartburn.) For others, nausea is the primary symptom of gastritis.

Some people have frequent stomach pain, with bouts of gastritis almost as predictable as morning sunrise. Others only have it now and then.

But how can you *prevent* the inflammation of your stomach lining? The large majority of cases are caused by either infection with a bacteria called *Helicobacter pylori* or by the repeated use of nonsteroidal anti-inflammatory drugs (NSAIDs).

H. pylori is an obstinate infection that resists the body's defenses and survives in the human stomach for a lifetime. Studies suggest that people unwittingly ingest a few of these organisms by having some sort of contact with an infected person's waste, says George Nikias, M.D., a gastroenterologist at Hackensack University Medical Center in New Jersey. So it is important to practice good sanitation, especially if you are the caretaker for children or older adults.

To avoid the other cause of gastric inflammation—NSAIDs—it is important to pay attention to over-the-counter medicines such as aspirin, ibuprofen, or naproxen (Naprosyn). Any of these medications can cause the form of inflammation known as chemical-induced gastritis. If that is the most likely cause of a bothered belly, here are some ways to prevent future episodes.

GET THE RIGHT DRUG. If you have to take nonsteroidal anti-inflammatory drugs regularly, ask your doctor about changing your medication. One type of NSAID may cause gastritis, but another might not. You and your doctor have to find the right drug for you, says Dr. Nikias.

GET THE RIGHT DOSE. The higher the dose of a nonsteroidal anti-inflammatory drug, the more likely it will cause gastritis. Work with your doctor to find the lowest dosage that controls your symptoms, suggests Dr. Nikias.

TAKE H$_2$, TOO. If you are taking NSAIDs, talk to your doctor about whether or not you should also take acid-suppressing drugs known as H$_2$-blockers (histamine-blockers) or proton-pump inhibitors (PPI). "These can protect you from drug-caused chemical gastritis," says Dr. Nikias. They are available both over the counter and in stronger formulations by prescription.

GO FISHING. Fish—or more precisely, the omega-3 fatty acids in fish oil—may be a good preventive against chemical gastritis. There is some evidence that fish oil helps spark the production of the prostaglandins, substances that help protect the lining of the stomach. "I think it is certainly worthwhile to try it," says Eugene Oliveri, D.O., professor of medicine at Michigan State University College of Osteopathic Medicine in East Lansing and a gastroenterologist in Milford.

While you can get some omega-3's from cold-water fish like salmon, mackerel, and tuna, the most convenient source is probably fish-oil capsules. Concentrated omega-3 fish-oil supplements are widely available at health food stores and most drugstores. To help ease the inflammation of gastritis, try a daily dose of two or three fish-oil capsules at 1,000 milligrams each, suggests Dr. Oliveri. Space them out throughout the day and take them as long as you are taking the NSAIDs.

WATCH OUT FOR INDULGENCES. Alcohol and tobacco can aggravate gastritis and its symptoms, especially if you are taking NSAIDs, says Dr. Nikias. So you might help your intestinal health if you cut out smoking or drink less alcohol.

GINGIVITIS
Getting to Glorious Gums

Gum disease, known to dentists as gingivitis, is one of those afflictions that drives doctors and dentists crazy. Why? Because in most cases, it is entirely preventable. If you take good care of your teeth and gums, you will probably never have to deal with the pain, the expense, or the other problems to which gum disease can sometimes lead.

Gingivitis gets its start when bacteria move into the area around your gums. If the bacteria are not cleaned out, they can move below the gum line and start to form a thin film. Within a few days, you have a buildup of a multi-bacterial gunk called plaque. Add some minerals from your saliva to the mix, and you end up with a hard-to-remove substance called tartar.

In some people, years of plaque and tartar buildup can lead to a bacterial infection of the gums. Their gums, which had been pink, firm, and healthy, become red and puffy, and they bleed easily when brushed. For some people, the infection can move from the gums down into the

---

Are More Than Your Teeth at Stake?

Some recent research suggests that gum disease could actually put your life at risk. Preliminary studies have found a link between gum disease and both heart disease and stroke.

One possible explanation is that the harmful bacteria that form into plaque in the mouth activate white blood cells, which in turn release clotting factors that play a role in both heart disease and stroke.

---

connective tissue and bone that hold the teeth in their mouths. And as if that's not bad enough, gingivitis might grow into dreaded periodontitis, which can eventually cause tooth loss.

Be a Hygiene Fiend

The central gum-disease prevention premise is good dental hygiene, which means keeping your teeth and mouth clean.

This is nowhere near as simple as it sounds. The mouth is a paradise for bacteria and germs. All the nooks and crannies between your teeth are perfect bacteria hiding spots. When you add in all the food that gets chomped and stuck between your molars, it is easy to see why mouth maintenance is no snap. But here are some ways to brush up on gum care.

WORK THE ANGLE. When you brush your teeth, don't hold the bristles of your toothbrush flat against your teeth, suggests Irwin Mandel, D.D.S., professor emeritus, former director of preventive dentistry, and director of clinical research for dentistry at Columbia University School of Dental and Oral Surgery in New York City. Tip them toward the gum line of your teeth at a 45-degree angle so that as you brush, the bristles gently massage and probe the space where your teeth and gums meet. Get the bristles ever-so-slightly under your gum line, he says.

ROTATE YOUR BRISTLES. Dr. Mandel suggests that instead of using the back-and-forth brush maneuver, move the brush in small circles over the surface of your teeth. He recommends that you start with the outer surfaces, then move to the inner surfaces, before finishing with the chewing surfaces of your teeth.

BRUSH YOUR TONGUE, TOO. Bacteria can hide anywhere in your mouth, including on your tongue. For high-level hygiene, be sure to brush your tongue, says Dr. Mandel.

GET VERTICAL. If you have difficulty getting at the backs of your front teeth, put your toothbrush in a vertical position and rotate the brush in tiny circles, suggests Dr. Mandel.

TAKE YOUR TIME. The average American brushes his teeth in 45 to 60 seconds. That's just not long enough. To do it right, it requires two to three minutes, says Dr. Mandel.

TWICE IS NICE. Many dentists believe that brushing after every meal is optimal for tooth and gum protection. But don't worry if it is inconvenient. "If you brush thoroughly and correctly in the morning and before you go to bed at night and floss at least daily, you don't have to brush after every meal," says Dr. Mandel. "Just rinse your mouth out with some water after you eat."

BE A SOFTIE. There seem to be as many models of toothbrushes as there are of cars. But you don't really need anything fancy if you have good brushing habits and use the right brushing technique. The only absolute requirement for a toothbrush is that it has soft bristles. Hard bristles can hurt your gums and teeth, according to Dr. Mandel. Be sure to change your brush once its bristles start to look beaten up, he adds.

Make an Appointment to Prevent Gingivitis

"The difference between brushing your teeth and really getting them clean can be the instruction you get from a dentist or dental hygienist," says Irwin Mandel, D.D.S., professor emeritus, former director of preventive dentistry, and director of clinical research for dentistry at Columbia University School of Dental and Oral Surgery in New York City. A dental professional can guarantee that you are cleaning your teeth correctly by watching you brush and floss in the office—and then showing you exactly what you might be doing wrong.

And a dentist or dental hygienist can also help prevent gingivitis by removing any plaque or tartar that you may have missed, especially in the hard-to-get-to areas below the gum line, says Dr. Mandel. You and your dentist should discuss the frequency of your visits, he says. It can vary from 3 to 6 to every 12 months, depending on how well you brush and floss—and how quickly your teeth build up plaque and tartar.

PICK THE RIGHT PASTE. Toothpastes are mostly a matter of personal preference, but Dr. Mandel says that one paste is especially effective in preventing gingivitis. It is called Colgate Total, and it contains ingredients that help prevent decay, plaque, and tartar. It also directly fights the inflammation of gingivitis. "This is probably the most effective multi-benefit toothpaste," says Dr. Mandel. To help prevent gum disease, he also favors Crest Gumcare, he says.

SPIT OUT THE RINSE. Don't waste your money on the anti-plaque, gingivitis-fighting rinses that are on the market. "They have little or no benefit," says David Kennedy, D.D.S., a dentist and the president of the Preventive Dental Health Association in San Diego. Their bacteria-killing ingredients only stick to the teeth and gums for about a minute.

The Flossing Follow-Up

Okay, you have just brushed your teeth for a good three minutes. You even used the rotation stroke. Your mouth feels as clean as a whistle. But it's not time to stop yet. Now, you have to prevent bacterial buildup between your teeth, in those teensy spaces where the brush bristles couldn't reach.

It's dental floss time. Here is a step-by-step strategy from Dr. Kennedy.

1. Break off 24 to 36 inches of floss and wind most of it around one of your middle fingers.
2. Wind the remaining floss around the same finger of the opposite hand. Dr. Kennedy suggests that as you use the floss and notice it is shredding, unroll a little bit off one finger and roll it up on the other.
3. Pinch the floss between your thumbs and forefingers. Using a gentle rubbing motion, guide the floss between your teeth. Never snap the floss into the gums. Not only does it hurt, but it can cause unnecessary bleeding.
4. As the floss reaches your gum line, curve it into a C shape against one tooth. Carefully slide into the space between the gum and the tooth.
5. Press the floss tightly against the tooth. Delicately rub the side of the tooth, moving the floss away from the gum with upward and downward motions. "You are basically using it like you use a towel to dry your back, only

you are scraping scum off the tooth," says
Dr. Kennedy.

6. Repeat these instructions on the rest of your
teeth. Don't forget the back side of your last
tooth. There is no in-between at your last tooth,
but it is still a side that you need to clean, says
Dr. Kennedy.

As for the type of floss to use, Dr. Kennedy says that
one type isn't better than another. "Find the floss that works
with *your* mouth."

Calcium and C for Gum Disease

Though having a clean mouth is the most important preventive step you can take to thwart gum disease, it is not
your only defense. Your diet may be a strong shield as well.

Our gums are tissues, which means they need certain
nutrients to stay healthy. Specifically, your gums require a
protein called collagen, the basic building block of all our
tissues. Vitamin C is central to our body's collagen production. There is scientific evidence that vitamin C strengthens
weak gum tissue and makes the gum lining more resistant
to penetration by bacteria and therefore less prone to swelling, bleeding, and tooth loss.

To prevent gum disease or keep it from getting worse,
Dr. Mandel suggests eating lots of fresh, vitamin C–laden
fruits and vegetables, especially broccoli, peppers, pineapple, oranges, and grapefruit.

Supplementation is an option when you don't get at
least 100 milligrams of vitamin C in your diet every day,
says Dr. Mandel. You might try one of these two vitamin C
anti-gum-disease strategies suggested by Mary Dan Eades,
M.D., vice president of the Colorado Center for Metabolic Medicine in Boulder. Which one you choose is up
to you.

An Apple a Day Recipe

Winning-Smile Fruit Salad

Vitamin C helps to give your gums that healthy glow. This kiwifruit salad has more than a day's supply of vitamin C and a creamy honey-orange sauce to boot. To peel a kiwifruit, cut off the ends and run a spoon around the inside of the peel until the peel slips free from the fruit.

8 kiwifruits, peeled and sliced
2 cups seedless red grapes
1 can (15 ounces) mandarin orange slices, drained
1 cup nonfat vanilla yogurt
1 tablespoon thawed frozen orange juice concentrate
1 tablespoon honey

In a large serving bowl, combine the kiwifruits, grapes, and oranges.

In a small bowl, whisk together the yogurt, juice concentrate, and honey. Spoon the sauce over the fruit.

Makes 4 servings. Per serving: 236 calories, 1 g. fat, 280% of Daily Value of vitamin C

Time-release capsules. Take one or two 500-milligram vitamin C capsules two times a day—in the morning and at night

Crystalline vitamin C. This type of vitamin C comes in powder form. It should be available at health food stores. Dr. Eades suggests mixing a half-teaspoon of the powder with a sugar-free citrus drink and swishing it around in your mouth for a minute or so before swallowing it. Make sure to rinse your mouth out with water after you take that vitamin C dose.

A couple of vitamin C cautions: Doses exceeding 1,200 milligrams a day may cause diarrhea in some people. Also, stay away from chewable vitamin C. It has been shown to erode tooth enamel.

Calcium is important for strong, healthy bones, including strong, healthy jawbones. If we don't get enough of it, gum disease can progress to tooth loss. Be sure that you are eating foods that are good sources of calcium. Try skim milk, nonfat yogurt and cheese, broccoli, Swiss chard, and salmon, suggests Dr. Mandel.

In addition, be careful not to overdo soft drinks, says Dr. Mandel. Soft drinks often have a lot of phosphorus, a mineral that can actually leach calcium from your bones.

A Moist Mouth for a Good Defense

Saliva is one of our best mouth cleansers. If you are short of it, you will probably have more bacteria in your mouth. More bacteria means more plaque, which means a greater likelihood of gum disease. Here are two tips to make sure that your mouth has all the moisture it needs.

CHECK YOUR MEDICINES. Lots of drugs—including some anti-hypertensives, anti-anxieties, antidepressants, and antihistamines—can cause dry mouth. If you feel that your mouth is not quite as well-lubricated as it should be, ask your doctor if a medication might be causing it, advises Dr. Mandel.

MAKE YOUR MOUTH WATER. Foods with strong flavors or foods that contain a lot of fiber stimulate saliva production. Sugarless gum, with its sweet burst of flavor, will help your mouth produce the extra saliva that helps keep your teeth and gums clean, says Dr. Mandel. Or try an apple: The action of chewing for a period of time will have your salivary glands working to get your mouth back to normal in no time.

GOUT
Make It "Toe" the Line

Your big toe is the South Pole of your body. Rather than being a temperate 98.6°F, it is a chilly 93°F down there. So maybe it is not surprising that crystals sometimes form in this anatomically arctic region.

The crystals aren't ice, though. They are composed of uric acid, a by-product of normal metabolism that is supposed to stay in liquid form but sometimes becomes a solid. Since your body regards those crystals as intruders, white blood cells rush to the area and release enzymes that are like attack dogs, specially trained to chew up trespassers. Unfortunately, those enzymes are indiscriminately vicious. Besides attacking the crystals, they also attack the joint of the toe, which becomes red, swollen, and tender—so painfully tender, in fact, that even the weight of a bedsheet can be excruciating. And that is when you feel the effects of gout.

Clutter in the Joints

Gout is actually a form of arthritis. In addition to hammering big toes, it can also attack ankles, elbows, wrists, and other joints. Wherever it finally settles, gout gets going because your body produces too much uric acid or because your kidneys don't excrete enough to clean it from your system. A person can have excessive uric acid levels for years and never have an attack, and then something—chilled feet, too much alcohol, a stubbed toe—can trigger the first acute episode of the disease. If it is your first attack, the pain usually lasts one to two weeks.

As far as risk goes, the person most likely to get gout is a man in his late thirties or forties, since men's bigger bodies produce more uric acid. If you are an overweight male in that age bracket, you are even more susceptible. Risk goes up even more if you are taking certain medicines prescribed for high blood pressure.

If you have had one attack, you will probably have more. Around 70 percent of sufferers have their second attacks within the next year, and 95 percent have their second attacks within five years. The brief periods of pain are bad enough, but there is another reason to prevent gout attacks if you can. Repeated attacks can damage the joints so badly that some people are almost immobilized.

Fortunately, gout attacks are completely preventable, according to Ronenn Roubenoff, M.D., associate professor of nutrition and medicine at Tufts University and lab chief at the U.S. Department of Agriculture Human Nutrition Research Center, both in Boston. And if you have never had an attack before, you can take steps to help ensure that it never happens. Here are the keys to gout prevention, according to Dr. Roubenoff.

How to Prevent the Encores

Once you have had a first attack of gout, the best way to prevent subsequent attacks is with appropriate medical treatment, says Ronenn Roubenoff, M.D., associate professor of nutrition and medicine at Tufts University and lab chief at the U.S. Department of Agriculture Human Nutrition Research Center, both in Boston. If you do get treatment, the attacks are completely preventable. But sometimes physicians don't prescribe the correct preventive medications, he says. If you make sure that you get the proper preventive treatment, your first attack could be your last.

While anti-inflammatory drugs like ibuprofen can help defuse a gout attack, they won't prevent future trouble.

For long-term prevention, your doctor first needs to determine whether you are an "underexcreter" or an "overproducer" of uric acid. Ninety percent of gout patients are underexcreters and 10 percent are overproducers, and the preventive medications for these two types of people are completely different, says Dr. Roubenoff. To find out which one you are, your physician needs to test urine that

Guarding Against the First Attack

In most cases of gout, the reason for high uric acid levels is unknown. There are, however, certain avoidable risk factors that increase your chances of getting a first attack.

CHECK YOUR MEDS. "We have seen an increase in the prevalence of gout at the same time that we have seen an increase in the use of thiazide diuretics in the treatment of high blood pressure," says Dr. Roubenoff.

If you have been diagnosed with high blood pressure and your doctor has prescribed a thiazide diuretic to control was collected repeatedly over a 24-hour period. "This is a very simple test and is a must in the proper preventive treatment of gout," he observes.

If you are an underexcreter, the doctor will prescribe a uricosuric drug, which helps your body excrete more uric acid. If you are an overproducer, the doctor may recommend allopurinol (Zyloprim). Although the drug is very effective, some people have a violent allergic reaction that can be fatal, so you and your doctor need to evaluate the risks and benefits of this drug and decide if it is for you.

When you start taking either drug, the doctor should also prescribe another drug, colchicine(ColBenemid), to help prevent side effects. This medication is temporary, however, and after you have had normal blood uric acid levels for one year, you can stop taking the colchicine, says Dr. Roubenoff.

If you have already had one or more gout attacks and your doctor is not familiar with these medications, Dr. Roubenoff recommends that you see a specialist in rheumatology or arthritis who can help you make choices and prescribe these drugs, if necessary.

the problem, you should talk to your physician about switching to another medication. "Nowadays, there are many other drugs to treat high blood pressure, including beta-blockers, calcium channel blockers, and ACE inhibitors," Dr. Roubenoff says. If you are able to switch to one of these medications, you might avoid ever having a first attack, he points out.

KEEP THE POUNDS DOWN. If you are overweight, you are basically asking your kidneys to process a lot of extra uric acid to deal with the waste from a lot of added-on body cells.

When someone is overweight, the kidneys have to

The Anti-Gout Diet: Is It Worth the Effort?

Many foods contain a substance called purine, which increases the level of uric acid in the body. For years, it was suggested that people restrict their intake of these purine-containing foods in order to avoid gout attacks. But Dr. Roubenoff now feels that this approach does not work and, worse, can actually harm a person with gout because of nutritional depletions.

"I try not to restrict the diet of people with gout," says Ronenn Roubenoff, M.D., associate professor of nutrition and medicine at Tufts University and lab chief at the U.S. Department of Agriculture Human Nutrition Research Center, both in Boston. "The maximum effect that you can get with a really restrictive, low-purine diet is very small and will not prevent gout attacks." Dr. Roubenoff says it *is* a good idea for people with gout who are on preventive medication to restrict alcohol intake to two drinks per week. It is also important that you don't overeat and that you get six to eight glasses of water a day, he advises.

struggle to deal with the overload. That's why you may end up with gout. A good rule of thumb to determine your ideal weight is 100 pounds plus 5 pounds for every inch over 5 feet tall for women. For men, it is 106 pounds plus 6 pounds for every inch over 5 feet. The more you weigh over this level, the higher your risk for gout, according to Dr. Roubenoff. Even 10 or 15 extra pounds can increase your risk.

CRASH DIET? DON'T BUY IT. Low-calorie crash diets—like dropping to 1,000 calories a day—can change your metabolism so that you produce more uric acid. "Quick weight loss can cause a person to have their first attack of gout," says Dr. Roubenoff. Losing your extra weight is smart; losing it fast is foolish. Don't go on a diet of less than 1,000 calories a day without discussing it with your doctor, he advises.

KEEP YOUR TOOTSIES TOASTY. Since gout seems to have an affinity for chilly climes, "keeping the toes warm is very helpful for preventing gout," says Dr. Roubenoff. If you are walking outside on a cold day, make sure that your shoes are well-insulated.

WEAR THE RIGHT SIZE. Injuring the joint of your big toe can increase uric acid levels, either causing a first attack of gout or subsequent attacks, says Dr. Roubenoff. And you are setting up your big toe for some brutal battering if you wear a shoe that is too tight. When you try on new shoes, make sure that your toes can move freely. You may also feel a kind of burning sensation on the bottom of your foot if the shoe doesn't fit right. And if you own shoes that pinch your toes, get the jump on gout by giving them away.

AVOID THIN SOLES. Walking in shoes with very thin soles can also traumatize the toe joint, says Dr. Roubenoff. To be certain the shoes you buy have padding that's thick enough, walk on noncarpeted areas when you are trying them on for the first time. The shoe should be comfortable and have a little cushioning when you push down with your toes.

HAIR LOSS
Holding On to Your Tresses

Most of the time, we go through life with the usual ration of hair—approximately 100,000 or so, give or take. The average person loses 50 to 100 hairs a day. Virtually all of it grows back.

But sometimes, hair growth is disrupted, leaving your locks abnormally patchy or thin. And temporary hair loss can also occur, triggered by serious illness or by physical stress. In rare cases, women can temporarily lose up to 50 percent of their hair as a result of these causes. But the most common form of permanent hair loss is known as male pattern baldness in men and as female pattern hair loss in women. Both are believed to result from genetic predisposition or hormonal abnormalities. Diet, grooming habits, and medications can also wreak havoc with healthy hair.

Cut Your Losses

If you are losing your hair, it is a good idea to consult your doctor to rule out medical causes or prescription medication. "Certain prescription drugs can cause hair loss," says Peter Panagotacos, M.D., a dermatologist and an expert in hair restoration and hair-loss prevention in private practice in San Francisco.

One of the most likely culprits is Accutane, an anti-acne medication derived from vitamin A. Other possible suspects are the calcium blockers used to treat high blood pressure, such as nifedipine (Procardia) or verapamil (Calan), and many cholesterol-lowering drugs, such as clofibrate (Atromid-S). When your physician prescribes a drug, ask him if hair loss is a possible side effect, says Dr. Panagotacos. If it is, pay attention to whether or not you are losing more hair. Maybe another medication wouldn't have that effect.

Apart from screening your medications, there are a few other ways that you may be able to help prevent hair loss. Here is what experts recommend.

AVOID IRON-DEFICIENCY ANEMIA. "Iron-deficiency anemia is a common problem in menstruating women, who sometimes lose a lot of iron during their monthly cycle," says Shelly Friedman, D.O., medical director of the Scottsdale Institute for Cosmetic Dermatology in Arizona, president of the American Board of Hair Restoration Surgery, and a medical advisor to the American Hair Loss Council. "When that happens, hair can become very brittle, so it breaks easily, leaving you with a lot less hair." To prevent iron-poor hair, eat plenty of iron-rich foods like lean meats, pinto and kidney beans, and ready-to-eat cereals. Also, women should take iron supplements if their doctors approve. Men, however, should not take iron supplements because too much iron has been linked to a higher risk of heart disease and cancer in men.

STYLE GENTLY. Overuse of personal hairstyling equipment like a hot comb, curling iron, or blow-dryer can cause hair to become brittle and break off, says Kathleen Walsh, chief executive officer of PK Walsh, a women's hair replacement salon in Wellesley, Massachusetts. "When my daughter was a teenager, she used a hot curling iron that was also a brush, and she would use that with hair spray. By overworking her hairdo, she was literally pulling out her hair. When she finally stopped abusing her hair, it grew back."

COLOR WITH CAUTION. "Even the most skillful dyeing, bleaching, or perming of the hair damages the cuticle, the outside lining of the hair shaft," says Dr. Friedman. This damage makes hair very thin and brittle and prone to breakage.

To avoid the damage, ask your stylist to test a strand of your hair with the dye, bleach, or perming chemical *before* going ahead with the procedure to see how the hair will react, says Walsh. If the chemical causes too much damage, consult with the stylist about a different type of product or procedure. For instance, you might try highlighting instead of using an overall dye.

FOR MEN ONLY: CONSIDER TWO OPTIONS. Over-the-counter minoxidil lotion, which actually does work to prevent hair loss or to restore hair, is available in both 2 and 5 percent strength. The 5 percent lotion, however, is for men only as it may cause facial hair growth in women. Minoxidil, says Dr. Panagotacos, works by sparking withered or miniaturized hair follicles to return to their normal size and sprout wider, more youthful hair.

In addition to the 5 percent minoxidil lotion, men also have available the recently approved oral prescription medication finasteride (Propecia). "Minoxidil is like life support

Hair Loss 101: Three Reasons You *Don't* Go Bald

The myths about baldness are almost as abundant as the misconceptions. Here are three common falsehoods.

1. Every man on your Mom's side of the family is bald. Yes, genes do determine hair loss, says Peter Panagotacos, M.D., a dermatologist and an expert in hair restoration and hair-loss prevention in private practice in San Francisco. But, no, it is not inherited only through your mother. "You could end up being balder than anybody in the family, depending on what *combination* of genes you have for those particular traits," says Dr. Panagotacos. Blame your ancestors, if you will. But there is no way of pinning the blame on Mom's people, in particular.

2. You shampoo too much. "That's a truly bizarre myth," says Dr. Panagotacos. "There's no truth to that whatsoever."

3. Stress made you go bald. Severe stress, anything from surgery to childbirth to an IRS audit, will cause increased hair loss, says Dr. Panagotacos. This phenomenon, however, is merely an accelerated version of a process that is always occurring—the natural growth cycle of hairs—and most of those lost hairs will be replaced.

   The reality of stress-caused hair loss leads to the myth that "chronic daily stress will cause someone to go bald who wasn't genetically predisposed to go bald," says Dr. Panagotacos. "That is not going to happen. But their hair might get thinner faster."

for an ailing follicle, whereas finasteride may tell the follicle not to get old in the first place," says Dr. Panagotacos. "Minoxidil hides the fact that you are still going bald, while finasteride will actually prevent the baldness process." Finasteride is only available by prescription, so check with your doctor.

HANGNAILS
How to Keep Your Cuticles Happy

When skin is healthy and moist, it is a terrific protective pelt. It thwarts lots of potential invaders. But when our epidermal wall gets breached, we suddenly become vulnerable. Bacteria and fungi can find their way in through even the smallest skin cracks, such as those around our fingernails. Hangnails, those little pieces of torn skin around our cuticles, are more than painful. They are also tiny windows of opportunity for infection.

We get hangnails because the cuticles on our fingers are easily dehydrated. And when they dry up, the skin splits and peels away in those awful little strips. Moisture is the secret to preventing hangnails and the infections they admit.

Here are some tips to keep your cuticles smooth and protective.

USE CUTICLE OIL. The best anti-hangnail moisturizer is one made *specifically* for your cuticles, says Vicki Peters, president of the Peters Perspective, a consulting firm for the

Stop Nail Nibbling

Nail biting is a common cause of hangnails, says Jerome Z. Litt, M.D., assistant clinical professor of dermatology at Case Western Reserve University School of Medicine in Cleveland and author of *Your Skin: From Acne to Zits.* "When people bite their nails, they also bite the cuticle along the sides and bottom of their nails, and they develop hangnails. Then they bite off those hangnails, and the ripping and pulling with their teeth cause even more hangnails."

Breaking the nail-biting habit can be as tough as . . . well, nails. But women can help themselves kick the habit by getting a manicure, suggests Vicki Peters, president of the Peters Perspective, a consulting firm for the nail industry, located in Las Vegas, and author of *Salon Ovations Nail Q and A Book.*

"The manicurist can apply a protective coating such as an acrylic gel of fiberglass to your nails. This will protect, strengthen, and beautify the nails, helping them grow longer. And because your nails will look better and you have invested in the procedure, you will be less likely to bite your nails," says Peters.

Darlene Hewitt, a manicurist and nail technician in Toronto, recommends what she calls the rude approach to breaking the nail-biting habit. "Do you know everywhere your hands have been during the day and exactly what is on them? Studies show, for instance, that there are actually traces of fecal matter on the hot-water faucet handles in public bathrooms. Think about *that* the next time you are about to bite your nails. It might not be pleasant, but it might help you keep your nails out of your mouth."

nail industry, located in Las Vegas, and author of *Salon Ovations Nail Q and A Book*. She recommends a cuticle oil for home nail care rather than a cuticle cream because the oil will be better absorbed. And she says to look for a product with special added natural ingredients that will help hydrate the cuticle, such as jojoba oil, almond oil, or tea tree oil. These oils are available through your professional manicurist or beauty supply store. If you get lots of hangnails, use the oil up to three times a day for prevention, she advises.

OIL THEM NIGHTLY. Apply the oil right before you go to bed, says Peters. For best results, wear light cotton gloves at night when you have cuticle oil and lotion on your hands.

WASH AND OIL. When you use the oil just before bedtime, try to apply it right after you wash your hands and put on the cotton gloves after applying the oil. Applying moisturizer while your hands are still wet actually increases the penetration of the moisturizer, according to Diana Bihova, M.D., a dermatologist in private practice in New York City.

TO KEEP NAILS WELL, DRINK WATER. "The best preventive 'medicine' for hangnails is to drink 8 to 10 glasses of water daily," says Darlene Hewitt, a manicurist and nail technician in Toronto. "If you don't get enough water, your cuticles will dry out and crack, creating a hangnail."

AVOID FAST-DRYING POLISH. Ingredients in nail polish that help it dry faster can also dry your cuticles and cause hangnails, says Hewitt. She says to avoid polishes with the ingredients formaldehyde or toulene.

PROTECT YOUR TOES, TOO. Hangnails on toes are uncommon, though they do happen occasionally, particularly if you frequently wear opened-toe shoes. The extra exposure to air can dry your cuticles. To help prevent hangnails on your toes, don't forget to moisturize your feet along with the rest of your body when you get out of the shower in the morning, says Peters.

SNIP IT AT THE BASE. You can prevent a beginning

hangnail from getting worse if you take prompt action. Using cuticle scissors, cut the dried cuticle, says Paul Kechijian, M.D., clinical associate professor of dermatology at New York University Medical Center in New York City and a dermatologist in Great Neck, New York. This will minimize the chance of it catching on something during daily activities and will prevent further tearing.

HANGOVER
Drown This Sorrow with Water

If you are reading this chapter, there is probably no point in suggesting sobriety. You have probably over-imbibed before, and you know what it is like to experience a hangover. And if right now you have already had a few too many, you are hoping there is something in this book that can head off the horror of the hangover to come.

Prevention, like the cause, comes in a tall glass. If there is a hangover on the horizon and you hope to stop it, your best bet is to keep drinking—water, that is.

Here's Looking at H₂O, Kid

Despite the fact that hangovers have been studied up, down, and sideways, scientists still aren't exactly sure what causes them. One possible cause is acetaldehyde, a toxin produced when your body metabolizes alcohol. Other possible causes are some chemicals called congeners, which are created during the manufacture of alcohol, or the additives used to enhance flavor and stabilize color. "Some people are very sensitive to these additives," says John Brick, Ph.D., executive director of Intoxikon International in Yardley, Pennsylvania, a company that conducts alcohol and drug research, education, and training. Most likely, all of these substances play a role. But this much is clear: The leading cause of hangover is dehydration, he says.

When you are in the midst of a hangover, your mouth feels like the Kalahari Desert because your body is short of water. Here's why. Alcohol inhibits the release of vasopressin, a hormone that tells the kidneys *not* to take water out of the blood. So when you are drinking, your kidneys siphon off some water from the blood passing through. All those trips to the rest room leave your body literally high and dry. And if the vasopressin suppression weren't parching enough, alcohol also directly removes water from the brain cells, actually causing them to shrink. Now you know why the next day your head feels as though it were in a vise when you are having a hangover. Cell by cell, your poor parched brain is tightening up.

"For a large portion of the population, most of the symptoms of hangover are caused by the loss of water," says Dr. Brick.

Here are your best hopes for staving off the morning-after miseries.

SLURP BEFORE YOU SLEEP. No matter how many servings of alcohol you have had, it is never too late to hydrate.

"You can significantly minimize a hangover by drinking as much water as you comfortably can after you have been drinking and before you go to sleep," says Dr. Brick. Every extra glass of water adds extra insurance. If you can restore the water balance in your body, your head and stomach will thank you in the morning.

TRY AN ALTERNATIVE TO H₂O. If you just don't like drinking water, lucky for you (and your brain cells) there are alternatives. "A beverage like Gatorade or any of the mineral-enhanced drinks with potassium, sodium, and glucose added to them are fine," says Dr. Brick.

GET A GOOD NIGHT'S REST. "People who don't get enough sleep after drinking can end up with a sleep-deprivation hangover," says Dr. Brick. He recommends getting eight hours.

There is good reason to go for extra rack time—and it is linked to what is called rapid eye movement, or REM sleep. Alcohol interferes with your sleep. "Although many people find that they get to sleep faster with a drink, alcohol decreases REM sleep, which is necessary for dreaming. The more you drink, the less you dream," says Dr. Brick.

"Lack of REM can cause irritability and cognitive problems," Dr. Brick adds. You must sleep more to compensate for having poor quality sleep. So try to sleep late the next day. It will give you a chance to recover your lost REM sleep.

Some Possible Pre-Party Planning

Fortunately, very few of us plan to get drunk. But if you think about hangover avoidance before you head out for an evening's entertainment, these tips may be useful.

HEAD FOR THE HORS D'OEUVRES. Eating food before you drink slows the absorption of alcohol into the bloodstream and makes it less likely that you will end up intoxicated tonight and hungover tomorrow, says Dr. Brick. Start with snacks and *then* have a drink. Better yet, if you are susceptible to hangovers, make it a rule never to drink on an empty stomach.

SLOW DOWN. Drinking at a fast pace changes your brain cells in such a way that you are more likely to get a hangover, says Dr. Brick. Also, the faster you drink, the greater the possibility that you will end up extremely intoxicated—and feeling extremely bad the next day. So pace your drinking: As a general rule of thumb, have no more than one drink per hour. That one drink may be 1 1/2 ounces of hard liquor, 5 ounces of wine, or 12 ounces of beer, but no more. This will keep your intoxication and hangover at a minimum.

HAVE A WATER CHASER. The best way to avoid dehydration is to match your alcohol intake with water intake. For every glass of wine you have, have the equivalent amount of water. "This advice—a glass of water for every glass of alcoholic beverage—is easy to remember and will allow you to comfortably drink as much water as possible," says Dr. Brick.

One caution: This advice does not mean that you should down mixed drinks like scotch-and-water all evening. "That won't have the same effect," says Dr. Brick. You have to drink your water straight.

CHOOSE CLEAR "POISONS." Though the kind of liquor you drink has little effect on the dehydration issue, dark liquors tend to have more of the chemicals that may cause hangovers, including congeners, additives, and other chemicals. "As a rule of thumb," says Dr. Brick, "the darker the beverage, the more hangover-causing compounds are in it." (This rule only applies to distilled spirits, not to beer and wine.) He cites dark rum and whiskey as two of the biggest offenders.

HAY FEVER
Probing the Pollen Pollution Problem

Wouldn't you know it, hay fever is caused by males. True! It's the male cells of flowering plants, trees, grasses, and weeds that make up these pollen particles. Smaller than the width of a hair, capable of traveling 400 miles out to sea or 2 miles above the earth, pollen particles cause the symptoms of allergic rhinitis, more commonly known as hay fever.

Hay fever afflicts 35 million Americans every year.

In many parts of the United States, pollen of one kind or another can get sniffed up almost year-round. In early spring, most pollen allergies are caused by trees like oak, elm, and maple. In late spring and early summer, the pollen villains are grasses like timothy and bermudagrass. Weeds take their turn in late summer and fall.

In fact, the only type of pollen that doesn't take its turn is flower pollen. That's because these particles are too big to cause allergy reactions and because they are carried from plant to plant by insects rather than by the wind.

Even moving doesn't do much good because the most

common pollen plants are all over the United States. And besides, even if you do change location, it is quite likely that you will develop allergies to the local pollens in a year or two. Or you may cross-react to a pollen that is much like the ones you fled from. But no matter where you are, there are ways to keep out of pollen's way.

CLOSE UP BEFORE YOUR SHUT-EYE. Before you go to bed, shut all the doors to the outside as well as the windows in your room. "Pollen is created at night, especially in the wee hours of the morning, and pollen production usually stops around 7:00 to 8:00 A.M.," says Robert Plancey, M.D., assistant clinical professor of medicine at the University of Southern California in Los Angeles and an internist and allergist in Arcadia. "So you don't want to sleep at night with your windows or doors open."

Even the normal comings and goings should be done cautiously during pollen season. "A lot of times, I'll tell people to go in and out through their garage door because that way there are two sets of doors, an extra barrier between the open door and the outside air," says Dr. Plancey. When you are in the car, drive with your windows closed and adjust the ventilation so that the air is recirculated, he advises.

TRY STRIPPING. Sometimes, people will weather-strip their homes to keep pollen from coming in around cracks in doors and windows. "Also, having a high-efficiency particulate air (HEPA) filter on the central intake of the heating, ventilating, and air-conditioning unit can keep a lot of pollen from entering the house," says Dr. Plancey.

GET WASHED UP. Wash your face and hair when you come home to remove the pollen that may have collected on you while you were out, says Dr. Plancey.

PROTECT YOUR EYES. Pollen can blow directly into the eyes and cause an allergic reaction, says Dr. Plancey. Usually, the eyes make tears to rinse the pollen out, but if your nose is congested, the tears can't drain and the eyes begin to itch.

You can help prevent that local allergic reaction by closing your eyes and wiping the outer surface of the lids with a clean washcloth dipped in warm or cool water, according to Dr. Plancey.

"This cleansing can be done many times during the day to help remove excess pollen, and it is very effective at preventing symptoms," he says.

EXERCISE AS THE SUN GOES DOWN. Exercising or jogging in the early morning hours is a problem because that is when pollen counts are highest. It is better to do outdoor exercise in the early evening, when the pollen counts tend to be somewhat lower, says Dr. Plancey. Or exercise indoors if you are very pollen-sensitive.

AVOID YARD WORK. "Mowing the lawn or raking leaves is highly inadvisable for someone with a pollen allergy," observes Dr. Plancey. "Better to pay some kid in the neighborhood to do the job."

If you must do these chores yourself, use a mulching mower, which drops the grass in place rather than blowing it out or into a bag, recommends Paul Ratner, M.D., an allergist in private practice in San Antonio, Texas. "And be sure to wash yourself off after you are finished to get all the pollen off your body."

PLANT THE RIGHT LAWN. "I tell people to plant lawns that are not allergenic," says Dr. Plancey. "For example, Saint Augustine grass and dichondra, which grow in warm regions of the United States, tend not to be pollinating grasses. But ryegrass, bermudagrass, and bluegrass all pollinate and cause allergic symptoms. Ask your allergist which nonpollinating grasses grow in your area."

SET YOUR SNEEZES SAILING. The seashore is often touted as a pollen-free zone. Dr. Plancey says that is true— sometimes. "It depends on which way the wind is blowing," he points out. "With an onshore breeze, pollen-free wind comes in off the ocean, and you get relief. If the wind is blowing sideways or it is blowing offshore, it won't do you any good at all because you are still getting pollen-laden wind." So check the weather report for wind conditions before you head for the beach. If it's an offshore breeze, you can save yourself a lot of sneezing by staying home.

HEADACHES: TENSION, MIGRAINE, AND CLUSTER
Head Off the Pain

Almost everybody gets a headache now and then, and a small dose of over-the-counter painkillers is usually all you need to send it packing. But what if you get headaches once or twice a week, or even every day, a condition doctors call chronic headache? Does that mean something is wrong with you?

If you are bothered by chronic headache, there is about a 1 in 10 chance that some other condition is causing the pain. It could be something as minor as a cavity or something as serious as cancer. So you need to tell your doctor about it. But in 90 percent of cases, all that is wrong with you is your ancestry. "Chronic headaches are usually an inherited physical illness," says Lawrence Robbins, M.D., assistant professor of neurology at Rush Medical College of Rush University in Chicago, director of the Robbins Headache Clinic in Northbrook, and author of *Headache Help*.

What Are the Real Signs of Sinus Headache?

"Sinus headaches are much less common than most people and most doctors think," says Lawrence Robbins, M.D., assistant professor of neurology at Rush Medical College of Rush University in Chicago, director of the Robbins Headache Clinic in Northbrook, and author of *Headache Help.* "Not a day goes by that I don't see someone who has been diagnosed with a sinus headache who actually has chronic migraine or tension headaches— headaches that could have been prevented or treated had they been properly diagnosed."

Any kind of headache can hurt in the sinus area. But a true sinus headache is linked to a sinus infection. When a sinus infection is the culprit, you will notice that your mucus turns slightly green and the sinus area is tender. In addition, you actually feel sick in other ways.

So if you have been blaming your sinuses for recurrent headaches, try out the preventive measures for chronic tension or migraine headaches. You may be able to clear up the headaches without antibiotics or other measures that doctors commonly prescribe for sinus conditions. Just make sure that you are being treated for the condition you do have, says Dr. Robbins.

Even if every member of your family gets headaches, however, that doesn't mean you are helpless. You can still find ways to prevent the pain, says Fred Sheftell, M.D., director and co-founder of the New England Center for Headache in Stamford, Connecticut; national president of the American Council for Headache Education (ACHE); and co-author of *Headache Relief for Women.* "Picture a stick of dynamite," he says. "The stick itself is a person's inherited predisposition to headaches, the biology. But what usually lights the fuse of that stick of dynamite are specific lifestyle and environmental factors—for example, the food you eat, the amount of sleep you get, the lighting in your office—and these factors are often within your control."

Since headaches of any kind are often triggered by something, if you can identify the factors that trigger your headaches, you will hold one of the keys to headache prevention. But the type of prevention you choose depends largely on what kind of headache you are prone to get. According to experts, there are basically three different types of headaches: tension, migraine, and cluster. Each can be triggered by different factors, so your first step is to figure out what kind you get, and then probe some of the possible causes.

Relieve the Tension

Three out of four people who get chronic headaches are afflicted by tension headaches. And even if you don't get the chronic form, there is a good chance that you have experienced the ache sometimes. The pain usually circles the head like a headband, and it is dull and steady. Scientists used to think that tight muscles around the head and neck produced the headache, until research showed that 50 percent of people who get headaches didn't have that kind of muscular tension. Now, scientists think that tension headaches are sparked by a possible combination of many factors, including tight head and neck muscles and a disturbance in what Dr. Sheftell calls the pain regulation centers of the brain.

Here are some ways to free yourself from this ache, whether it is chronic or occasional.

BE HEADSTRONG. Exercise helps prevent tension headaches by relieving stress and keeping muscles more relaxed, says Dr. Robbins. It also boosts levels of the endorphins, natural painkillers manufactured by the brain.

"People who experience tension headaches will probably have fewer headaches after a few weeks of exercise," says Dr. Sheftell.

The best kind of exercise to prevent headaches is aerobic exercise, says Dr. Robbins. Take 15 to 20 minutes out of your day for brisk walking, bicycling, jogging, swimming, or any other activity that gets your heart beating faster. But moderate activity of any kind is also helpful, whether it is a leisurely stroll around the block or weeding your garden. "Any type of exercise that you are likely to do on a daily basis is a good exercise," he says.

TAKE A DEEP BREATH. OR TWO. They don't call it a tension headache for nothing; stress can really put the squeeze on your noggin. That's why experts say that learning a tension-taming relaxation technique is a must for headache prevention.

Perhaps the easiest way to relax is to take a few deep breaths. "Practicing deep breathing for a minute or so, three or four times a day, can relieve tension and prevent headaches," says Dr. Robbins.

To do this, sit in a comfortable chair, rest your hands lightly on your belly, and close your eyes. Now count to four, inhaling for the entire count, then exhale for another count of four. While you inhale, make certain that you are breathing into your belly and not your chest. Belly-breathing is deep, relaxing breathing that expands your diaphragm, so your belly actually swells out. Avoid lifting your shoulders or expanding your chest—that's a sign of shallow, tense chest-breathing.

SEE YOUR WORRY LINES FADE. While you are doing deep breathing, try this visualization from Dr. Sheftell: Imagine the muscles in your forehead as scrunched-up, jagged lines. Now imagine them turning into perfectly smooth, evenly spaced lines. "Doing this visualization during deep breathing works really well to both soothe and prevent headaches," he says.

VISUALIZE A BALMY SCENE. While you are deep

Preventing Menstrual Migraines

For thousands of women, the menstrual cycle means a monthly headache. But relief may come in a surprisingly humble bottle. Anti-inflammatory medications may scrub menstrual-related migraines before they even got started, according to Seymour Diamond, M.D., director of the Diamond Headache Clinic and national chairman of the National Headache Foundation, both in Chicago.

In one study, Dr. Diamond asked 400 women with menstrual migraines to take a nonsteroidal anti-inflammatory drug (NSAID), starting several days before their periods began and continuing through menstruation. The drugs he tested were naproxen (Aleve), the prescription medication nabumetone (Relafen), and ibuprofen. Since women who take birth control pills are even more prone to menstrual headaches, Dr. Diamond asked any women taking the Pill to start the NSAIDs on the 19th day of their Pill cycles and continue it until the day after their periods ended. Dr. Diamond reports that there were fewer menstrual-related migraines in about 80 percent of the women who tested the NSAID regimen.

"The change in hormone levels that occurs with menstruation is probably the most common migraine trigger there is," says Dr. Diamond. Using NSAIDs to block the migraines could help eliminate the need for the heavy-duty medications that are used once a migraine has started, he suggests. But if you have menstrual migraines, talk to your doctor before you self-medicate.

breathing, imagine that you are lying on a sunny beach with gentle waves of warm water lapping the shore, says Dr. Robbins. This visualization helps you focus on your breathing and banishes distractions.

TRY SOME HERBS. The herbs ginkgo and feverfew are

often used to prevent chronic tension headaches. Ginkgo increases circulation to the brain, while feverfew boosts serotonin, a brain chemical that can help to prevent chronic headaches. Dr. Sheftell recommends 40 milligrams of ginkgo, taken in supplement form three or four times a day. More than 160 milligrams can be harmful, he says.

Try a supplement form of 125 milligrams of freeze-dried feverfew containing caffeine or guarana, recommends Dr. Robbins. His studies show that the freeze-dried variety is the most effective. Don't use feverfew if you are pregnant or nursing.

HOLD YOUR HEAD HIGH. Are you sitting with a phone cradled in your neck for hours a day? Are you hunched over a keyboard at work? Both of these postures can strain the muscles in your head, neck, and shoulders, and those muscle aches could be setting the stage for a tension headache, says Dr. Robbins.

For those people who spend long hours on the phone, Dr. Robbins recommends headphones. If you are wedded to your keyboard, adjust the height of your desk and the height and tilt of your computer so that your posture is upright and your arms and shoulders are relaxed. Take frequent breaks—get up from your desk and move around a bit every 20 minutes or so, hc advises.

AVOID THE REBOUND. Headache medications, or analgesics, work by shrinking the blood vessels around your brain, relieving the pressure and the pain. But large doses of these medications can create a rebound effect. After the blood vessels shrink, they swell again, which means that the pain can return, causing you to take even more medication. "People with chronic headaches who overmedicate can go from having a headache once every three or four days to having headaches every day," says Dr. Robbins.

"That's why the first thing a person with chronic tension headaches wants to do is make sure that he is not experiencing analgesic rebound," says Dr. Sheftell. If you are taking analgesics every day, see your physician to work out a program that weans you off the medications.

"There are many people who have gone from, say, six Excedrin a day down to two a day, and their headaches have gone away," points out Dr. Robbins.

CAN THE CAFFEINE, TOO. Caffeine addiction is also a source of rebound headache pain. Your best bet, says Dr. Robbins, is to consume less than 200 milligrams a day—that's less than two cups of coffee or five cups of soda or brewed tea. Avoid the withdrawal headaches that are associated with cutting out caffeine by slowly tapering your caffeine intake over a two-week period, he advises.

Mute the Migraine

Although both men and women seem to be affected by migraines, the condition is more common in adult women. Female hormones can trigger migraines, though scientists don't know how. Unlike the headband-style pain of tension headaches, migraines usually hurt on only one side of the head. The throbbing pain can become so intense that it leads to nausea and vomiting. A migraine may end after four hours, but the bad ones can last two days. Any activity, from climbing a flight of stairs to bending over to pick something up, makes it worse.

People get migraines because they were born with more excitable brains, says Dr. Sheftell. The migraine trigger—a specific food, a lack of sleep, a really bad day at the office—causes nerve cells in the cerebral cortex of the brain to act abnormally, becoming "manic" and then "depressed." This process knocks down the levels of serotonin and endorphins, two body-soothing, painkilling brain chemicals. Deprived of those chemicals, blood vessels on the surface of the brain expand and become inflamed. Here's how to keep an excitable brain calm.

Foods That Trigger Migraines

The foods listed below are extremely common migraine triggers, says Lawrence Robbins, M.D., assistant professor of neurology at Rush Medical College of Rush University in Chicago, director of the Robbins Headache Clinic in Northbrook, and author of *Headache Help*.

The migraine usually occurs within three hours of eating the food, but some food triggers are inconsistent. "On one occasion you may have a headache caused by a particular food, but the next time you eat that food, a headache may not occur," he says. Remain aware that some headaches are triggered by specific foods. If you notice that certain foods are a consistent trigger, avoid them.

You will also want to avoid any dishes or products containing ingredients that trigger your migraines, Dr. Robbins says.

Monosodium glutamate (MSG). This is also labeled autolyzed yeast extract, hydrolyzed vegetable protein, or natural flavoring. Possible sources of MSG include broths

WATCH WHAT YOU EAT. Certain substances in food may trigger migraines. Avoid the amino acid tyramine, which is found in aged cheeses, red wine, and beer, says Dr. Sheftell. You will also want to stay away from nitrates, used to cure meats, and the Chinese food flavor enhancer monosodium glutamate (MSG). (When you order a Chinese meal, be sure to specify "no MSG.") Researchers have also fingered histamine, which is in salami, Cheddar cheese, and other varieties of aged cheeses. (For more information, see "Foods That Trigger Migraines.")

DON'T BE A FATHEAD. A scientific study reported in the medical journal *Headache* suggests that if you cut back on fat, you may cut back on migraines, too. When 54 peo-

or stocks, seasonings, whey protein, soy extract, malt extract, caseinate, barley extract, textured soy protein, chicken or pork bouillon, smoke flavor, spices, carrageenan, meat tenderizer, and seasoned salt. Other possible sources are TV dinners, instant gravies, and some potato chips and dry-roasted nuts.

Ripened, aged cheeses. These include Colby, Roquefort, Brie, Gruyère, Cheddar, blue, brick, mozzarella, Parmesan, boursault, Romano, and processed cheese. Fresh cheeses are less likely to trigger headaches, but some people do have a reaction to cottage cheese, cream cheese, and American cheese.

Meats. Hot dogs, pepperoni, bologna, salami, sausage, and canned or cured meats such as ham and bacon are all known triggers. Also, keep an eye on aged meats or marinated meats.

Some alcoholic drinks. Red wine and beer are known to trigger migraines.

Chocolate and citrus fruits. If you notice that you get a migraine after eating these foods, you may need to avoid them.

ple with regular migraines went on reduced-fat diets for a full month, their headaches were less frequent, less intense, and shorter in duration. The people in this group also found that they needed fewer medications than when they ate their regular fare. When they started adding the fat back in, they started getting more migraines again.

This study found success with cutbacks to an ultralow 20 grams of fat (about 10 percent of calories from fat) in people who had previously been eating 80 to 120 grams of fat per day. Getting down to that level might sound difficult, but this diet is very achievable, says the study's leader, Zuzana Bic, Dr.P.H., assistant adjunct professor in the division of hematology and oncology at the University of California, Irvine, and preventive care specialist at the Chao Family Comprehensive Counsel Center in Orange. The key to achieving that level, she says, isn't to replace fatty foods with nonfat processed options. Instead, replace fatty foods with fruits, vegetables, legumes, and grains. But before you go on such an ultralow diet, be sure to talk to your doctor to make sure that you get the nutrients you need from nonfat sources or from supplements.

TAKE YOUR VITAMINS. "I put my patients on a multivitamin/mineral supplement to help prevent migraines," says Dr. Sheftell. Once they are taking the daily supplement, he recommends additional daily dosages of other nutrients that help prevent the body changes that trigger migraines.

Dr. Sheftell starts his patients with 200 milligrams of riboflavin the first week, increasing to 400 milligrams the second week, because scientific research shows that high levels of riboflavin decrease the frequency of migraines. His patients also get 50 to 100 milligrams of vitamin B_6 daily. That boosts the levels of serotonin, a brain chemical that can help to prevent migraines. For women, Dr. Sheftell prescribes an additional 200 milligrams of magnesium, increasing to 400 milligrams if the migraines don't ease up. Studies show that women who get migraines may have lower brain levels of magnesium than women who don't. Be sure to check with your doctor before treating yourself with supplements.

Supplemental magnesium may cause diarrhea in some people, and people with heart or kidney problems should check with their doctors before taking supplemental magnesium. Over prolonged time, unstable gait and numb feet may occur while taking vitamin B_6 in doses above 50 milligrams.

He also recommends that women take 400 IU (international units) of vitamin E the week before and the week after their periods since a change in hormone levels can trigger migraines and vitamin E helps mute the negative effects of hormonal changes. If you are considering taking amounts above 200 IU, discuss this with your doctor first. One study using low-dose vitamin E supplements showed an increased risk of hemorrhagic stroke.

After six months of positive results, stop taking the supplements in order to reevaluate your need for them, says Dr. Sheftell. In many cases, people grow out of migraine occurrence. If your migraines return, begin the same treatment and then reevaluate again in six months. If you don't notice positive results within three months, discontinue use, he says.

TALK TO YOUR DOCTOR ABOUT ASPIRIN. Results published from an ongoing study of 22,000 male physicians showed that those doctors taking 325 milligrams of aspirin every other day reported 20 percent fewer migraines than those taking a placebo. But you need to check with your doctor before you start taking aspirin regularly since it can have some harmful effects on the stomach and liver.

NOSH ON TIME. Varying any type of habitual behavior can trigger a migraine, says Dr. Sheftell. Skipping a meal is perhaps the worst offender. In one study, more than 40 percent of migraine patients cited missing a meal as the single biggest cause of their headaches.

RISE AND SHINE REGULARLY. Sure, everyone likes to sleep in on Saturday morning, but that could invite agony if you are prone to migraines. Getting up later than usual can trigger a migraine. To prevent headaches, go to bed and get up at the same time every day, advises Dr. Sheftell.

DIM YOUR BRIGHTS. Bright lights can cause migraine headaches, says Dr. Robbins. Since overhead fluorescent lights cause glare, try to use lamps with incandescent bulbs. If you have to contemplate a computer monitor all day long, use a glare screen. And if you wear glasses, choose the kind that darken automatically in bright light.

Bust the Cluster

There is no pain worse. "Cluster headaches used to be called suicide headaches because the pain is so bad that suicide can seem like the only way out," says Dr. Robbins. "I've asked women who get cluster headaches and who have had a baby whether they would rather have the headache or go through childbirth, and they always say that childbirth is less painful."

These mega-headaches are called cluster because they come in bunches. You will be free of them for months at a time, and then for no reason that scientists can identify, you start to get them again.

When the headaches return, they stay a while. Once or twice a day, for about an hour each time, over a period lasting a month or two, you experience an excruciating pain in one eye. "People say that it is like being stabbed in the eye with a hot knife," says Dr. Robbins. About 1 out of every 250 men and 1 out of every 800 women experience this type of headache. If you are among them, here are some ways to avoid the known triggers.

BE A REGULAR GUY OR GAL. One of the most important measures for preventing an outbreak of cluster headaches is to keep a regular schedule, says Dr. Sheftell. "Get up at the same time every day, go to sleep at the same time every day, and eat your meals at the same time every day." If your eating and sleeping schedule gets jumbled up, you might trigger a cycle of cluster headaches, he says.

STAY ON THE WAGON. When you are in a cycle of cluster headaches, alcohol will trigger a cluster instantly, says Dr. Robbins. So if you have had one of these headaches and you are praying to avoid the next one, don't go near wine, beer, mixed drinks, or even food and medicine that contain alcohol. Once safely past the cluster cycle, it seems to be all right to resume moderate drinking, he says.

PREVENT THE PAIN. Two treatments are remarkably effective at stopping cluster headaches almost as soon as

Don't Scream for Ice Cream

Eating ice cream or anything cold in a hurry can cause a sharp pain in your head often referred to as an ice cream headache. The cold food cools the back of your throat faster than the tissue can tolerate it, says Fred Sheftell, M.D., director and co-founder of the New England Center for Headache in Stamford, Connecticut; national president of the American Council for Headache Education (ACHE); and co-author of *Headache Relief for Women*. His preventive advice: "Warm the food by keeping it in your mouth longer before swallowing."

they start, thereby preventing an hour or so of terrible pain. One is breathing oxygen from a tank. "Sixty percent of people with cluster headaches get complete relief within a few minutes by breathing oxygen at the rate of eight liters a minute," says Dr. Robbins. The other treatment is the prescription drug sumatriptan (Imitrex).

"I've seen a lot of people with a cluster headache take Imitrex through a nasal spray, and within five minutes their pain goes away." If you have had cluster headaches before, talk to your doctor about being prepared next time with either of these two prescription treatments.

HEARING LOSS
Advice Worth Listening To

Until a hundred years or so ago, the loudest noise that earth's inhabitants were likely to hear would be the roar of a waterfall, the sound of musket fire, or maybe a church bell rung too loud and too often by an overly zealous parishioner. The blare of rock music and roar of jet engines just were not part of the sonic landscape.

All that changed with the industrial age. When locomotives, jackhammers, and amplifiers came along, the soundtrack of life increased far beyond anything nature had to offer. And the more intensely people were assaulted by noise, the less they ended up hearing.

That is because mega-decibel mayhem—a roaring lawn mower, trucks whizzing by, a rock concert—destroys nerve endings in the inner ear. At a certain point, usually around age 60, you may find yourself constantly asking people to repeat what they said. Or you may have to turn up the TV volume so much that your spouse complains. Or you begin to notice a constant ringing in your ears, signaling the onset of a hearing problem called tinnitus.

Hearing loss has several possible causes, but the number one cause is loud noise. It is also the most preventable cause.

In some parts of the world, people don't have hearing loss with age, says audiologist Kathleen Hutchinson, Ph.D., associate professor of audiology at Miami University of Ohio in Oxford. "That's because they are not exposed to excessive noise levels."

Here is how to protect your ears and keep your hearing intact.

IF IT HURTS, PUT IN THE PLUGS. There is an easy way to know whether the concert, the snowblower, or the barking bloodhound next door is affecting your long-term hearing: If your ears hurt, chances are that your hearing is being hurt, too—even if the person next to you is perfectly comfy, says hearing expert Harold Reuter, M.D., clinical assistant professor in the department of otorhinolaryngology at Baylor College of Medicine in Houston. His advice is to keep moldable silicone or foam earplugs handy and pop them in whenever you wince. These plugs are available at drugstores. Or pick up a pair of ear-muff-style ear protectors, which are available at sporting goods stores or in catalogs.

DON'T MAKE YOUR EARDRUM A BULL'S-EYE. Many people who shoot firearms for sport or target practice carelessly damage their ears. Even small-caliber weapons can cause gradual hearing damage. "Hunters and marksmen forget that gunshots are extremely intense," says Stephen W. Painton, Ph.D., associate professor of communication science and disorders at the University of Oklahoma Health Sciences Center in Oklahoma City. "Every time they shoot without hearing protection, they come away with a little temporary hearing loss, and soon it becomes permanent." Always wear earplugs or ear protectors when you shoot, he warns.

GET FIT TO PROTECT YOUR EARS. Everyone temporarily loses a bit of hearing after being exposed to noise. But a scientific study conducted in the department of communication at Miami University of Ohio showed that people who were physically fit had only half that loss compared with people who weren't fit. Researchers discovered this by having 28 people take hearing tests. The people in the group had varying levels of fitness, and those who were the least fit had the most hearing loss following noise exposure. Highly fit people, on the other hand, showed the least amount of hearing loss. And the highly fit folks weren't triathletes, just people who exercised briskly three or four days a week.

"Exercise may allow more oxygen-rich blood to be pumped to distant small areas, such as the inner ear," says study co-author Helaine M. Alessio, Ph.D., associate professor of physical education and sport studies at Miami University of Ohio. But there might be another reason: Exercise produces an increase in certain stress proteins, and these defend the organs of the inner ear against stressors, so the organs and tissues maintain their integrity longer.

HEARTBURN
Hold the Line on Stomach Acid

By any standard, digestive juices are totally unappetizing. Stomach fluid is a caustic cocktail of acid, food-dissolving enzymes, and other chemicals that bite. And the acid mix is meant to stay in your stomach, where a protective coating of mucus stops it from destroying your stomach lining. All perfectly normal. But sometimes, that juice sneaks into the esophagus, the tube from the mouth to the stomach. If enough juice lingers long enough, it burns the esophageal lining.

Block That Burn

Today, what is typically called heartburn sets more than 15 million Americans on fire. A lot of those folks probably use antacids to douse the flames. But you don't have to wait for a three-alarm esophagus to take action. You can prevent heartburn. Here is a roundup of current medical advice

---

Is It Heartburn—Or Your Heart?

Heartburn is often experienced behind the breastbone, in the same general area as the heart. That is why even doctors cannot always tell the difference between heartburn and heart attack without the use of sophisticated medical equipment.

If you have risk factors for heart attack, like obesity, a family history of heart problems, high blood pressure, or diabetes, be extra cautious when you notice chest pain, warns M. Michael Wolfe, M.D., chief of the section of gastroenterology at Boston University and Boston Medical Center.

Unusual pain around the heart or pain accompanied by nausea, vomiting, weakness, breathlessness, fainting, or sweating may signal a heart attack. And since every minute following a heart attack is crucial, head to the emergency room if you are unsure.

---

from M. Michael Wolfe, M.D., chief of the section of gastroenterology at Boston University and Boston Medical Center.

SUPPRESS ACID AT THE SOURCE. The newest approach to preventing heartburn involves a class of over-the-counter drugs called H_2-blockers (histamine-blockers), formerly available only by prescription. As their name implies, H_2-blockers block the stomach's ability to produce acid. (In contrast, antacids work after the fact by neutralizing existing acid.)

Currently, the Food and Drug Administration (FDA) has approved four H_2-blockers for preventing heartburn. They are Pepcid AC, Axid AR, Tagamet HB, and Zantac 75. Whichever brand you choose, don't expect relief for about 45 minutes. Taken as directed and for less than two weeks, H_2-blockers are safe and effective with very few side

An Apple a Day Recipe

Stomach-Soothing Salad

Sea vegetables like kelp and nori (the green wrapper used in making sushi) can help reduce the stomach acids that cause heartburn. Here, the sea vegetable hijiki and a fresh ginger dressing create the ultimate stomach-soother. Look for dried hijiki and tahini (sesame butter) in health food stores, Asian markets, and the international aisle of some supermarkets.

SALAD
- ½ cup crumbled dried hijiki or arame
- 2 tablespoons soy sauce
- ¼ cup rice vinegar
- 1 head Boston lettuce, torn into bite-size pieces
- ½ bunch of watercress
- 2 red radishes, sliced
- 1 cup alfalfa sprouts

DRESSING
- ¼ cup tahini (sesame butter)
- 1 tablespoon soy sauce
- 3 tablespoons water
- 2 tablespoons lemon juice
- 1 teaspoon grated fresh ginger
- 1 clove garlic, minced

To make the salad: Place the hijiki or arame in a medium bowl. Cover with water and let soak for 20 minutes, or until soft. Remove with a slotted spoon and place in a small saucepan. Allow the soaking water to settle, then add 1 cup of the clear part of that water to the pan. Discard the gritty remainder. Add the soy sauce and vinegar to the pan. Cover and simmer for 15 minutes. Drain, cool, and coarsely chop.

In a large salad bowl, toss the lettuce, watercress, radishes, and sprouts. Top with the hijiki.

> *To make the dressing:* In a small bowl, combine the tahini, soy sauce, water, lemon juice, ginger, and garlic. Serve with the salad.
>
> **Makes 4 servings.** Per serving: 135 calories, 10 g. fat

effects. If your symptoms persist for more than two weeks, see your doctor.

Pregnant women, children, and people with ulcers or kidney problems, however, should still consult their doctors before using any heartburn drug. And before you take an H_2-blocker, read the label's fine print about drug interactions, especially if you are on any prescription medication like blood thinners (Coumadin), seizure-disorder medications (Dilantin), or oral asthma medications (Ventolin).

SAVOR SOME SEAWEED. This unusual food found in health food stores and Asian markets in the form of kelp, wakame, nori, and other varieties can help form gels that bind up stomach acid, says Arthur Jacknowitz, Pharm.D., chairman of the clinical pharmacy department at West Virginia University School of Pharmacy in Morgantown. Simply cut it into strips and add to soups, salads, or stews.

Caution: If you are sensitive to sodium or have high blood pressure, rinse or soak sea vegetables before using them.

FORGO THESE FOODS. Certain foods relax the valve at the lower end of the esophagus, allowing acid to seep into the tube. Other foods stimulate excess acid production in the stomach. Still others contain lots of acid to start with. If you are prone to heartburn, here is the menu from which you don't want to order.

- Alcohol
- Carbonated drinks

Double-Whammy Drinks

Revelers, beware. While a festive drink may please your palate, certain combos (like citrus or tomatoes and alcohol) may rev up an uncomfortable episode of heartburn. If heartburn plagues you, there are a number of alcoholic beverages that you should probably avoid, according to M. Michael Wolfe, M.D., chief of the section of gastroenterology at Boston University and Boston Medical Center. Here is his list of potential undesirables.

- Peppermint schnapps
- Bloody Marys
- Mimosas
- Eggnog
- After-dinner coffees with cream and liquor

- Chocolate or caffeine, and any food or beverage containing them
- Citrus fruits
- Coffee and tea (both caffeine-containing and decaf)
- Fatty foods
- Garlic and onions
- Mint in any form, including tea, gum, jelly, candies, and breath fresheners
- Spicy foods
- Tomatoes
- Whole-milk and whole-milk dairy products

"MINI-MIZE" YOUR RISK. The bigger the meal, the more likely some stomach juice will spurt into your esophagus. Eating smaller, frequent meals, called mini-meals, can help prevent heartburn, says Dr. Wolfe.

DRINK WATER WITH YOUR MEALS. It rinses acid out of the esophagus and dilutes acid already in the stomach.

RELIEVE THE PRESSURE. Anything that puts pressure on your stomach right after a big meal can drive stomach acid upward into your esophagus. If you are planning to indulge in a sizable feast such as a traditional Thanksgiving dinner, avoid wearing clothes that are too tight. And don't exercise vigorously or carry anything heavy (like weights) for at least two to three hours after eating a big meal, says Dr. Wolfe.

STEER CLEAR OF THE COUCH AND BED. If you lie down within two hours after eating, heartburn is likely to take a nap with you. The horizontal position allows acid to flow out of the stomach and into the esophagus. For the same reason, schedule your supper well before bedtime so that you aren't headed for bed immediately after you eat.

STROLL AFTER DINNER. Walking after a meal gets gravity to do its part in keeping stomach acid where it belongs. And you can do it right after eating if you stroll at a leisurely pace.

AND CHEW SOME GUM, TOO. One of the best ways to prevent heartburn is to coat and protect your esophageal lining with saliva, and a great way to do that is to chew gum. Choose a sugarless variety if you want fewer calories, and remember to avoid the mint flavors. Also, be careful not to chew too much gum, cautions Dr. Wolfe. Three sticks of common sugarless gum can give you gas and diarrhea.

STOP FUMING. In case you needed another reason to avoid cigarettes, keep in mind that smoking inhibits saliva, stimulates stomach acid, and relaxes the protective muscle between the esophagus and the stomach. (All bad.) So ban the smoking, and you will be good to your esophagus.

HEART DISEASE
Aiming for Zero Risk

Imagine cutting your risk of heart disease to *zero*. Impossible? Not for most of us. With reams of data collected during decades of research, scientists have a pretty good idea why some people get heart disease and some don't. It all boils down to risk factors. As it turns out, almost all of those risk factors are within your control, and the one that isn't (family history) usually can be minimized by controlling the others.

Who says? One of America's foremost heart doctors, William P. Castelli, M.D., former director of the famed Framingham Heart Study and medical director of the Framingham Cardiovascular Institute in Massachusetts. As director of the longest-range research project designed to assess risk factors for coronary artery disease, Dr. Castelli has also applied what he has learned. At age 66, he is still holding heart disease at bay, unlike every other male member of his family, who started showing signs in their forties.

The secret? "Know, monitor, and change controllable

A Woman's Option: Hormones for Heart Health

Beginning at menopause, a woman's rate of heart disease slowly rises. By the time a woman reaches age 75, her rate is the same as that of a man. But women have a prevention tool that isn't available to men, and it is called estrogen. The incidence of death from heart disease in postmenopausal women who take estrogen during hormone-replacement therapy (HRT) is about *half* that of women who have never used it, says one of America's foremost heart doctors, William P. Castelli, M.D., former director of the famed Framingham Heart Study and medical director of the Framingham Cardiovascular Institute in Massachusetts.

Research shows that estrogen can reduce blood pressure, keep blood vessel walls from collecting plaque, and prevent blood vessels from constricting. Some scientists speculate that these benefits may prove to be even more important than estrogen's well-documented effect on cholesterol levels: It can raise high-density lipoprotein and lower low-density lipoprotein by as much as 15 percent. The experts also acknowledge that HRT is not right for every woman. The decision must be based on a careful evaluation of each individual's risk factors for heart disease and other health considerations.

Even when women do decide to take HRT, they must be closely supervised by a physician. Dosages and treatments often need adjustment for women to maximize benefits and minimize side effects, says Dr. Castelli.

risk factors," says Dr. Castelli, recently retired from the Framingham study. "If all Americans did this, heart disease would be eradicated, just as polio was."

CEASE SMOKING NOW. Smoking is the number one

risk factor for heart disease. If you smoke, you practically double your risk of a heart attack.

WALK TWO MILES A DAY. "Not exercising is almost as great a risk factor as smoking," says Dr. Castelli. For optimum heart protection, get into the habit of walking at least two miles a day or engaging in at least 30 minutes of moderate aerobic exercise. If you haven't exercised at all in the last year, however, begin slowly and with your doctor's okay. If you have had a heart attack, you should make sure that you are in a good cardiac-rehab program, monitored by your doctor.

DECREASE CALORIES TO MAINTAIN A HEALTHY WEIGHT. For maximum heart protection, you should weigh the same as you did at age 21, assuming that you were a good weight when you were younger, says Dr. Castelli. But weight alone doesn't predict heart disease risk. Fat distribution plays a role, too. "Tummy fat is the most dangerous kind of fat," says Dr. Castelli. "Even if you are not significantly over-weight, fat deposited on your belly can greatly exaggerate your heart disease risk. If a paunch hides your belt or if you can feel fat on your belly, you will know that you are at risk."

If you are overweight, modify your diet and exercise regimen until you achieve a one-half to one-pound weight loss weekly. (For tips on the best ways to lose weight and keep it off, see the prevention advice in Overweight on page 593.) The Framingham Cardiovascular Institute starts all patients on a 2,000-calorie diet, which is less than what most of us are eating to begin with. This calorie limit makes it easier to use the new Nutrition Facts labels, for which all values are based on 2,000 calories.

BEWARE OF LOW-FAT, HIGH-CALORIE FOODS. Though saturated fat (animal and tropical oils) and cholesterol may be public enemies number one and one-A, calories are a danger, too. "Low-fat and fat-free foods lull people into a false sense of security," says Dr. Castelli. We often eat these foods freely and end up gaining weight. Fat-free cookies and chips are not for people trying to lose weight. Think fruits, vegetables, and whole-grain products. You will get thin and reap more nutritional benefits.

DECREASE OVERALL DIETARY FAT. Defatting your diet helps you not only lower blood-fat levels but also shed pounds. To limit total fat, steer clear of bakery goodies, snack foods (such as chips and packaged cookies), and deep-fried foods (especially fast foods).

REDUCE SATURATED FAT TO NO MORE THAN 20 GRAMS DAILY. And make that amount 10 grams if you have already suffered a heart attack. "These are absolute maximums," says Dr. Castelli. "Anything less is better." To limit saturated fats, avoid butter and dairy products like whole and 2% milk, high-fat cheeses, and high-fat ice cream. Limit meat servings to three to four ounces daily. Choose only select grade meats, trim all visible fat, and prepare them by broiling or grilling. Even low-fat cheese should be limited to an ounce or two daily. When you do eat cheese, decrease your meat allowance by the same number of ounces that you increased your cheese.

LOWER YOUR BLOOD PRESSURE. When blood courses through blood vessels at excessive pressures day after day, it damages their surfaces. This makes them more prone to collecting fatty debris, which in turn can lead to the development of blood clots and possibly a heart attack or stroke. To lower your blood pressure, take these steps.

- Lose weight. "Losing as little as 5 to 10 pounds normalizes blood pressure in many people," says Dr. Castelli.
- Decrease sodium intake. Although not everyone is sensitive to salt's blood-pressure-raising ability, there is no way to predict who is. That is why Dr. Castelli recommends that everyone cut sodium intake to just 1,250 milligrams per day. The easiest

way to do this, he says, is to cut down on processed, canned, and convenience foods, and don't use salt in cooking or at the table.

• Find an outlet for your stress. Stress negatively impacts many body systems, blood pressure in particular. Dr. Castelli advises his patients to identify a stress-reduction strategy that works well for them— meditation, deep breathing, regular exercise, massage, to name just a few—and to stick with it.

Cholesterol and Related Blood Tests

When it comes to preventing heart disease, the measurement of cholesterol is a well-known measure of risk. That is why the National Cholesterol Education Program (NCEP) encourages you to know your numbers—your total cholesterol and high-density lipoprotein (HDL) cholesterol. You can find out those numbers with one quick blood test. And once you know what they are, you can take comparative measurements to find out whether your risk of heart disease is going up or down, which is a quick way to find out whether your preventive tactics are working.

Here are some ways to get cholesterol working in your favor.

CUT YOUR TOTAL CHOLESTEROL. For maximum protection, total cholesterol should be under 150—much lower than 200, which the NCEP suggests as a safe limit. "Thirty-five percent of people who have heart attacks actually have total cholesterol between 150 and 200," Dr. Castelli explains. "But people with total cholesterol levels under 150 just don't get heart disease." So if your cholesterol is under 150, you needn't concern yourself with the numbers for HDL and low-density lipoprotein (LDL) cholesterol. If your cholesterol is over 150, you need to take a look at your other blood-fat scores to determine how much of a risk you face.

Go for the French Factor

For years scientists have wondered why the rate of heart disease is so much lower in France than in the United States. This is especially remarkable given the fact that the French eat diets dripping with saturated fats, consuming almost four times more butter than Americans, for example. Now, studies suggest that the secret French factor may be flavonoids (pronounced FLAY-vuh-noyds), natural compounds found in the red wines beloved by the French. "We're pretty sure that it is the flavonoids that have a clear protective effect," says John Folts, Ph.D., professor of medicine and the head of the coronary thrombosis research laboratory at the University of Wisconsin Medical School in Madison. This extended family of compounds comes in almost all fruits and vegetables. Here are the best sources and simple ways to maximize flavonoids in your diet.

Favor the flavonoid superstars. The highest levels of flavonoids are found in onions, kale, green beans, broccoli, endive, celery, cranberries, and in the peel and white pulp of citrus fruit. Medium levels can be found in red wine, tea, lettuce, tomatoes, red peppers, broad beans, strawberries, apples, grapes, grape juice, and tomato juice.

Bag it. To brew tea with the most flavonoids, use tea bags instead of loose leaves, says Dutch researcher Michael Hertog, Ph.D., an epidemiologist at the National Institute of Public Health and Environmental Protection in

---

As for LDL cholesterol, this is the "bad" cholesterol component, the one that clings to artery walls and blocks blood flow. So, generally speaking, the lower your LDL number, the better. Your target should be 130 or below, or under 100 if you have had a heart attack.

If your total cholesterol or LDL cholesterol score is too high, you should restrict the amount of saturated fat

The Netherlands, who has compiled tables of flavonoid content in foods. The tea in bags is crushed into tiny pieces, making more surface area for flavonoids to dissolve into the hot water. Steep your tea for five minutes, Dr. Hertog advises.

SPARE THAT SKIN. Flavonoids in apples and other fruits are concentrated in the skin, which means that you will be tossing out some heart protection if you peel an apple before eating it. Though a wax coating is applied to about 35 to 40 percent of commercially shipped apples to retain moisture, health authorities (including researchers at the National Cancer Institute) say that the coating is safe. And if you just don't like that coating on your apple, you can remove it by scrubbing the fruit with lukewarm water and a soft vegetable brush.

TAP ORANGES' SECRET SOURCE. Bet you have been tossing out the flavonoids in oranges without knowing it. In citrus fruit, flavonoids cluster in the peel and in the white, pulpy parts. Peels are too bitter to eat (except in marmalade). But for a flavonoid fix, you can eat the albedo, the mild-tasting white material just under the outer peel and the core at the center of oranges, says Dr. Folts.

TRY ONIONS WITHOUT TEARS. Onions are a top source of flavonoids. But if you get tears when you chop them, try chilling onions in the freezer for 20 minutes to one hour before they hit the cutting board. The chilling treatment reduces irritating fumes.

you eat to no more than 20 grams per day. But that is a maximum. The less, the better. People who have already had a heart attack should limit saturated fat to just 10 grams daily, says Dr. Castelli. To further boost your cholesterol-lowering potential, eat foods high in soluble fiber, such as oat bran, beans, peas, and pearl barley. Tofu is also another heart-healthy food.

HIKE YOUR HDL. Higher is definitely better when it comes to this cholesterol number. In fact, Dr. Castelli recommends having an HDL level above 45, a bit higher than the 35 recommended by the NCEP. That is because this cholesterol, also known as the "good" one, appears to pick up cholesterol from deposits in your arteries and carry it to the liver for elimination.

If your total cholesterol is over 150, you also need to keep your eye on the ratio of total cholesterol to HDL cholesterol. This ratio outpredicts all other cholesterol numbers. If you divide your total cholesterol by your HDL cholesterol and score under 4, it means that you probably have enough good cholesterol on board to usher out the bad. In fact, a score under 3 may afford you protection similar to having total cholesterol below 150.

To raise your HDL score, prolong your exercise, but first ask your doctor what is safe for you. Instead of walking two miles per day, for example, you might want to try three miles. But stay away from speed, says Dr. Castelli. "Long, slow distance is best and safer."

If your ratio of total to HDL cholesterol is greater than 4, raising your HDL through exercise and lowering LDL through dietary changes should normalize it.

SLICE YOUR TRIGLYCERIDES. Too-high triglyceride levels are another factor associated with a greater risk of heart disease, according to Dr. Castelli—especially when the count reaches 150 or above. This is even true in some people with total cholesterol levels of 150 or below. (If you have already had a heart attack, you need to take an especially aggressive stand against these troublemakers by aiming for a target of 100 or below.)

If your triglyceride score is too high, restrict saturated fat. Restrict your intake of alcohol and refined carbohydrates such as candy, white bread, cookies, and cakes as well. Weight loss is particularly important in normalizing triglycerides.

How to Defuse Heart-Hurting Anger

Anger is probably as much of a risk factor for coronary disease as cholesterol, smoking, high blood pressure, and a sedentary lifestyle, says Redford Williams, M.D., professor of psychiatry and director of the Behavioral Medicine Research Center at Duke University Medical Center in Durham, North Carolina, and author of *Life Skills*. It is not the occasional moment of rage that ruins your heart, it is when you regularly explode outward or constantly hold it inside and stew. That can send your levels of stress hormones like cortisone and adrenaline as well as your blood pressure into the stratosphere.

Dr. Williams suggests that you learn to disarm the anger by asking yourself three questions.

1. Is the situation that is causing my anger important to me?
2. Is my anger appropriate to the objective facts of the situation?
3. Is there anything that I can do to modify the situation that is causing my anger?

A "no" answer to any of these questions means that this is not anger that is signaling you to take action. A "no" means that you need to chill out and tell yourself that it is not that important. Distract yourself, meditate, do whatever it takes to calm down and get your mind off the bothersome situation. If you answer yes to them all, Dr. Williams suggests confronting the situation in an assertive way. "Don't explode at the ticket clerk," he says. "Just ask directly for what you want."

HEART PALPITATIONS
Maintaining the Beat

We rarely pay attention to the steady thumping of our hearts. But there are exceptional times when the heart suddenly draws attention to itself. It thumps like a tom-tom or flutters like a pigeon fleeing traffic. Sometimes, it can even go on strike for a moment. What is going on?

An occasional irregular beat or so—technically known as a heart palpitation or arrhythmia—is generally quite common and usually quite harmless, says Paul N. Hopkins, M.D., associate professor of internal medicine at the University of Utah Cardiovascular Genetics Research Center in Salt Lake City.

But Dr. Hopkins warns that heart palpitations aren't always innocent. If they occur more than once a week or make you feel light-headed, they may signal a possible heart problem that should be checked by a doctor. And if you have a history of heart disease, call your doctor at once because arrhythmia may trigger a heart attack, he says.

Serving Your Heart

Fish oil can decrease the risk of fatal heart palpitations, according to a U.S. Physicians' Health Study of more than 20,000 doctors.

"I would definitely recommend increasing the dietary intake of fish or taking fish-oil supplements to anyone who has a history of arrhythmia," says Paul N. Hopkins, M.D., associate professor of internal medicine at the University of Utah Cardiovascular Genetics Research Center in Salt Lake City.

Eating fish as seldom as once a week significantly reduced the risk of sudden cardiac death in this study. Participants ate canned tuna fish, dark-meat fish (mackerel, salmon, sardines, swordfish, and bluefish), and other fish and seafood (shrimp, lobster, scallops). But even if you don't eat fish that often, you can get the same level of protection by taking fish-oil capsules, says Dr. Hopkins. Check with your doctor for the recommended dosage.

That said, there are some easy things that you can do to help prevent palpitations. Here is what doctors recommend.

CANCEL THE COFFEE AND COLA. Beverages like coffee and black tea, which are high in caffeine, stimulate the sympathetic nervous system that manages the heart rate. "It is best to avoid coffee and other caffeine-containing substances if you have heart palpitations," says Dr. Hopkins. Colas usually contain caffeine, and so does chocolate, though far less.

CLEAR THE SMOKE. Need another reason to quit cigarette smoking? The nicotine is a more damaging stimulant than caffeine. Tar and carbon monoxide from the smoke will also harm your heart, says Dr. Hopkins.

DECLINE THE WINE. "Alcohol makes every kind of irregular heart rhythm worse," says Dr. Hopkins. Eliminate the alcohol, and you may be able to prevent or reduce the symptoms of palpitations.

AVOID SECONDS. The dinner was so delicious that you would like a second helping. Be kind to yourself and your heart by eating more slowly, savoring each bite, and limiting the portions in your meals, says Dr. Hopkins. "Overeating decreases the blood supply to the heart as the blood flows into the intestinal tract," he says. "And that decreased supply can significantly increase the risk of arrhythmia." This advice is especially directed at people with a history of heart disease to avoid life-threatening arrhythmia.

HEAD FOR BED. Getting at least six or seven hours of uninterrupted sleep nightly keeps your heart on a regular pace and keeps you refreshed. "Being exhausted can bring on heart palpitations," says Dr. Hopkins.

SOOTHE YOUR STRESS. Excess stress can trigger irregularities in the heartbeat, says Bruno Cortis, M.D., a cardiologist in Chicago and author of *Heart and Soul: A Psychological and Spiritual Guide to Preventing and Healing Heart Disease*. He advises people who experience occasional heart palpitations to practice an antistress relaxation technique such as deep breathing every day.

"Take full, slow breaths from the belly and exhale," says Dr. Cortis. "Deliberate control of breathing forces everything in the body, including the mind, to assume the same controlled, relaxed state."

PACE YOURSELF. If you don't exercise regularly and you have a history of heart palpitations, a bout of sudden exercise such as shoveling snow or running to catch a bus can cause arrhythmia. If you have a history of heart palpitations or heart disease and a desire to get in better shape, Dr. Hopkins recommends that you take the slow, steady course to fitness. Begin an exercise program under medical supervision at a cardiac rehabilitation program.

SCRUTINIZE YOUR MEDICINE CABINET. Without your realizing it, your medicine cabinet may harbor medications containing stimulants that can cause heart palpitations. Dr. Hopkins recommends checking labels on all decongestants, asthma medicines, and over-the-counter diet pills to see if they contain the powerful stimulant ephedrine, or the less powerful stimulants pseudoephedrine or phenylpropanolamine. And avoid any *ma huang* herbal preparation because it contains ephedrine as well. Also check for caffeine, which is included in many medicines.

HEAT RASH
Letting Those Poor Pores Breathe

You probably haven't had a diaper rash lately. But if some sensitive sections of your skin stay wet and warm too long, you are likely to end up with an adult version of the same problem, the itchy, stinging, burning, tiny red bumps that doctors call miliaria rubra. By adulthood, this form of diaper rash gets called heat rash or prickly heat.

The exact mechanism by which heat and moisture team up to trigger this minor skin problem is still being debated by scientists. But one of the latest theories says that a breed of bacteria that lives on the skin (usually without causing any problems) produces a microscopic slime when your skin stays wet and hot for too long. While this is happening, the heat is also swelling your sweat glands, opening them up to invasion. So the surface slime plugs up the swelled sweat glands, causing the rash. Other scientists think that anything that irritates or clogs the sweat glands can cause the rash.

But whatever the cause of heat rash, the key to preventing this itchy annoyance is to treat your sweat glands right. Following are four pore-friendly actions.

PUT ON YOUR COOLEST CLOTHES. "Heat rash is often caused by tight clothing," says Ralph C. Daniel III, M.D., clinical professor of dermatology at the University of Mississippi in Jackson and a dermatologist in Jackson. When it is hot and humid—typical weather for Mississippi—he says to wear loose-fitting clothing that breathes and that has a light weave. Cotton is a prime candidate.

If you are prone to heat rash, avoid tight nylon and silk clothing, cautions Dr. Daniel. Those fabrics are tightly woven and don't provide the wicking action of cotton.

HANG UP THOSE JEANS. If it is a warm, humid day, you might want to pick another pair of pants other than jeans. "Jeans have a very tight weave and are more likely to cause heat rash," Dr. Daniel says.

STRIP OFF YOUR SWEATS. "If you exercise in a T-shirt and it gets sweaty, try to take it off as soon as you can—and definitely as soon as you have finished exercising," says Christen M. Mowad, M.D., assistant professor in the department of dermatology at the University of Pennsylvania in Philadelphia and co-author of a scientific study on the causes of heat rash. "One type of person who often gets heat rash is a runner who sweats a lot and wears a T-shirt. The T-shirt gets wet, he keeps it on, and the skin on his back develops a rash." The solution is to always have an extra, dry T-shirt around and change into it when the first one gets wet.

LOSE WEIGHT. If you are "wearing" too much fat, you can also find yourself with heat rash. Being extremely overweight is a major risk factor for the problem, says Dr. Daniel. The areas of the body where skin is constantly pressing on skin or where a skin fold covers skin generate lots of heat and moisture that can't escape.

Avoid the Morning Rash

What you do during your morning bathroom routine—in the shower and after—can help prevent heat rash.

USE AN ANTIBACTERIAL SOAP. Some dermatologists don't like to recommend antibacterial soap, such as Lever 2000, because it can dry the skin, causing all kinds of problems. But if you are prone to heat rash, you may want to give an antibacterial soap a try, says Dr. Mowad. It will help reduce the bacteria that can cause the rash.

RINSE IT OFF. No matter what kind of soap you use, rinse well before getting out of the shower, says Dr. Daniel. A soap residue on your skin can plug sweat glands.

GET DRIER THAN DRY. You should dry yourself extremely well after the shower, says Dr. Daniel. Leaving extra moisture on your skin is not helpful.

PAMPER YOURSELF WITH POWDER. Talcum powder or any moisture-absorbing powder will help dry the areas of your body that are prone to heat rash. Sprinkle some in your armpits and groin and dust your back with it. Some women need to powder under their breasts to avoid getting heat rash. But women should avoid powdering the genital area. Studies show that there may be an increased risk of ovarian cancer among women who routinely dust this area with talcum powder after bathing.

DOUBLE-CHECK YOUR DEODORANT. If you are prone to heat rash in your underarms, the problem might be the deodorant you are using, says Dr. Daniel. Antiperspirants can clog sweat glands and scented deodorants can irritate them. Switch to an unscented deodorant that doesn't contain an antiperspirant ingredient.

Cool Ways to Block It

Heat rash is from the heat, of course. So beat the heat before it gives you a bit of a beating.

DON'T GET SUNBURNED. Most people know about skin cancer risks and avoid getting sunburned for that reason. But there is another reason as well to block those rays. Sunburn causes swelling at the openings in the sweat glands, making it more likely that they will end up plugged, says Dr. Daniel. And plugged glands invite heat rash.

TURN ON THE FAN. If you don't get warm and sweaty in the first place, you are much less likely to get heat rash. So when it is hot and humid outside, turn on the air conditioner or fan and stay indoors.

DON'T COUNT ON COOL WATER. Watch out for long, cool baths, says Dr. Daniel. It may feel great on a hot summer day, but a bath does not prevent heat rash. When skin gets waterlogged from soaking in a bath, the pores where the sweat comes out become stopped up, he explains. That gets your skin set for another bout of heat rash.

HEEL PAIN
Prevention Can Be a "Shoe-In"

A heel can hurt for a lot of reasons—arthritis, a fracture, or a sore heel pad, to name a few. But by far, the most common cause of heel pain *and* the most common foot problem seen by podiatrists is plantar fasciitis (pronounced PLAN-tar fas-sy-EYE-tiss).

The plantar fascia are bands of ligaments that stretch from the ball of the foot to the heelbone, holding the muscles at the bottom of the foot in place. If these ligaments are repeatedly stretched too far or twisted too much, such as when your shoes don't provide the right support or when you are exercising too hard, they tug at the heelbone, causing a bruise and inflammation that *really* hurts.

If that stretching or twisting continues, extra calcium can accumulate at the site of the bruise and cause additional pain, a problem called a heel spur. Don't be surprised if that heel pain gives you a wake-up call the moment you step out of bed. Typically, the pain is most intense in the morning when the ligaments are tight. You will probably find that the pain eases as the ligaments warm up, but it begins to bite at your heels again as you walk around during the day.

Your heels don't have to treat you like a heel. With the right shoes and appropriate exercise, you can stomp out trouble before it begins.

BE IN A STABLE RELATIONSHIP—WITH YOUR SHOES. "The best way to prevent heel pain is to wear a stable shoe," says Lawrence Z. Huppin, D.P.M., a podiatrist at the Foot and Ankle Center of Washington in Seattle. That excludes a lot of slip-on dress shoes that don't provide a lot of stability and support. Moccasins, sandals, slippers—and other types of shoes that slip on rather than tie—can allow your foot to overpronate, or turn too far inward and flatten as you walk. This stretches the plantar fascia, leading to heel pain.

An experienced clerk in your shoe store may be able to guide you to shoes that are stable and provide good support. If no one is available to help you, have a look at the store's selection of running shoes. "Running shoes are usually very stable," says Richard Braver, D.P.M., a sports podiatrist and director of the Active Foot and Ankle Care Center in Englewood and Fair Lawn, New Jersey. He also recommends any athletic shoe that has a removable insert. If you want to wear sandals, he says that Birkenstock and Teva types are the ones that provide the most stability.

KEEP THEM ON. "Not only do you need to wear a stable shoe, you need to wear it in the house," says Douglas Hale, D.P.M., a podiatrist at the Foot and Ankle Center of Washington.

If you are in the habit of shedding your footwear for socks or slippers as soon as you get home, you may want to change your ways. Stable shoes won't protect your feet from heel pain unless you wear them all the time. "If you can fold your shoe in half and the toe touches the heel, then the shoe is too unstable," he adds.

CUSTOMIZE FOR EXERCISE. Tennis players shouldn't wear running shoes. Fitness walkers shouldn't stride out in shoes made for the racquetball court. The shoes may feel comfortable enough, but when you wear the wrong shoes for an activity, you sacrifice stability, says Dr. Braver. "Wear the proper shoes for your fitness activity."

KEEP YOUR FASCIA FLEXIBLE. If your plantar fascia are tight, you will be more likely to get heel pain, says Dr. Braver. "The more flexible you can make the plantar fascia, the less pulling there will be on the heelbone." To keep the area loose, take off your shoes and roll the bottom of your foot over a golf ball or foot massager (a set of rolling balls, usually made from wood). Foot massagers are available at many stores that sell health and beauty products. Do this for a few minutes once or twice a day, when you can get away with it at the office or at home.

NOTCH UP THE ACTION GRADUALLY. You can damage the plantar fascia if you try to do too much too soon in a fitness routine. "I often see women who start out attending aerobic classes two or three times a week, and then, when they decide they need to get fitter faster and start attending five, six, or seven times a week, they end up with heel pain," says Dr. Huppin. Start any fitness routine at a level where you are comfortable and pain-free, then increase the amount of activity by no more than 10 percent per week, he advises.

CUSHION YOUR PAD. If your heel pain is not caused by plantar fasciitis, it could be the pad of fat underneath the heel that is feeling some damage. "People who are overweight or people with high arches naturally put more pressure on their heels with every step," says Dr. Braver. That extra pressure eventually starts to hurt the pad. He recommends wearing a shoe that cups the heel more to prevent the fat pad from spreading out when the foot hits the ground. Most athletic shoes have contoured heel cups. In dress shoes, he recommends the brands Naturalizer, Red Cross, Rockport, Florsheim, Comfortech, or Easy Spirit because of their extra heel padding.

STRETCH YOUR CALF. Heel pain can also be caused by a tight Achilles tendon, which attaches your calf muscle to your heelbone. "I have people stretch their calf muscles three or four times a week before they go to bed to help prevent heel pain," says Arnold Ravick, D.P.M., a podiatrist at Capital Podiatry Associates in Washington, D.C. Here's how to do it.

Stand facing a wall, with your feet flat on the floor, your forearms on the wall, and your forehead resting on the backs of your hands. Bring your right foot forward until your toes are almost touching the base of the wall, and bend your right knee. Keep your left leg straight with the heel flat on the floor. Keeping your toes pointed straight ahead, move your hips a little toward the wall. You should feel a full stretch in the calf and ankle of the left leg. Hold the stretch for 30 seconds. Change position and repeat to stretch out the other leg.

During the stretch, you can also tone the Achilles tendon. When you are leaning against the wall, slightly bend the knee of the back leg, keeping the entire foot on the floor. This gives the lower leg a stretch, which helps keep the ankle stable.

HEMORRHOIDS
Stop the Swelling Before It Starts

Hemorrhoids aren't caused by sitting too much. And they are not caused by being overweight. Nor are they caused by stress, spicy foods, or smoking, according to Steven D. Wexner, M.D., chief of staff at the Cleveland Clinic Florida in Fort Lauderdale and professor of surgery at the Cleveland Clinic Foundation Health Sciences Center at Ohio State University in Cleveland.

Yet all of these factors have been blamed for causing hemorrhoids. The truth is that most often, those annoying, sometimes painful, swellings of anal tissue can be traced to a diet that is short on fiber and fluid.

Here is the hemorrhoid chain of events. If you don't get enough fiber, your stool tends to be small and hard. And if your stool isn't bulky enough, the colon can't get a grip on it and move it along the path to elimination. Consequently, you have to strain during bowel movements. So straining connected to constipation is thought to be one of the most common causes of hemorrhoids, says Dr. Wexner.

An Apple a Day Recipe

Sittin' Pretty Breakfast Cereal

Swiss breakfast cereal is loaded with fiber-rich oats, which may help keep your seat smooth and hemorrhoid-free. Plus, you can change the fruit to suit your tastes. Use oranges, grapefruit, pineapple, grapes, or strawberries in place of the tangerines. Substitute pears or peaches for the apples.

1⅓ cups rolled oats	2 tangerines, peeled
2⅔ cups water	and sectioned
¾ tablespoon nonfat plain	2 unpeeled apples,
or vanilla yogurt	chopped
1 tablespoon honey	

Place the oats in a large bowl. Add the water and let soak for 1 hour or overnight. Stir in the yogurt, honey, tangerines, and apples. Divide among 4 serving bowls.

Makes 4 servings. Per serving: 323 calories, 4 g. fat, 10 g. dietary fiber

"Prolonged, chronic straining while attempting to defecate may possibly create pressure in blood vessels and predispose a person to swollen hemorrhoids," says Dr. Wexner.

The best way to head hemorrhoids off at the pass is to add fiber to your diet. "If you eat adequate amounts of fiber, you will ensure that you have large, soft, easy-to-pass stool," says John G. Lee, M.D., a gastroenterologist and assistant professor of medicine at the University of California, Davis. That will decrease the straining during bowel movements and decrease the chances that you will get inflamed hemorrhoids.

To help you take the preventive track, here are some stool-moving notes on fiber from Drs. Wexner and Lee.

SEE TO YOUR CEREAL. Choose the right breakfast cereal, and you may be purchasing daily insurance against hemorrhoids. Brands like Fiber One, All-Bran, and 100% Bran are loaded with dietary fiber.

BECOME A FRUIT FANATIC. Fresh fruits are also a good source of fiber. Apples, apricots, oranges, pears, and berries are especially good. Be sure to eat the skin of apples and apricots to maximize the fiber factor.

BE A MELON MANIAC. The type of fiber in melons, soluble fiber, is especially good for preventing hemorrhoids. Soluble fiber absorbs water as it moves through your system. The water makes your stool both heavier and larger. This helps move the stool through your colon quickly and without strain.

SNACK ON RAISINS. These wrinkled-up grapes are handy fiber servings. Substitute them for other between-meal snacks.

GET VIGOROUS ABOUT VEGETABLES. Many fresh vegetables are loaded with fiber. Among the best sources are broccoli and corn, especially white corn. Other excellent garden crops that are loaded with fiber include artichokes, green peas, and sweet potatoes.

BE A BEAN COUNTER. Beans are sources of fiber as well. Eat kidney beans, chickpeas, lima beans, and black beans to bulk up your stool and avoid the straining that leads to hemorrhoids.

AIM FOR GRAINS. Oat bran is famous as a fiber source, and wheat bran is even better. Breads and cereals are great sources. Just be sure you get foods containing wheat germ or whole wheat. If the wheat has been processed—as in white bread, for example—you get far less fiber. When you check for labels on bread, look for the words "whole wheat" or

Preventing the "Workout" Hemorrhoid

If you have already had a bout of swollen hemorrhoids, strenuous exercise can cause a flare-up, says Lester Rosen, M.D., a colorectal surgeon in private practice in Allentown, Pennsylvania. On the other hand, you don't want to stop exercising just because you have had hemorrhoids. Here are two ways to avoid future problems.

WARM UP TO A TOPICAL. To relieve itching and burning that may make you uncomfortable during your workout or any other time, Dr. Rosen suggests using a hydrocortisone hemorrhoid agent. Among the brands available are Anusol-HC and Preparation H hydrocortisone cream. Apply these preparations two or three times a day for up to three weeks, but don't use them any longer, he advises. They can break down delicate tissues.

RETHINK YOUR ROUTINE. "If you are doing squats, especially with weights, as part of your exercise routine, you may want to consider finding a substitute," says Dr. Rosen. Squats can put the kind of direct pressure on the lower rectum that can trigger a swelling. And avoid exercise routines that involve prolonged sitting, such as long bike rides, he cautions. No matter how you work out, take frequent breaks and wear comfortable, nonirritating clothing, he advises.

"whole-wheat flour" at the top of the ingredient list. Other grains that are rich fiber sources include bulgur and barley.

JUST ADD WATER. Fiber builds bulkier, softer stools by absorbing water into the intestinal tract. By drinking plenty of water, you speed up the digestive process and avoid swollen hemorrhoids.

"Most people drink only two to three glasses of water a day, and that's not enough," says Dr. Wexner. He recommends a daily intake of at least 64 ounces of water or juice.

Great Sources of Fiber

Getting plenty of fiber in your diet is the best way to prevent swollen hemorrhoids, say experts. Here are some of the best sources.

FOOD	PORTION	GRAMS OF FIBER
General Mills Fiber One Cereal	1 oz.	12.3
Kellogg's All-Bran Cereal	1 oz.	9.2
Nabisco 100% Bran Cereal	1 oz.	7.8
Lentils	½ cup	7.8
Black beans	½ cup	7.5
Figs, dried	3	6.9
Refried beans, canned	½ cup	6.7
Kidney beans	½ cup	6.5
Chickpeas	½ cup	6.2
Navy beans	½ cup	5.8
Guava	1	4.9
Artichoke hearts	½ cup	4.5
Lima beans	½ cup	4.5
Peas, green	½ cup	4.4
Pears, dried halves	3 halves	4.3
Succotash	½ cup	4.3
Raspberries	½ cup	4.2
Bulgur	½ cup	4.0
Oatmeal	½ cup	3.9
Pear	1	3.9
Blackberries	½ cup	3.8
Post Raisin Bran Cereal	1 oz.	3.8
Sweet potato	1	3.4
Spaghetti, whole-wheat	½ cup	3.2
Orange	1	3.1
Apple	1	3.0
Apricot, dried, halves	½ cup	2.9
Barley, pearled	½ cup	2.9

That's eight eight-ounce glasses. "That amount of fluid will work with the fiber to create a soft stool," he says.

SUBTRACT THE FAT. "Along with getting more fiber and water, you also should cut down on saturated fat, which can cause a harder stool," says Dr. Wexner. "That means eating less red meat, fewer high-fat dairy products, and fewer processed baked goods."

TAKE A STROLL. Thirty minutes or so of aerobic exercise a couple of days a week can help prevent constipation, which means that it can also help prevent swollen hemorrhoids, says Dr. Lee. Go for a brisk walk, ride a stationary bike, or swim some laps.

HEPATITIS
Keep Your Liver Virus-Free

Nestled safely beneath the diaphragm in the upper right side of your torso, the liver is your silent buddy in health protection. Larger than any other internal organ—even larger than your brain—your liver performs over 500 tasks. One of its main functions is to filter your blood, scrubbing out anything that might be harmful—like alcohol or pollutants—and getting rid of those infiltrations by turning them over for waste disposal.

Should your liver become infected, it becomes inflamed. The result—hepatitis—can wreak havoc with your health, causing flulike symptoms, jaundice, and sometimes even liver failure.

Five different viruses can cause hepatitis. But you can easily outwit the three major strains and help prevent their delivery of liver problems. Your liver will thank you.

Simple Protection against Hepatitis A

The virus hepatitis A originates in feces and is transmitted through person-to-person contact or via contaminated food and water.

You are at highest risk for hepatitis A if you travel to areas where there are high rates of hepatitis A and sanitation is inadequate. Among the areas where you might be at risk are Central or South America (including Mexico), Southeast Asia, and China. Here is how to protect yourself when you are at home or away, says Miriam Alter, Ph.D., chief of epidemiology in the hepatitis branch of the Centers for Disease Control and Prevention.

DOUSE YOUR DIGITS. Wash your hands after every trip to the bathroom and after changing a diaper. Also, wash your hands before meals and snacks—no exceptions.

WATCH WHAT YOU DRINK. Stick to bottled soda, juice, and water. And if you are drinking bottled water in a foreign country, make sure that the cap has remained sealed. You want a container of water that was bottled at the source, not refilled with tap water. Avoid having ice in your drinks because it may be made from contaminated water.

PEEL YOUR FRUIT YOURSELF. If you peel fruit carefully, you will remove the virus with the skin. The fruit underneath is fine as long as you don't eat it with tainted fingers. So wash your hands after you peel any raw fruit.

EAT WELL-COOKED MEAT AND VEGETABLES ONLY. Avoid raw or undercooked seafood as well since it may have been harvested from contaminated water.

GET VACCINATED. Don't leave home without getting a vaccine. Hepatitis A vaccines are available for long-lasting protection for persons two years of age and older. The vaccines are very safe with the most common side effect being soreness at the site of injection. It is important to be vaccinated at least four weeks before traveling. Immune globulin, a preparation of antibodies, may be used for children under two years of age, for anyone desiring short-term protection, or for prevention of infection after exposure. Talk to your doctor about what is right for you.

Steer Clear of Blood—and Hepatitis B

Each day, as many as 14 Americans die from illnesses related to the hepatitis B virus (HBV), which infects up to 320,000 people each year. But many of those infected with this virus don't even realize that they are. Hepatitis B targets the liver, but the B-type virus is more aggressive than A and more likely to cause chronic or even fatal liver problems.

Hepatitis B is spread primarily by sexual contact with an infected person. HBV is also spread among people who share needles and drug paraphernalia while injecting illegal drugs and from an infected mother to her baby at birth.

The Centers for Disease Control and Prevention recommends that anyone at risk should be immunized. Three shots in six months will give you a lifetime of protection. High-risk groups include anyone who engages in anal sex, men and women who have sex with more than one person, and health-care workers.

"Basically, any sexually active adult who wants to avoid getting hepatitis B should be immunized," says Gary Noskin, M.D., associate professor of medicine in the division of infectious diseases at Northwestern University Medical School in Chicago.

Hepatitis C: Not from Casual Contact

As many as four million people in the United States could be infected with hepatitis C, which, like other forms of the virus, can cause chronic liver problems. Most people who contract hepatitis C do so by sharing needles while injecting illegal drugs. The virus may also be transmitted through sexual contact.

Assuming that a person has never experimented with self-injection, the remaining preventive measures are safe work practices and safe sex, according to the National Institutes of Health. If you handle blood or blood products in the workplace, be sure to follow good infection-control measures. Also, unless you are involved in a long-term one-on-one relationship and you are certain that you and your partner are both monogamous, use a latex condom during intercourse.

HICCUPS
Get the Hic Out

Seems like everybody has their favorite treatment for hiccups: Eat a teaspoon of dry sugar. Gently pull on your tongue. Drink a glass of water as fast as you can. But what if those annoying and seemingly useless "hics" and "hucs" have started to bother you a little too often and you would like to *prevent* hiccups? Well, even though scientists haven't figured out exactly what causes a hiccup, they have figured out some ways to make the spasm less likely to occur. Here are some recommendations from Jack A. DiPalma, M.D., professor of medicine and director of the division of gastroenterology at the University of South Alabama College of Medicine in Mobile.

PUT YOUR FORK IN FIRST GEAR. Eating too fast causes you to swallow air, which may irritate the diaphragm, the all-encompassing umbrella of muscle that is under the lungs and above the cavity that houses your stomach, intestines, and other organs. When the diaphragm gets irritated, it goes into a spasm, which sets off the hiccups. The

A Cure for GERD

GERD is gastroesophageal reflux disease, better known as severe heartburn. When acid seeps upward into the esophagus—the food tube leading to the stomach—you will experience heartburn symptoms such as a burning sensation behind your breastbone and the sour taste of stomach acid in your mouth. And sometimes this upward invasion of stomach acid leads to another problem—long bouts of hiccups.

"Over a dozen scientific studies have reported a link between GERD and hiccups," says Jack A. DiPalma, M.D., professor of medicine and director of the division of gastroenterology at the University of South Alabama College of Medicine in Mobile.

If you hiccup a lot and are prone to frequent attacks of heartburn, talk to your doctor about medications that can treat the problem, suggests Dr. DiPalma.

slower you eat, the less likely hiccuping will occur. "Slow down at meals by chewing thoroughly and carefully," says Dr. DiPalma.

CONSTRAIN YOUR SIPPING. Another way to break the back of hiccups is with a straw.

If you have had frequent, long bouts of hiccups and you want to make sure it doesn't happen again, take along extra straws wherever you go—and always use one when you drink cold beverages. A straw helps because it limits the amount of air you swallow.

HOLD THE BUBBLES. Soda and beer can spark a bout of hiccups because the carbonation sets off those unwanted diaphragm spasms. "Carbonated beverages that are cold are the worst," says Dr. DiPalma. So if you need a soda now and then, let it warm up a bit. And skip the ice.

GO FOR "JUST RIGHT." Any food or drink that is too

hot or too cold can set off a bout of hiccups because foods at extreme temperatures stimulate irritation. For smoother, hic-free dining, let that piping-hot casserole cool down a few minutes.

DON'T PLUMP UP YOUR TUMMY. Overeating may cause a bout of hiccups by irritating the diaphragm. Never eat to the point where you feel too full, says Dr. DiPalma.

BE A TEETOTALER. Cartoon characters like Andy Capp *always* go "hic" when they are drunk. In real life, some people start hiccuping at the first sip of alcohol.

"If you find that you have bouts of hiccups when you drink that are protracted, I would recommend abstinence from alcohol," says Dr. DiPalma.

KEEP YOUR LUNGS OPEN. Smoking can cause hiccups if you are prone to them because it causes you to swallow air, and nicotine is an irritant that lowers the pressure of the esophageal sphincter. The esophageal sphincter is the muscle, linking the esophagus to the stomach, that keeps stomach acid from coming back up into the esophagus. It is not the prime reason to stop smoking, of course, but certainly a side benefit of stopping. (For a stop-smoking strategy, see "Stop in the Name of Your Lungs" on pages 524–25.)

CHECK YOUR MEDICINES. If you have started to take a new medicine and notice that you are hiccuping a lot more, you may be suffering from a minor-league side effect.

Anti-anxiety medications like diazepam (Valium), for example, can sometimes cause the problem. If you think a medication is making you hiccup, ask your doctor about prescribing an alternative.

HIGH BLOOD PRESSURE
The Lowdown on Prevention

It seems as though a lot of Americans are living the high life, a life that leads to high blood pressure, that is. Only about half of us have what doctors call optimal blood pressure—a reading of no more than 120/80 (the top number is your systolic pressure, which is how hard your heart has to pump to circulate your blood, and the bottom figure is your diastolic pressure, which is the pressure between heartbeats). About one out of every four adults has a reading of 140/90 or higher, which counts as high blood pressure. And another one-quarter of the population is somewhere in the midrange, which means that they are probably at risk of developing it. As people age, the situation gets worse. Nearly half of all older Americans have high blood pressure.

Those percentages prophesy bad news. High blood pressure (hypertension) makes us five times more prone to strokes, three times more likely to have a heart attack, and two to three times more likely to experience heart failure.

Prevent the Mild from Getting Worse

Often, doctors don't start giving treatment to people who have mild high blood pressure, according to William B. White, M.D., professor of medicine and chief of the section of hypertension and clinical pharmacology at the University of Connecticut Health Center in Farmington. "They wait until the hypertension is worse."

Unfortunately, even mild high blood pressure increases your risk of stroke and heart attack, according to Dr. White. What doctors call mild high blood pressure means that your systolic reading is between 140 and 159 and your diastolic pressure is between 90 and 99. So anything between 140/90 and 159/99 is classified as mild or Stage I hypertension.

Dr. White thinks that doctors fail to see Stage I hypertension as a significant problem if a person is otherwise vigorous and healthy. "They think, okay, this person is 40 and pretty healthy with a blood pressure of

One-third of the folks who have high blood pressure don't know it because you never feel any direct pain from high blood pressure. But over time, the force of that pressure damages the inside surface of your blood vessels like tunnel walls getting scarred by BB pellets. Fatty debris sticks easily to rough walls, vessels narrow, and clots can form. When clots break loose, they can cause a heart attack or stroke. Even if that doesn't happen, the buildup of pressure causes the heart to labor and strain.

But high blood pressure isn't inevitable, say experts. "Reducing salt intake, adopting a desirable dietary pattern, losing weight, exercising, and moderating alcohol can all help prevent high blood pressure," says Lawrence J. Appel, M.D., associate professor of medicine, epidemiology, and

140/90," he says. "And the patient thinks that he is healthy because he doesn't have something bad enough to get medicine for."

But mildly elevated blood pressure is likely to become even higher over time, Dr. White points out. Five years later, the patient's blood pressure might be 160/110. "During that interval, some damage may have occurred, such as cardiac changes associated with blood pressure elevation or some kidney problems," he says.

Other doctors advocate intervention when blood pressure is high-normal, with a reading of 130 to 139 systolic and 85 to 89 diastolic. "If blood pressure is 135/85, the risk of cardiovascular disease is increased," says Ray W. Gifford Jr., M.D., professor of internal medicine at Ohio State University College of Medicine in Columbus and consulting physician in the department of nephrology and hypertension at the Cleveland Clinic Foundation in Cleveland. "That's the time to get to it. There is really good evidence that you can prevent high blood pressure then, before it gets worse," he says.

international health at the Johns Hopkins University Medical Institutions in Baltimore. Let's look at those preventive factors, and a few more, one by one.

Weight loss is an excellent starting point if you want to prevent high blood pressure. "Being overweight is linked to an increased risk of developing high blood pressure, and losing weight decreases the risk," says James Hagberg, Ph.D., professor of kinesiology at the University of Maryland in College Park. In one study, 15 overweight people with normal blood pressure who lost an average of 13 pounds over a three-month period had a 12-point drop in their systolic pressures and an 8-point decrease in their diastolic pressures. Meanwhile, here are some other steps that you can take to help keep the pressure off.

Control Your Salt Intake

Salt is sodium chloride. If you are sodium-sensitive, it means that your blood pressure rises in reaction to increased salt intake. "All people are, more or less, sodium-sensitive," says Norman Kaplan, M.D., professor of internal medicine in the hypertension division at the University of Texas Southwestern Medical School in Dallas. "It varies a great deal among individuals. Some people are exquisitely sensitive. If they touch salt, their blood pressures go way up. For a few others, their intake hardly seems to matter." But everyone who doesn't have high blood pressure would be wise to moderate their intake as a preventive measure, he advises.

And we live in a sodium-dense world. The average American consumes between 3,000 and 6,000 milligrams of sodium each day, Dr. Kaplan observes. That's quite a few shakes beyond the 2,400 milligrams that the National Academy of Sciences suggests as a maximum intake for just about everyone. A level teaspoon of salt contains about 2,400 milligrams of sodium. So if your current intake is 3,500 milligrams or less, you can get yourself to the adequate-intake zone by getting rid of about a half-teaspoon of salt each day. Here is a plan to help you do just that.

DON'T REACH FOR IT. "Salt poured on food is the thing that people have the most immediate control over," says Dr. Kaplan. If you customarily sprinkle salt over every entrée, try to shake the habit. You might miss the saltiness at first, but if you substitute spices or just savor the hidden flavors a little more, you can easily get used to less sodium.

SAY YES TO NO-SALT COOKING. "Begin eliminating some salt from your cooking," says Harvey B. Simon, M.D., professor of preventive cardiology at Harvard Medical School. "Look upon your low-salt cooking as a great opportunity to experiment with new flavors and seasonings. Your tastebuds will love you."

Label Shakeout

Here is a simple guide to deciphering food labels to help you figure out how much salt is really in the food you just bought.

Sodium-free. Less than 5 milligrams per serving. No need to restrict yourself since 400 servings a day would still keep you at 2,000 milligrams of sodium.

Very low sodium. There are 35 milligrams or less per serving. You are still in the safe zone, but be sure to note how much is in a serving and stick to one serving.

Low sodium. One serving contains 140 milligrams or less. Don't get reckless. A few servings can add up in a hurry, especially if that sodium is in a condiment like salad dressing.

Reduced sodium. Three-quarters less sodium than is typical for that food. Fact is, many foods are typically high in sodium, so reducing that amount may not be as helpful as you think.

Also, any type of salt is high in sodium, no matter how it is described on the label. Don't be fooled by labels like sea salt, onion salt, brine, garlic salt, and seasoned salt. All are filled with sodium, just like normal everyday table salt.

CLOSE DOWN THE SALT MINES. Start to limit the foods that Dr. Kaplan calls salt mines, such as potato chips, pickles, salami, and many processed foods. "All we are talking about here is taking a few of life's pleasures away," he says.

Salty snack foods like potato chips are a crunchy way to overdose on sodium. "You would need to eat 10 whole potatoes to get the amount of sodium in just 10 potato chips," says Dr. Simon.

But you can also find a high sodium content in canned goods, some frozen foods, baked goods, and many staples at fast-food restaurants. When you are shopping, be sure to read food labels to find your way past the salt mines in the supermarket. (For more information on how to determine the salt content of foods from food labels, see "Label Shakeout.")

Add Vitamins and Minerals

It is not only what you take out of your diet that can help you prevent high blood pressure, it is also what you put in. One of the most important dietary factors is potassium. Other nutrients that can help protect you are calcium, magnesium, and folate. Here are some hows and whys for getting these benefits into your diet.

PILE ON THE POTASSIUM. "You can think of potassium as the opposite of sodium," says Dr. Simon. Low potassium intake can raise blood pressure, but this doesn't mean that huge amounts of potassium are needed.

The Daily Value for potassium is 3,500 milligrams, "but it is safe to consume more than that, unless you have kidney disease or you take spironolactone (Aldactone) or other medications that cause the body to retain potassium," says Dr. Simon. Bananas are an easy source of potassium, so don't hesitate to add them to your cereal in the morning. Other fruits and vegetables are also potassium-rich, including dried apricots, dried prunes, spinach, boiled potatoes with skin, boiled lima beans, baked sweet potatoes with skin, cantaloupe, and winter squash.

ADD SOME MORE "-UMS." Along with potassium, calcium and magnesium may also help prevent high blood pressure, says Dr. Simon. Though scientists can't explain why, people with high blood pressure tend to have less of these minerals in their systems than do people with normal or low blood pressures.

To be certain that you are getting enough calcium, be sure to include skim milk, nonfat yogurt and cheese, and broccoli in your diet. Other sources include canned salmon with bones, sardines with bones, corn tortillas processed with lime, and calcium-fortified orange juice. Good food sources of magnesium include brown rice, avocados, spinach, haddock, oatmeal, baked potatoes, navy beans, lima beans, broccoli, nonfat yogurt, and bananas.

PROTECT YOUR PRESSURE WITH FOLATE. The B vitamin folate may help prevent high blood pressure. And you can easily get more of it in your diet if you read the labels on bread and cereals and look for the brands that are fortified with folate.

Folate is believed to lower a blood factor called homocysteine. Researchers theorize that high levels of homocysteine may reduce the stretchability of arteries. When arteries are too stiff to help move blood around effectively, the heart has to work even harder. This pushes pressure ever upward, explains Kim Sutton-Tyrrell, Dr.P.H., an epidemiologist at the University of Pittsburgh.

With plenty of B vitamins, researchers hope, the arteries might be able to remain more elastic—at least enough to help prevent high blood pressure. Until the results are in, "people should be paying a lot of attention to what they are eating and should be making sure that they are getting enough foods with these types of vitamins in them," says Dr. Sutton-Tyrrell.

In a study led by Dr. Sutton-Tyrrell, researchers found that people with one kind of high blood pressure problem had higher homocysteine levels than those with normal blood pressures. But the study didn't show how much folate it might take to lower homocysteine levels.

For general health, the Centers for Disease Control and Prevention recommends getting 400 micrograms of folate daily. So it is wise to start filling up on the most chock-filled folate finds. Along with fortified breads and cereals, be sure to pick up some asparagus (250 micrograms per cup), brussels sprouts (125 micrograms per cup), or any variety of beans (100 to 300 micrograms per cup).

DASH to the Produce and Dairy Sections

DASH stands for "Dietary Approaches to Stop Hypertension," and it is the name of a large scientific experiment that tested whether a healthy way of eating could lower high blood pressure. The study found that people with high blood pressure who consumed 8 to 10 daily servings of fruits and vegetables and approximately 3 daily servings of low-fat dairy products, and limited the total fat in their diets to 25 percent of calories had a significant drop in blood pressure.

"Following the DASH combination might also be an effective nutritional approach to preventing high blood pressure," says Lawrence J. Appel, M.D., a DASH investigator and associate professor of medicine, epidemiology, and international health at the Johns Hopkins University Medical Institutions in Baltimore.

Save Yourself from Stress

Yes, stress means "pressure." When you are stressed, your body pumps out hormones that make your blood vessels contract and your heart race, a combination of reactions that can launch your blood pressure into the high-risk regions. That's why learning to recognize stress and doing something about it can help prevent high blood pressure, says Patricia Liehr, R.N., Ph.D., associate professor of nursing at the University of Texas, Houston School of Nursing, and a stress-management consultant at the Hermann Hospital Wellness Center, also in Houston. To feel less stressed, here are some ways to calm down.

Talk yourself out of high blood pressure. Speaking very fast and very loudly raises blood pressure, says Dr. Liehr. "People who have this habit of speech can use it as a sign to stop and consider their stress levels. Often, they are trying to make a point and trying to make sure that everybody else gets their point." If you notice yourself speaking this way, stop a moment and take a deep breath. Then take another breath or two while you focus on your breathing.

The next time you speak, talk more quietly. Slow down by putting a "period" of space after every sentence. You will still be able to make your point, says Dr. Liehr. In fact, softer speech is often more emphatic, but your blood pressure is less likely to rise to high-risk regions.

PUT YOURSELF IN A STORY. "A lot of people judge themselves quite harshly," says Dr. Liehr. "They are never satisfied with who they are or anything they do, and they are constantly criticizing themselves. All of this is very stressful." One way to learn to accept yourself is to see your entire life as a story, she says. "Look at your story just as you would a novel or a movie and embrace your story. Embrace who you are."

TAKE A DEEP BREATH. One of the best ways to short-circuit stress is to spend time every day focusing on your breathing, says Dr. Liehr. "When you are stressed, your breathing becomes very shallow, and that becomes a pattern." If you breathe deeply, however, you can reset your nervous system at a calmer level. Spend five minutes every morning and evening just taking slow, deep breaths, she advises. "Just pay attention to the breath going in and out. If other thoughts enter your mind, simply return your attention to the breathing."

A Reason to Stop Rude Awakenings

For some people, it is what's going on at night, not during the day, that could be pushing their blood pressures to the upper limits. And this nocturnal stress has nothing to do with leaky faucets, noisy neighbors, or worries about bills. It is about breathing during sleep—and how lapses in it may cost you more than a few winks.

When your breathing during sleep stops for 10 seconds or more—and this happens at regular intervals—researchers call it sleep apnea. Scientists know that these pauses in breathing send your blood pressure and heart rate skyward. These spikes might cause changes in hormones, blood vessels, and nerve tissues that could keep the pressure up for good.

In a scientific study, blood pressure was measured every 20 to 30 minutes for 24 hours in 53 people with sleep apnea. The researchers discovered that blood pressures in these people were consistently higher than they were in 53 people who simply snored (the mildest

Try Some New Habits

You probably heard it first in your high school health class: Drinking and smoking too much are bad for your health. And if you listened to your high school gym instructor, you heard how good it is to exercise.

Well, it turns out that their arguments for good health are also persuasive reasons to help prevent high blood pressure. Here is what doctors have to say about drinking, smoking, and exercising.

CUT DOWN ON ALCOHOL. Alcohol may make you feel relaxed, but it gets your blood pressure pretty uppity. Exactly how this happens isn't known, but drinking may form of sleep-disordered breathing) and in 41 smooth sleepers. So strong is the link between apnea and high blood pressure that apnea is now considered an independent risk factor for high blood pressure.

"Sleep apnea may turn out to be one of the mechanisms behind essential high blood pressure," says study leader Khin Mae Hla, M.D., professor in the departments of medicine and preventive medicine at the University of Wisconsin School of Medicine in Madison. If you know that you have sleep apnea, you may want to take steps to control it as a way of helping to prevent high blood pressure, too. For instance, "losing weight is one way of trying to improve sleep-disordered breathing, and that might also improve blood pressure," says Dr. Hla.

The current state-of-the-art diagnostic test for sleep apnea is to get an overnight full-sleep study, which is available through sleep disorders clinics in major medical centers. Once sleep apnea is diagnosed, a sleep specialist may recommend a number of different tactics to treat apnea.

stimulate the kidneys to keep more salt and water in the blood, or it may constrict your blood vessels. "If you drink more than two drinks a day, you raise your blood pressure," says Dr. Kaplan. "And the more you drink, the worse it gets." Keep in mind that 1 1/2 ounces of hard liquor, 5 ounces of wine, or 12 ounces of beer equals one drink.

SNUFF OUT THE SMOKES. "If you are smoking, quit," says Dr. Kaplan. "Every time you light up, it raises your blood pressure 10, 15, 20 points and lasts for 15, 20, 30 minutes. If you light up 30 times a day, your blood pressure can be up a lot."

LIMBER UP TO KEEP PRESSURE DOWN. Scientific research shows that regular exercise is still one of the best ways to help prevent high blood pressure, says Dr. Hagberg.

A long-term study of alumni from the University of Pennsylvania found that those who were involved in vigorous physical activity in the years after college decreased their risk of developing high blood pressure by 20 to 30 percent. In another study, people with a family history of high blood pressure were divided into two groups: one group exercised and the other didn't. After five years, 19 percent of the nonexercise group had high blood pressure, as compared to only 9 percent of the people in the exercise group.

Aerobic exercise has been shown to reduce the level of blood pressure in people if it is done for 40 minutes, three times a week or more. Dr. Hagberg says it is likely that the same type of exercise can prevent high blood pressure. So do some aerobic activities like walking, bicycling, and swimming if you want to help prevent high blood pressure.

HIVES
Hunting for Triggers

There are hundreds of different substances and situations that can trigger hives (known as urticaria), those itchy, red bumps with a whitish center that pop up on your skin. Aspirin is a trigger for some people. Peanuts, for others. Some swimmers get hives after plunging into a cold pool. Even the hot sun on your face or other exposed areas can set things off.

When your skin gets exposed to the trigger—whatever it is—your body releases histamine or other types of immune system chemicals that produce the hive. A single hive might last a few minutes or as long as a couple of hours. But sometimes the hives come and go over a period of about six weeks. These *acute* hives, doctors say, are usually caused by a single trigger, which can be easy to identify. But if you continue to have hives for longer than six weeks, you have a condition called *chronic* hives, or chronic urticaria. When hives continue this long, there are often multiple triggers, which can be extremely difficult to identify.

"Identifying and avoiding triggers is one of the best ways to prevent urticaria," says Vincent S. Beltrani, M.D., associate clinical professor of dermatology at the Columbia University College of Physicians and Surgeons in New York City and a dermatologist in Poughkeepsie. When searching for some triggers that may be causing your hives, you will want to begin with the following places.

QUESTION YOUR CABINET MEMBERS. Aspirin and other nonsteroidal anti-inflammatory drugs (NSAIDs) like ibuprofen and naproxen (Aleve) are a common cause of hives. Discontinue the product and never use it again, advises Dr. Beltrani. Work with your doctor to find pain-relieving medications that may not trigger hives.

REMIND YOUR DOC. A number of prescription medications can trigger hives, including opiates like codeine (found in Tylenol with Codeine) as well as penicillin and other antibiotics. "People with chronic hives need to be very cautious with the penicillin family of drugs," says Dr. Beltrani. "It is the most common drug trigger."

You should also watch out for diuretics, says Ernest N. Charlesworth, M.D., clinical associate professor of medicine and dermatology at University of Texas Medical School at Houston and a staff allergist and dermatologist at Brenham Clinic Association in Brenham. Most diuretics are prescription drugs, but certain over-the-counter drugs like cough medicines, laxatives, and pain medications, for example, can also cause hives. If you realize that a medication is causing hives, talk with your doctor about prescribing an alternative, he says.

FIGURE OUT THE OFFENDING FOOD. Most food-caused hives pop up within 20 minutes of eating, providing a clue that something in your meal was the trigger, says Dr. Beltrani. Peanuts, shellfish, eggs, milk, soy, wheat, and fish cause more than 90 percent of food-triggered hives, he says.

Other foods that typically cause hives in adults are cheese, sausage, beer, wine, and strawberries, says Dr. Charlesworth. Once you have identified the trigger foods or food group, cut them out of your diet and see whether the hives go away, he says.

BLOCK THAT SUN. People with solar urticaria—hives triggered by the ultraviolet (UV) radiation of sunlight—should be certain to always wear a sunscreen, says Dr. Beltrani. Either type of UV radiation—UVA or UVB—may cause urticaria, but some people react to both kinds of rays. You can be tested by a dermatologist to find out which kind of radiation is causing your problem. Wearing the right sunscreen to block your trigger (UVA, UVB, or both) may prevent these hives from appearing, he says.

PUT THE COLD ON HOLD. Some people break out in hives when any part of their bodies—skin, mouth, or throat—is exposed to a sudden drop in temperature of 30°F or more. To find out if you have cold urticaria, put an ice cube on your forearm for 15 to 20 minutes, then remove it. If cold is a trigger, the hive will pop up 10 to 15 minutes after you have removed the cube.

People with cold urticaria should not eat ice-cold food or drinks. The soft tissue of their throats can swell, block their airways, and result in suffocation. And they should never jump into a cold swimming pool. The sudden release of histamine from the contact with the cold water can be so severe that it can also cause anaphylactic shock, a body-wide swelling that can also lead to asphyxiation. (For more information, see "When Hives Are a Red Alert.")

CALM YOURSELF. Your mother-in-law is coming for dinner *and* to deliver her monthly critique of your housekeeping skills. You greet her at the front door with a big smile—and a faceful of hives. Stress and anxiety don't trigger that emotional reaction, but they do generate chemicals called neuropeptides that make you more sensitive to factors that trigger hives. Obviously, you can't avoid stress. But if you notice that your hives often pop up when you are in stressful situations, Dr. Charlesworth says that you should

When Hives Are a Red Alert

If a cluster of round, red, itchy hives is inside your mouth, on your palms and soles, on the top of your scalp, and in the genital area, they may be telling you that you are about to have life-threatening anaphylactic shock.

Whatever is creating the reaction can cause your body to release greater-than-normal amounts of histamine. Swelling ensues—inside the body as well as externally. If the swelling reaction narrows your airways, you risk suffocation.

If you have chronic hives, talk to your allergist or dermatologist about providing you with an EpiPen, a device that injects you with adrenaline, says Vincent S. Beltrani, M.D., associate clinical professor of dermatology at the Columbia University College of Physicians and Surgeons in New York City and a dermatologist in Poughkeepsie.

You will need to carry the EpiPen with you at all times, Dr. Beltrani advises. And if you have a sudden outbreak of hives, use the EpiPen immediately to rush adrenaline into your system and block the life-threatening rush of histamine. If you don't have the EpiPen with you, call 911 or have someone drive you to an emergency room right away.

learn a relaxation technique, such as the following deep-breathing exercise, that can help you keep your cool and keep hives to a minimum.

Sit upright in a comfortable chair with your feet flat on the floor. Slowly breathe in, letting your belly expand. Picture your lungs filling from the bottom to the top. Hold your breath for a few seconds, then slowly exhale, emptying your lungs from top to bottom. Repeat several times.

MAKE AN ANTI-HIVE FASHION STATEMENT. Some hives

are caused by pressure on the skin. To help prevent them, stay away from tight waistbands and skintight exercise clothes, says Dr. Charlesworth.

PREVENT THEM WITH A PRESCRIPTION. Most hives are sparked by the release of the cellular chemical histamine, so the best type of drugs to prevent hives are the antihistamines. Chronic hives will disappear by themselves, with or without medication, says Dr. Beltrani. "Medicines are used to keep you comfortable until your mast cells (the cells that release histamine) stop twitching," he says. These drugs are most effective when taken round the clock, following your doctor's instructions, until no hives are seen for at least 96 hours.

There are many different kinds of antihistamine; the "best" is the one that works for you. If you have chronic hives, you and your doctor should come up with a program, trying different medications to see which one is most effective. Mixing different antihistamines can be more effective than just increasing the dose of a single medication, says Dr. Beltrani. Since some antihistamines cause drowsiness so severe that it can be dangerous to drive a car, ask your doctor about nonsedating antihistamines. If your hives are not controlled with a nonsedating antihistamine, your doctor may add a more potent (sedating) antihistamine like hydroxazine (Vistaril) or doxepin (Doxepin HCl), he says.

IMPOTENCE
Simple Ways to Safeguard Your Sex Life

Coleslaw and yogurt may have limited shelf lives, but your sex life has no expiration date. For men, it may come as a surprise (and relief) to know that many men remain potent until age 70 and beyond. In the Massachusetts Male Aging Study, for example, researchers took blood samples, medical histories, and information on personality and sexual activity from nearly 1,300 men between the ages of 40 and 70. Nearly half of the men said that they had had no problem maintaining or having an erection in the previous six months. Clearly, loss of potency isn't automatic as men age.

Keeping a healthy sex life from losing its freshness is not as difficult as most men may think. A study conducted at the Boston University Medical Center on male sexuality has found that many roadblocks to good sex that were once blamed on aging may be brushed aside with simple lifestyle changes. In many cases, the difficulties reported seemed to result from modifiable factors—meaning, they can be prevented.

A Maintenance Manual for Potency

Like keeping a smooth-running sports car in tip-top condition, the key to a healthy sex life is maintenance. Here are some of the maintenance ideas that could help prevent impotence, as suggested by the Boston University Medical Center study.

WORK OUT, EAT RIGHT. Low levels of high-density lipoproteins (HDLs) seem to be linked to sexual dysfunction. In the Massachusetts study, men being treated for heart disease, diabetes, and high blood pressure were up to four times more likely to become completely impotent in later life than men without those problems. "These are problems that regular exercise and a healthy diet can really combat," says Kenneth Goldberg, M.D., founder and director of the Male Health Institute in Irving, Texas.

CHECK THE MEDS. If you're taking medication for other health problems, these drugs might be affecting your sex life. Impotence is much more common among men who are taking medications, especially for blood pressure, heart disease, and diabetes. "Talk to your doctor about drug substitutions," says Dr. Goldberg. Some medications may have no substitute, but if your doctor can recommend a drug that won't impair your sex life, you may want to substitute it.

DROP SOME EXCESS. Since overweight is a factor that raises your risk of all the impotence-related diseases, shedding pounds is an important preventive measure. And the components of a weight-loss program—a healthy diet and regular exercise—can help preserve blood flow, a big factor for good sex. "Most of the problems noted in the study were vascular in nature—that is, impaired blood flow contributed to impotence," says Irwin Goldstein, M.D., professor of urology at the Boston University School of Medicine and co-director of the New England Reproductive Center–Medical Center in Boston. So avoiding fatty, cholesterol-boosting foods may not only keep you from expanding your

Is the Bicycle an Anti-Sex Machine?

Bicycling can pump up your heart and lungs, deflate your spare tire, and give you quads that rival the Colossus of Rhodes. But if you're a guy, frequent or long-distance cycling can also shift your erections into low gear.

An estimated 100,000 men are impotent because of damage to the penis from a bicycle seat or from the top tube of a bike frame, says Irwin Goldstein, M.D., professor of urology at the Boston University School of Medicine and co-director of the New England Reproductive Center–Medical Center in Boston. He says that he is seeing a parade of men who have lost their sexual function from riding too much.

The nerves and blood vessels responsible for erections are funneled through an area called the perineum, which lies between your sit bones (the bony protrusions of the pelvis that you sit on). When you are sitting on a chair, your weight is supported by these protrusions. When you are riding a bicycle, Dr. Goldstein says, your weight is concentrated between them. "Fifty percent of the penis is actually inside the body. Riding over extremely bumpy terrain, as you would on a mountain bike, will traumatize

waistline but may also help prevent the blocking of the penis's arteries.

DESTRESS FOR SEX. The mind, not just the penis, may be one of the most important factors for preventing impotence. In the Massachusetts Male Aging Study, depression, anger, and submissiveness were strongly linked to increased sexual difficulties. Among men who reported feeling the most angry, 35 percent were unable to maintain an erection and have intercourse at least some of the time, the cavernosal arteries, which run into the penis supplying it with blood."

If you are a man who enjoys bicycling and wants to continue to ride, follow these rules to protect your potency, according to Dr. Goldstein.

LEVEL YOUR SADDLE. Or point the nose a few degrees downward to ease the pressure on your crotch.

LOWER YOUR SEAT. Your knees should be slightly bent when your feet are at the bottom of each pedal stroke. This allows your legs to support more of your weight.

BE WARY OF AERO BARS. These are the handlebar extensions that triathletes use. They encourage riding on the nose of the saddle, which increases crotch pressure.

TRY DIFFERENT SADDLES. Find a model that has a space in the middle where your penis will rest and sides that will support your buttocks.

EVERY 10 MINUTES, STAND UP TO PEDAL. This will encourage blood flow.

USE YOUR LEGS AS SHOCK ABSORBERS. When riding over bumps, level the pedals and rise out of the saddle.

DON'T IGNORE NUMBNESS. If you experience genital numbness while riding, it is a sure sign that you are pinching the nerves and arteries of the perineum. Adjust your bike before you do further damage.

and nearly 20 percent were completely unable to achieve an erection.

"This may suggest that dealing with stress is important," says Dr. Goldberg. When we get excited or stressed-out, our nerves release a form of adrenaline that has been shown to stop an erection in its tracks. "The adrenaline seeps into your system and is released into the penis any time you are anxious," he says. "Stress reduction, through relaxation, exercise, or both, is a must." After all, Dr. Goldberg notes, did you ever notice that sex is better when you are on a vacation? "That's not coincidence," he says. A good erection requires that you lighten up.

KICK THE SMOKES. We know what smoking does to the lungs and heart, but the Massachusetts Male Aging Study makes the erection connection. The probability of complete impotence was 56 percent for current smokers, compared with 21 percent for nonsmokers. "Tobacco can also cause circulatory problems, reducing blood supply to your penis and destroying tissue flexibility," says Dr. Goldberg.

RECHARGE THE BATTERIES. The more erections you have, the more you are likely to have them. Erections supply your penis with the stuff it needs most, oxygen-rich blood circulation. Research suggests that if a man's penis doesn't get enough oxygen through circulation, permanent damage to blood vessels or penile muscles may occur. "This is not the sole reason why men become impotent, though. So men shouldn't feel that not having frequent erections will ultimately lead them to becoming impotent," says Dr. Goldberg. "But there is increasing evidence that having more of them helps—you might call it the 'use it or lose it' syndrome."

Young men spend about two to three hours a night having full erections while sleeping. As men push 50, though, this declines, so less oxygen gets to the penis, which may reduce the quality of erections during the day. To keep your potency up to par, provide yourself with an insurance policy by trying to have at least three waking erections each week. "Of course, if you have other risk factors—you smoke or have high blood pressure, diabetes, or high cholesterol—you should target those problems first. Then perhaps having more erections can help," says Dr. Goldberg.

INCONTINENCE
A His and Hers Guide to Bladder Control

When little boys and girls leave home for day care or kindergarten, they soon learn that there is a time and a place for everything. Milk and cookies—10:00 A.M., at the table. Nap—10:30 A.M., on the mats. "Making number one"—in the bathroom, at the rest break. When accidents happen, they are equally embarrassing to boys and girls.

Grown-up boys and girls have mastered the basics of number one. On the average, an adult excretes $1^{1}/_{2}$ quarts of urine a day—usually, in the bathroom. Occasionally, though, the bladder releases small amounts of urine accidentally. What we have here is a plumbing problem, but sometimes it can be preventable.

Urinary incontinence affects both men and women, but for different reasons. And while certain solutions can help both men and women, others are for women only.

In men, incontinence is usually a symptom of some underlying condition. It ranges from feelings of urgency to leakage to complete loss of control. Causes are a bladder

Relief Work

Feel a sneeze coming on? Cross your legs. For years, women with incontinence have noticed that they leak less urine when they cross their legs before they laugh, cough, or sneeze. Now, research verifies this bit of practical wisdom.

In one study, researchers found that women with stress urinary incontinence lost 9½ times less urine when their legs were crossed compared to when they weren't. That could be the difference between having to change clothes after a cough or just getting rid of a slightly damp pad, says Jan E. Baker, an advanced practice registered nurse in the department of obstetrics and gynecology at the University of Utah Hospital in Salt Lake City, who co-authored this study. Subtly slipping one knee over the other may boost the power of the pelvic muscles enough to overcome the downward force of the laugh, cough, or sneeze, making it more difficult for urine to escape through the urethra.

muscle that doesn't work properly, an enlarged prostate gland, or diabetes, among other conditions.

In women, normal wear and tear—coupled with neglect and giving birth to a bouncing baby or two—can damage nerves, weaken the muscle, and compromise connective tissue and ligaments that affect urination. The weakness may not become apparent for years after the damage is done.

In women, stress incontinence—meaning that urine is released during lifting, laughing, sneezing, or exercising—is the most common sign that the pelvic floor is losing ground. This area of muscles stretches like a hammock from the pubic bone to the spine, and it helps support the bladder. When this area gets slack, urine control becomes less than ideal. "It is one of the secrets of motherhood. A third of women who deliver vaginally develop stress incontinence," says Linda Brubaker, M.D., associate professor and director of urogynecology at the Rush–Presbyterian–St. Luke's Medical Center in Chicago. (A urogynecologist is a gynecologist who specializes in disorders of the pelvic floor.) "Some of these women recover naturally, some don't. Many recover partially or completely with extra therapy," she explains.

To help control incontinence, doctors recommend regular exercise of the pelvic-floor muscles with workouts called Kegels (pronounced KEE-guls). Developed back in the 1940s by California physician Arnold Kegel, they involve repeatedly squeezing the muscles supporting the bladder. (For women, this can feel like clenching a tampon.)

"Kegels aren't a cure-all," says Nicolette S. Horbach, M.D., a urogynecologist in private practice in Annandale, Virginia. "But studies show that, when practiced correctly and faithfully, Kegels do make a difference for most women with mild incontinence." Here's how to do Kegels.

ISOLATE THE PELVIC-FLOOR MUSCLES. This is critical to learning how to do Kegels correctly. For women, the simplest way is to lie down, put a finger or two inside your vagina, and squeeze as if you were trying to stop the flow of urine. If your fingers feel pressure from the side vaginal walls, that means you are using the right muscles.

Men and women can identify the muscles while urinating. See if you can stop or slow the flow of urine by squeezing, says Stephen B. Young, M.D., associate professor and director of urogynecology at the University of Massachusetts Medical Center in Worcester. This should be a one-time test only; repeatedly interrupting urination can aggravate urinary problems.

If you have any doubt about where these muscles are, ask your gynecologist (if you are a woman) or your urologist (if you are a man) for help during your next exam.

For women: Once you have found the muscles, squeeze and count to three slowly. Let go and relax. Repeat three to five times. As in any exercise regimen, you can build endurance. Gradually hold a little longer until you can hold the squeeze for 10 seconds, says Katherine Jeter, Ed.D., retired executive director of the National Association for Incontinence, a nonprofit consumer organization in Union, South Carolina.

Work your way up to 10 repetitions for 10 seconds, three times a day, adds Dr. Brubaker.

For men: Doctors suggest that men do three sets of five Kegels a day for a week. Once you have found the muscles, squeeze and hold for about 10 seconds.

Gradually add 5 repetitions to each set, working up to 30 repetitions, three times a day, says Dr. Young. Your ultimate goal is 60 to 90 repetitions, three to five times a week for maintenance, he explains.

FIND THE RIGHT TIME. Since doctors advise doing pelvic exercises three times a day, you could practice them either before or after mealtime, says Jane Marks, R.N., clinical coordinator for the continence program at the Johns Hopkins Geriatric Center in Baltimore.

"I tell women to do them in the shower or standing at the sink while brushing their teeth," says Kathe Wallace, a urogynecologic physical therapist in private practice in Seattle.

ANTICIPATE THE BIG LAUGH. Over time, especially in women, the pelvic muscles tend to sag and do not provide enough support to prevent incontinence during certain activities. Many women particularly run into trouble holding their urine when laughing and when nose blowing, sneezing, or coughing.

By performing a pelvic-muscle contraction whenever you anticipate extra pressure on your pelvic muscles, you may be able to avoid leakage, advises Dr. Jeter. Here's how.

Weight a Minute

For women who need additional help to strengthen their pelvic-floor muscles, special tamponlike vaginal "weights," called cones, are available. (Your doctor can help you determine if you need this.) A set contains five cones that vary in weight. As your muscles get stronger, you progress to a heavier cone. To keep the cone from slipping out of the vagina, you must keep squeezing your pelvic muscles continuously for several minutes.

"The weights are very convenient," says Linda Brubaker, M.D., associate professor and director of urogynecology at the Rush–Presbyterian–St. Luke's Medical Center in Chicago. "You can pop them in when you are showering and blow-drying your hair. After 15 minutes, you have done your pelvic-floor exercises for the day." The weights cost about $100 and are available by writing to *The Self-Care Catalog* at 104 Challenger Drive, Portland, TN 37148-1716.

Sitting up in a chair with hands on your abdomen, cough normally. You should be able to feel your abdomen tighten and jut out a bit against your hands, presumably increasing the pressure on the pelvic floor. Next, counter that pressure. Breathe in through your nose. Tense your pelvic muscles and hold on. Cough. Relax. And again. "If you practice this, it will finally become automatic to squeeze before you sneeze, laugh, or cough," says Dr. Jeter.

Preserving the Pelvic Floor

Beyond Kegels, here are other actions to guard against incontinence.

DROP EXCESS WEIGHT. One study comparing over-weight women to non-overweight women observed that incontinence was more common in overweight women than in their slim sisters, according to Dr. Jeter.

DON'T SMOKE. "Smokers have been found to be predisposed to problems with pelvic weakness," says Dr. Horbach.

LIFT WITH CARE. Straining to lift a jammed window or schlepping a stack of encyclopedias to the attic can create incredible stresses on your pelvic floor, says Dr. Brubaker. "When you lift a heavy object, you momentarily push the pelvic muscles down very forcefully beyond the normal range of motion," she explains. That's called an increase in intra-abdominal pressure. And the cumulative effect of years of repetitive motion that creates this kind of pressure can certainly take its toll. Don't be shy. Ask for help if you need to hoist anything heavy. Or contract your pelvic muscles and hold it as you lift.

GO LOW IMPACT. Doctors are the first to admit that they are just not sure how jogging and high-impact aerobic exercise affect the pelvic floor. The trauma of repetitive jolting may damage the nerves and muscle. So if you have particular problems or concerns about incontinence, consider low-impact over high-impact exercise, Dr. Brubaker advises. To burn calories and challenge the cardiovascular system, you can walk, bike, or swim. Other ways to work out include getting on a stairclimber or rowing machine or pumping those arms in a low-impact aerobics class, she adds.

KEEP REGULAR. "Early research suggests that straining because of chronic constipation may damage pelvic muscles as well as the nerves that supply those muscles," says Dr. Horbach. To help avoid constipation, adopt a high-fiber diet, get regular (low-impact) exercise, and drink eight eight-ounce glasses of water a day.

INSOMNIA
What's Wrecking Your Shut-Eye?

Shakespeare called it the "chief nourisher in life's feast." Keats referred to sleep as the "soft embalmer of the still midnight." And according to Ralph Waldo Emerson, "health is the first muse, and sleep is the condition to produce it."

Though not M.D.'s, Shakespeare, Keats, and Emerson knew well the value of sleep. A sleeping body looks pretty inert, but sleep keeps your body functioning at its peak.

"Sleep quality affects your immunity, cardiovascular health, growth rate, and a lot of other things conducive to a long life," says Bob Ballard, M.D., director of the National Jewish/University of Colorado Sleep Disorders Center at the National Jewish Medical and Research Center in Denver. "Illness and sleep patterns go hand in hand. When you don't get enough sleep, you are more prone to illness because there is a circadian rhythm in keeping immunity strong. Your body needs to rest through sleep in order to stay healthy."

Lying still doesn't nourish your brain the way sleep does. "When you sleep, your brain has a chance to calm down from the day and recharge itself," says Alex Clerk, M.D., director of the Stanford University Sleep Disorders Clinic. "Brain waves slow down, at least in the early stages of sleep, and the various connections to the brain are more or less rejuvenated. Most experts will tell you that we don't fully understand the exact function of sleep. We know that it is beneficial. We know that we need it. And we know that you can prevent some of the problems associated with bad sleep."

Approximately 40 million Americans experience sleep disorders and sleep deprivation. The cost of this is apparently a lot easier to count than sheep. According to the National Sleep Foundation, sleep deprivation was behind the Exxon Valdez oil spill, when the wavering attention of a super-tanker captain resulted in $10 billion worth of damage to the environment. It was a contributing factor of the Chernobyl nuclear accident and Three Mile Island near miss. And falling asleep while driving causes an estimated 100,000 accidents each year; about one in four American drivers will fall asleep behind the wheel at least once in their lifetimes.

If, night after night, you toss and turn for hours, take longer than normal to fall asleep, or wake up too early, your body and brain won't function at their peak. Here is how to manage your days and nights to prevent insomnia. If you can ward off the things that stop you from sleeping well, there is a good chance that you can snooze.

Help for the Wired and Worried

The biggest reason for our nighttime problems, according to most experts, is the stress caused by our daytime problems.

"About half of the time, insomnia is caused by stress," says Peter Hauri, Ph.D., director of the insomnia program and co-director of the Mayo Clinic Sleep Disorders Clinic in Rochester, Minnesota. "Most of the sleep problems, obviously, are because of negative stress—anxiety, depression, worries, and the like. But even good stress can keep you from getting good sleep. As many brides will tell you, the night before the wedding is not a time for good sleep."

That's why stress prevention translates into sleep promotion. When you experience stress, your body releases adrenaline and other hormones that put you in an increased arousal state, says Michael Thorpy, M.D., associate professor of neurology at Albert Einstein College of Medicine of Yeshiva University and director of the Sleep/Wake Disorders Center at Montefiore Medical Center, both in Bronx, New York. Your heart rate speeds up, and as your pulse quickens, both mind and body become more alert, revving up for the fight-or-flight response that served our ancestors well during their hunting-and-gathering days. But these days, or nights, stress can make you hunt and gather the TV remote for the late, late show as you try to get through another sleepless night.

Few people live stress-free lives. But here are some tips to keep stress from ruining your sleep.

SET UP A WORRY TIME. One way to ease your troubled mind before hitting the sheets is to set aside a specific worry time to address the stresses that plague you at bedtime. "I recommend that you sit down for 30 minutes, two or three hours before going to bed, and let your mind wander about all the stresses in your life," says Dr. Hauri.

"Write down each problem on a piece of paper, and once you have collected them all, write down an action plan that you can do to solve each problem. If you can't solve an entire problem immediately, can you solve one small part of it? If not, write, 'This is out of my hands and is in so-and-so's court.' Setting aside this nightly worry time can not only help you plan a specific course of action but also help you separate the stresses that are worth worrying about

Less-Than-Miraculous Melatonin

You have probably heard that when it's taken in pill form, the supplement melatonin is an all-natural nightcap.

Praised in major magazines and books, melatonin is a synthetic form of a hormone produced in the brain's pineal gland that helps set and control your natural body clock. When released by your brain, melatonin helps you fall asleep each night. As an over-the-counter pill or lozenge, melatonin has been ballyhooed as doing everything from overcoming jet lag and sleep problems to setting back the aging process.

Following the publication of several books on melatonin and a *Newsweek* cover story praising the wonders of the supplement, melatonin became a hot-selling item at health-food fairs. But it remains controversial.

Few argue that these supplements can prevent and treat jet lag and can help some people prevent insomnia. But long-term use of melatonin may produce unanticipated effects, according to some experts.

"The problem is the use of these supplements has gone ahead of the research done on its safety," says Alex Clerk, M.D., director of the Stanford University Sleep Disorders Clinic. "Since it is sold as a dietary supplement, melatonin doesn't need FDA approval, so we really don't know exactly what people are taking."

from those that you can do nothing about and aren't worth keeping you awake," he says.

THINK BORING THOUGHTS. Ever wonder why counting sheep is so effective at getting us some Zzzs? Because it is so boring. "The goal for people who can't fall asleep because of stress is to replace those stressful thoughts that are keeping them awake with something that is comforting and even monotonous," says Dr. Ballard. "It is good to have people

Even for preventing sleep problems, melatonin supplements aren't universally effective, says Dr. Clerk. "Really, the only people who benefit from melatonin supplements are those who suffer from extreme jet lag and people who are night owls, who go to sleep very late and tend to sleep late in the morning."

Melatonin also seems to help some older people, according to Dr. Clerk. Since the brain's production of melatonin decreases with age, the supplements help make up for some of that deficiency. For other people just trying to get better sleep, the supplements may be more dangerous than helpful, he observes.

The bottom line is that if you want to take melatonin supplements as a remedy for insomnia, do it under a doctor's supervision. A doctor may want to test you for a melatonin deficiency, but the problem is that this test is not widely available, according to Irina Zhdanova, M.D., Ph.D., a research scientist in the department of brain and cognitive sciences at the Massachusetts Institute of Technology in Cambridge. Also, because melatonin is not regulated by the Food and Drug Administration, you can't be sure that you are getting pure melatonin, she explains. If you should start experiencing headaches, dizziness, or nightmares, stop taking the melatonin.

recite their favorite poem before going to bed." Not into poems? Try counting down from 100 to 1 or name the states and capitals.

TIGHTEN UP TO LOOSEN UP. Storing up tension? A relaxation technique that works well is progressive muscular relaxation, according to Dr. Thorpy. "You tighten and then relax various muscles in your body. It is best to start with your feet, gradually working toward your head. Count to 10 as you first tighten the muscles, then count to 10 again as you let them relax. The point is to first feel the tension as you tighten them, and then the release as you relax."

Do this relaxation technique several times during the day, and then again before going to bed, as a way to relax your body and ease your stress, suggests Dr. Thorpy.

GET A POST-WORK WORKOUT. Regular aerobic exercise is a great way to manage stress, but timing is crucial if you are having trouble sleeping at night. "For people with stress-related insomnia or poor sleep quality, the best time to exercise is about four to six hours before you go to bed. So for most people, that's immediately after work," says Dr. Hauri. "That's because exercise has a stimulating effect that lasts for several hours. But when it wears off, you feel relaxed."

NAP NOT. If you like a daytime nap but have trouble with insomnia at night, maybe there is a simple solution: Nix the nap.

"For most people, napping isn't a good idea because it can throw off your body clock," says Dr. Hauri. "No one knows why, but about one of five people sleep better at night when they have had a nap during the day. But four out of five people sleep worse."

Prep for Slumber

Check into any good hotel, and the rooms are designed for perfect sleeping—large beds, "blackout" light-blocking shades on the windows, and individual climate controls. Yet many travelers report getting less than four-star shut-eye while staying away from home.

"It's natural to not sleep well in a strange environment," says Dr. Hauri. "It stems from how we, as humans, are built. Back in prehistoric times, we didn't know what dangers faced us when we were in a strange environment, so we were more alert and less likely to feel relaxed. And it continues today."

But what about when you are not sleeping well in the comfort of your own home? Doctors suggest that you take stock of your bedroom and look for reasons why you are not snoozing well. If you fix some of those sleep blockers and make your bedroom conducive to sleep, you just may prevent insomnia. Here's how.

HIDE THE CLOCK. The average person wakes up about five times during the night. Most fall back to sleep. People with insomnia do not.

"A big problem for many people is that when they wake up, they look at the clock to see what time it is," says Sonia Ancoli-Israel, Ph.D., professor of psychiatry at the University of California, San Diego, School of Medicine; director of the Sleep Disorders Clinic at the Veterans Affairs Medical Center in San Diego; and author of *All I Want Is a Good Night's Sleep*. "Looking at a clock wakes you up more," she observes. You have to turn your head and focus your eyes enough to see what time it is, which is often enough to take someone from that state of semi-sleep to full wakefulness. "So the first thing I recommend is to hide the clock or at least turn it around so that its face is toward the wall," she says.

Many sleep specialists say that the clock interferes with sleep in other ways as well. "Anyone who needs an alarm clock in the bedroom to wake up each morning is probably not getting enough sleep," adds Dr. Thorpy. "One key to avoiding sleep deprivation is to train yourself to wake up without the aid of an alarm clock."

STAY COOL. A warm bath can help promote sleep. Studies show, however, that people tend to sleep better when the temperature is slightly on the cool side, says Gary Zammit, Ph.D., director of the Sleep Disorders Institute at St. Luke's–Roosevelt Hospital in New York City. "Ideally, it should be slightly cooler than what is comfortable for you during the day." So if you keep your home thermostat at 68°F during the day, turn it down a couple of degrees at night.

KEEP YOUR HOME WELL-HUMIDIFIED. During the winter months, a heated bedroom can make breathing difficult for snorers and other mouth breathers, so they wake up several times during the night for water, says Dr. Clerk. "Humidity is very important, especially if you snore, because when you are breathing through your mouth, it gets dry. Having more moisture in the air can help." A commercial humidifying system is the easiest way to add moisture to your house.

USE THE BED FOR SLEEPING. Period. One reason some people can't fall asleep or stay asleep in their beds is that they have become accustomed to using them for other things, such as paying bills, knitting, watching TV, or reading. "You should use your bed for sleep and sex only. But use it for sex only if it is relaxing and rewarding," says Dr. Ancoli-Israel. "The idea is to associate the bed with sleeping, not with doing chores or other activities."

That's why some sleep experts recommend that you don't keep a TV in your bedroom. "Of course, some people find that watching TV helps relax them, so they are better able to fall asleep," says Dr. Hauri. "But I advise against watching any show that is likely to aggravate them."

LEAVE THE BEDROOM. Time-honored advice says that if you are tossing and turning to no avail, get out of bed and move to another room. And it works.

Read or watch videotapes (watching a TV show could remind you of what time it is). Try to stay awake as long as you can. "The harder you try to avoid sleep, the faster it will come," says Dr. Hauri.

Watch Your Sips and Smokes

If you enjoy a cup of espresso, a couple of glasses of wine, or a cigarette with dinner or afterward, these pleasures could contribute to sleep problems. In different ways, caffeine, alcohol, and tobacco all disrupt trouble-free rest. To prevent sleep disruptions, here is what experts advise.

PUT A CAP ON THE COFFEE HABIT. "Studies show that caffeine does affect the quality of most people's sleep, and the bottom line is that anyone who has any sort of sleep problem should ideally avoid caffeine altogether, but especially within four hours of going to bed," says Dr. Thorpy. "Besides the stimulating effect, caffeine increases tension and anxiety, which may spill over into the night and contribute to the inability to fall or stay asleep."

DON'T LOSE WITH BOOZE. "Alcohol does help you fall asleep because it is a sedative, but studies show that sleep becomes more disruptive—what we call fragmented sleep," says Dr. Thorpy. "There may be an increased chance of having nightmares for people who drink significant amounts of alcohol within four hours before going to bed."

Small amounts of alcohol, he adds, don't seem to pose these problems. "But we're talking about less than one ounce, what you would get in a very small shot glass. Anything else seems to have a detrimental effect."

AVOID THE SMOKE SIGNALS. "Nicotine disrupts sleep because it is a central nervous system stimulant," says Dr. Ancoli-Israel. "So people who smoke before bed tend to have a harder time falling and staying asleep."

All experts recommend that you quit smoking for overall good health. Just to prevent insomnia, though, sleep specialists say that you should avoid smoking within four hours of bedtime, reports Dr. Thorpy.

Snooze News on Snacks

Some food for thought: A light snack before bedtime may be a nutritionist's nightmare, but it can mean sweet dreams for you. "The relationship between food and sleep isn't very clear because nobody studies that area," says Dr. Hauri. "But some earlier studies show that a little snack before bedtime can help you fall asleep."

Some people believe that it is because foods such as milk, turkey, and bananas contain tryptophan, an amino acid that induces sleep. So one reason you may feel tired after Thanksgiving dinner could be the tryptophan in all that turkey. But that's probably not the only reason. "It could be because there seems to be a relationship between the stomach and the brain—when the stomach is satisfied, the brain is more relaxed and better equipped to sleep," says Dr. Hauri. Whatever the reason, here is what experts say you should and shouldn't eat to help prevent insomnia.

SNACK, DON'T FEAST OR STARVE. When you are having trouble falling asleep, many experts recommend a light snack—ideally, a bowl of cereal with skim milk. The protein in the milk increases the activity of neurotransmitters, chemical messengers in the brain that induce sleep, says Dr. Hauri. He also recommends a slice of chicken or turkey, or a banana, all containing tryptophan.

AVOID SPICY FOODS. Don't reach for that leftover Mexican food. "Spicy foods can irritate the stomach and keep you awake," says Dr. Hauri.

DON'T CRASH-DIET. "Any changes in your food intake can make a difference, so if you start a food-restrictive diet, it may prevent you from falling asleep more easily," says Dr. Thorpy. If you must diet, don't skip meals, skimp, or starve yourself. Instead, follow a plan that centers on small, healthful meals throughout the day. Substitute healthier fare for high-fat, high-calorie foods whenever possible.

Are Your Meds Meddling?

Illness is another enemy of the sandman. Scores of conditions manage to keep people awake with pain, stuffy nose, and difficulty breathing. So we turn to medications to curb our pain and hopefully get our bodies the rest they need. And what happens?

Many prescription medications tend to either keep us awake at night or make us sleepy during the day, says Dr. Ballard. So do many over-the-counter drugs. Also, many medications interfere and can disrupt what is called rapid eye movement (REM) sleep, the part of your sleep cycle when you do most of your dreaming. So even if you manage to get to sleep, these drugs may interfere with restfulness.

But how can you prevent drug-related insomnia if you must take medication? Doctors offer this advice.

FOR OTCs, SEEK SUBSTITUTES. Some over-the-counter (OTC) pain relievers such as Excedrin can have a negative impact on your sleep. That's because aspirin and acetaminophen—their active ingredients—are often paired with caffeine. In fact, the amount of caffeine may be as much as you would find in nearly two cups of coffee. "The best thing to do is read the label to see if caffeine is listed," says Dr. Hauri. Then look for substitute pain relievers. "There are plenty of over-the-counter pain relievers that don't contain caffeine, including ibuprofen products," he adds.

TALK TO THE PHARMACIST. Before you use a medication, Dr. Ballard recommends that you talk to your pharmacist about ingredients that could contribute to sleep problems. Cold remedies and other decongestants may not list caffeine as an ingredient on the label, but they still contain other substances that act as central nervous system stimulants and that could interfere with sleep. So you don't want to take them near bedtime.

During the day, on the other hand, sleep-inducing medications could augur ill for your nighttime rest. "A lot of antihistamines and other allergy medicines have a sedating effect during the daytime, which could interrupt sleep at nighttime," says Dr. Ballard. The solution for that problem could be on the same shelf. "There is a whole new generation of allergy medicines sold under brand names such as Seldane and Hismanal that don't have the sedating effects."

OPT FOR LONG-LASTING DRUGS. The more doses of a drug you take, the more likely you are to feel its impact, either sedating or stimulating. "A lot of medications—both prescription and over-the-counter drugs—have very short half-lives and can give you a hangover effect," says Dr. Ballard. "But you are less likely to feel these effects if you take a longer-lasting medication."

INTERMITTENT CLAUDICATION
Kick the Causes

When the blood vessels in the legs are narrowed and choked with cholesterol and other fatty materials (the disease process known as atherosclerosis), you have a condition called peripheral arterial disease. That is when the calf muscles can't get enough oxygen. So whenever you try to walk much farther than a block or two, your calves start to hurt. You get a cramplike, aching sensation that stops you in your tracks. It might let up after a couple of minutes of rest, but when you start walking again, the pain comes chasing after.

Five million Americans, most of them in their fifties or older, are nagged by this circulatory ball-and-chain. And the most likely reason is tobacco. "Smoking is a more malignant risk factor for intermittent claudication than it is for heart disease," says William Hiatt, M.D., professor of medicine in the section of vascular medicine at the University of Colorado Health Sciences Center and executive director of the Colorado Prevention Center, both in Denver. The entire body gets suffocated as carbon monoxide from

An Apple a Day Recipe

Folate-Filled Casserole

The greens and beans in this simple casserole add plenty of folate to your diet. Best of all, it is easy to make and tastes great.

2 teaspoons olive oil
1 teaspoon red-pepper flakes
2 cloves garlic, minced
2 medium bunches Swiss chard, cut into 2" strips (12 cups)
1 can (19 ounces) cannellini beans, rinsed and drained

2 large tomatoes, chopped
1 tablespoon chopped fresh sage or thyme or 1 teaspoon dried sage or thyme
½ cup unseasoned dry bread crumbs
½ cup grated Parmesan cheese

Preheat the oven to 350°F.

Warm 1 teaspoon of the oil in a large nonstick skillet over medium heat. Add the red-pepper flakes and garlic. Cook for 2 minutes, or until garlic is soft. Add the chard and cook for 3 minutes, or until just wilted. Add the beans and cook for 5 minutes, or until heated through. Remove from heat and stir in the tomatoes and the sage or thyme.

Coat a 1½-quart baking dish with nonstick spray.

Spread the mixture in the prepared baking dish. Sprinkle with the bread crumbs and Parmesan. Drizzle with the remaining 1 teaspoon oil. Bake for 30 minutes or until lightly browned and bubbly.

Makes 4 servings. Per serving: 276 calories, 7 g. fat, 51% of Daily Value of folate cigarettes shoves aside the oxygen in red blood cells. Exactly why smoking hits blood vessels harder below than above the belt isn't clearly understood, says Dr. Hiatt. But studies have shown that 90 to 95 percent of people with the disease are smokers. "The best way to prevent this disease is to not smoke or to quit smoking," concludes Dr. Hiatt.

But a few other cautions are in order, too. Here is what Dr. Hiatt advises.

CONSIDER FOLATE. High levels of the body chemical homocysteine are a risk factor in intermittent claudication, says Dr. Hiatt. And when you increase the level of the B vitamin folate in your diet, you can lower homocysteine levels. Good food sources of folate include beans, broccoli, spinach, orange juice, and fortified cereals.

CUT CHOLESTEROL AND TRIGLYCERIDES. "Try to raise high-density lipoprotein (HDL) cholesterol and lower triglycerides," says Dr. Hiatt. HDL cholesterol is the "good" kind that helps usher "bad," artery-clogging low-density lipoprotein (LDL) cholesterol out of the body. And triglycerides are a blood fat with the same mean streak as LDL.

The best way to affect both of these blood fats at once is to lose weight if you are overweight. "Even losing as little as 5 to 10 pounds will significantly lower triglycerides and LDL cholesterol," says Dr. Hiatt. (For tips on managing your weight, see Overweight on page 593.)

GET ACTIVE. Regular exercise, like brisk walking four or five days a week, is a good way to both positively change your blood fats and lose weight. Try to get out for a 20- to 30-minute stroll as often as you can.

IRRITABLE BOWEL SYNDROME
Calming the Colon

The word *irritable* doesn't do justice to this digestive ailment. *Infuriated* or *long-suffering* seem like more appropriate adjectives for the bowel of someone with irritable bowel syndrome, or IBS. Just reading a list of the possible symptoms can start to make you feel a bit queasy.

You can have diarrhea or constipation (or the two can alternate), and your stools can be hard and lumpy or soft and watery. Your body's "call to nature" can be an abrupt shout—so abrupt, in fact, that you just might not make it to the toilet in time. And even after you defecate, your rectum may feel as though it hasn't been emptied completely. To top it all off, you may have abdominal pain, cramping, and bloating. You may have one of those symptoms, a few of them, or all of them. You may have them nonstop, frequently, or every now and then.

Approximately 5 million Americans have IBS. The condition prompts approximately 3.5 million doctor's office visits per year with 20 to 50 percent of all visits to gastroenterologists. The condition is found in more women than in men.

While doctors don't know why people develop IBS, some experts think that it is triggered by an intestinal infection or a severely stressful life event. Whatever the cause, the troubling results are spasms in the colon, the large section of the intestine before the rectum and the anus. And doctors also know that people with IBS have a higher-than-normal sensitivity in the colon or rectum from gas, stool, or spasms. For someone who has IBS, any activity in the colon can be painful.

If you find that you are having symptoms and you feel uncomfortable on a regular basis, see your doctor for a diagnosis, says Douglas A. Drossman, M.D., professor of medicine and psychiatry in the division of digestive disease at the University of North Carolina (UNC) at Chapel Hill and co-director of the UNC Functional Disorders Center. With a positive diagnosis of IBS, he might prescribe an anti-spasmodic medication such as hyoscyamine sulfate (Levsin) or dicyclomine (Bentyl). And some doctors recommend very low doses of tricyclic antidepressants such as amitriptyline (Elavil) or fluoxetine (Prozac), which can help calm the gastrointestinal tract in some people who have severe IBS.

But whether or not you have been given a prescription, there are many other things that you can do to help combat the symptoms. "Most people with IBS can prevent their symptoms if they eat properly and take a few other measures," says William B. Salt II, M.D., clinical associate professor of medicine at Ohio State University in Columbus, educational director in gastroenterology at the Mount Carmel Health Hospital, and author of *Irritable Bowel Syndrome and the Mind-Body, Brain-Gut Connection.*

"You can prevent the symptoms of IBS by undertaking a program of prevention," adds gastroenterologist Marvin M. Schuster, M.D., professor of medicine and psychiatry at the Johns Hopkins University School of Medicine and director of the Marvin M. Schuster Center for Digestive and Motility Disorders at the Johns Hopkins Bayview Medical Center, both in Baltimore. "Just doing two or three preventive measures may not be effective. But when you add the fourth, then the symptoms may be prevented." And perhaps the best way to start your personal prevention program is to find out which foods and lifestyle factors are the main triggers of your colonic spasms. Here is what experts recommend that you do.

JOT IN A JOURNAL. "We ask new patients with IBS to keep a symptom diary for about a month," says Dr. Drossman. "Every time they have symptoms, they write down the food or meal they ate before the onset of symptoms, and what they were doing and feeling when the symptoms began. This way, people can begin to discover—and eliminate or reduce—the foods and lifestyle factors that trigger their symptoms."

SCUTTLE THE SPASMODICS. The symptom diary can help you figure out the foods that cause your symptoms. Some foods, however, are much more likely to spark spasms than others, and you should pay particular attention to how you feel after you eat them, says Dr. Salt. They include dairy products, wheat, corn, and gas-producing foods like beans, cabbage, brussels sprouts, broccoli, and asparagus.

GET SOME ORAL FIBER. "One of the best ways to prevent the symptoms of IBS is by adding extra fiber to the diet," says G. Nicholas Verne, M.D., assistant professor of medicine in the division of gastroenterology, hematology, and nutrition at the University of Florida College of Medicine in Gainesville. He recommends that people with IBS take a fiber supplement. Divide the amount recommended on the label into three daily doses, he advises.

"Many people with IBS can prevent their symptoms with nothing more than a fiber supplement. It reduces spasms in the colon and normalizes bowel movements,

IBS: Your Mental Watchdog

Why are the bowels of people with irritable bowel syndrome (IBS) so sensitive? The answer is in their brains.

"Under certain conditions, people with IBS have dramatically different types of brain activity than people without the problem, and this brain activity can be responsible for some of their discomfort and pain," says gastroenterologist Marvin M. Schuster, M.D., professor of medicine and psychiatry at the Johns Hopkins University School of Medicine and director of the Marvin M. Schuster Center for Digestive and Motility Disorders at the Johns Hopkins Bayview Medical Center, both in Baltimore.

This fact was discovered by a scientific study in which two groups of people—one with IBS and one without— were given brain scans indicating the level and exact location of brain activity. During the scan, the bowels of each group were distended with air. In the non-IBS group, the brains became active in a location where there are natural painkillers, so pain from the distension was suppressed. But in the IBS group, the brains became active in a different area, an area in the front of the brain that is known for being hyper-vigilant, says Dr. Schuster. "This means that people with IBS are super-sensitized to the activity in their bowels rather than being naturally narcotized, or deadened, to the pain."

whether they have constipation, diarrhea, or both," says Dr. Verne.

DON'T CHEW AS MUCH FAT. Fat in the diet is usually a major trigger of symptoms in people with IBS, says Dr. Salt.

"People who have sick guts just don't tolerate fat very well," adds Dr. Schuster. That's because fat sends a signal from the stomach to the colon called the gastrocolic reflex. In people with IBS, that reflex can spark cramping, pain, and the urgent need to defecate. Fat is also hard to digest, so it can cause bloating and nausea in those with IBS.

"To prevent symptoms from fat, I recommend that people with IBS limit their daily fat intake to between 20 and 50 grams daily," says Dr. Salt. You can figure out the fat grams in packaged foods by reading the Nutrition Facts labels on their containers. For nonpackaged foods, your best bet is to go to a bookstore and purchase any one of the dozens of fat-gram counters.

CUT BACK ON CAFFEINE. Caffeine is a big-league trigger of symptoms, especially abdominal cramping and diarrhea, says Dr. Salt. "Caffeine is highly stimulating to the digestion of normal individuals, and if you have IBS, it can be a disaster. So I get people with IBS to 'decaffeinate' themselves."

The most common sources of caffeine in the diet are coffee, tea, and regular cola. To quit or reduce caffeine, Dr. Salt recommends that you reduce your intake of coffee, tea, and caffeine-containing colas by five ounces every five to seven days, until you are drinking no more than 100 to 120 milligrams of caffeine a day. That's the amount in one 6-ounce cup of percolated coffee, two 6-ounce cups of instant coffee, two 6-ounce cups of black tea, three 6-ounce cups of green tea, or two 12-ounce servings of cola.

High doses of caffeine are also found in many over-the-counter painkiller and weight-loss medications as well as "alertness" drugs that are meant to fight off drowsiness. If you are taking any of these, check the labels to see if they have caffeine. And if they do, ask your pharmacist about an alternative medication.

TAKE A DEEP BREATH. Stress and emotional upset are common triggers of IBS symptoms, says Dr. Salt. He recommends using a body-calming, tension-busting relaxation technique to soothe that stress. "Practicing a relaxation technique is very important in the prevention of IBS symptoms," he says. The best time and place to practice that technique? Not on a quiet mountain, but in the midst of a stress barrage, like when you are caught in a traffic jam or right before an important meeting.

For immediate stress relief, Dr. Salt suggests deep breathing. Inhale through your nose, counting to four, hold for a count of seven, then exhale through your mouth for a count of eight. Repeat four times. Even if you are not under a lot of stress, practice this technique once or twice every day.

WATCH WHAT THE DRUGS DRAG IN. Some over-the-counter and prescription drugs can trigger symptoms. Among over-the-counter drugs, aspirin and ibuprofen-containing painkillers may create trouble for patients with IBS, says Dr. Verne. "I tell all my patients to avoid these and use acetaminophen."

Antacids are another big offender. "Over-the-counter antacids can cause diarrhea in patients with IBS," says Dr. Salt. High levels of the mineral iron, often from iron supplements, are sometimes a problem, causing constipation or, in some people, diarrhea. Among prescription drugs, antibiotics and blood pressure and heart medications can be very aggravating, says Dr. Salt.

"A doctor who prescribes medication for you should be aware that you have IBS," says Dr. Verne. If the doctor is aware of possible digestive side effects, he will be able to prescribe a drug with no or minimal impact on your condition.

JET LAG
Secrets to Getting in Sync

Long flights interrupt your natural biological rhythms. For some people, crossing time zones is the biggest problem—a direct flight to insomnia, headache, diarrhea, and a 747-size case of fatigue.

Travelers can figure on about one day of jet lag for each time zone crossed. So recovering from a flight to Europe or Asia may take up to a week. And experts say that it is generally worse when you are traveling west to east, so it may be harder to recover when flying from Japan to New York than from New York to Japan.

"There are multiple 'zeitgebers' (time-givers) or cues that influence your internal body clock," says Charles F. Ehret, Ph.D., senior scientist emeritus at Argonne National Laboratory in Clarendon Hills, Illinois, who has studied the effects of jet lag for nearly 50 years and wrote *Overcoming Jet Lag*. "Time-givers include when and what you eat, your exposure to light or darkness, intake of substances like caffeine, and the amount of exercise you get."

Program Your Body with Food

Although the specifics vary among travelers, depending on flight departure, arrival, and destination, here is how you can minimize jet lag on your next extended trip by eating strategically, according to Dr. Ehret.

REGULATE. When you know you are flying, you already know how crucial it is to take your time schedule seriously. To avoid jet lag, adjust your eating schedule, too. "It is ideal to have strictly controlled mealtimes," explains Dr. Ehret. As best you can, eat breakfast, lunch, and supper at the same time for several weeks before the trip.

FEED YOUR METABOLISM. Protein stimulates adrenaline, an energy-producing hormone, while carbohydrates stimulate hormones that help you sleep. So while a combination of protein and carbs should be eaten at each meal, go heavier on energy-stimulating proteins at breakfast and lunch and eat more carbohydrates at dinner. Knowing these chemical effects of food can help you regulate your body clock. For example, if you are trying to trick your body into sleeping through lunchtime while in flight, get mellowed by a carbohydrate breakfast. If you plan on dashing to boarding gates in the middle of the night, get primed by a meaty or beany dinner beforehand.

Good choices for breakfast and lunch include yogurt, cottage cheese, cereal, lean meat, and vegetables. For dinner, focus on pasta and other grain products.

EAT LIGHT PRE-FLIGHT. Under Dr. Ehret's plan, *feasting* means eating as much as you want, while *fasting* means cutting your usual calorie count in half. The day of departure should be a fasting day. During that day, you should still eat at mealtimes but go for half-size portions.

RESUME REGULAR MEALS. The next feast (full-portion meal) after you get on the plane should be in sync with the next feast at your destination. When you get on the plane, go ahead and set your watch to the next time zone. If

Melatonin, The Traveler's Aid

For years, a small fraternity of seasoned business travelers has been taking a pill that supposedly helps them sleep on airplanes and overcome the effects of jet lag. The pill is a synthetic form of melatonin, a hormone produced in the brain when it is time to sleep.

Taken at, say, 4:00 P.M., melatonin will advance the body clock, in effect, making you drowsy earlier. In contrast, if it is taken at 7:00 A.M., it tricks your body into believing it is still dark out and time to keep on snoozing, theorizes Quentin Regestein, M.D., director of the Sleep Clinic at Brigham and Women's Hospital in Boston. So depending on where you are going and when you are leaving, melatonin is used to help synchronize the body's natural body rhythms in a matter of hours when traveling across several time zones. In effect, it speeds up a process that would otherwise take days, he explains.

"There are strong indications that melatonin can be of value for jet lag," says Dr. Regestein. And if you want to *gradually* shift your sleep patterns, you can start taking it a number of days before your flight. If you were flying from

the next meal in Paris is breakfast, and you have planned ahead, you can take along enough food for a light breakfast and have it at breakfast time on your new Paris schedule. If there is an in-flight lunch or dinner planned, you can ask the attendant to hold the meal for you until it is the right time to dine.

According to Dr. Ehret, most airlines will accommodate you if you call ahead with your meal schedule.

New York to London, for example, it is helpful to adjust your sleeping schedule to make up for the five-hour time difference. That means a week before the trip, you might start taking melatonin progressively earlier each night to create an earlier bedtime.

But before you buy a bottle for your next flight to Europe, consult your doctor. Most researchers say that the typical health-food-store tablet contains more melatonin than you need, which can mean drowsiness during the day, actually prolonging jet lag, says James D. Frost, M.D., a jet lag specialist and professor of neurology at Baylor College of Medicine in Houston.

And some experts believe that there is good reason to bypass this remedy entirely. Experts can't yet guarantee that it is safe, says Dr. Regestein. Unlike aspirin or other over-the-counter drugs, melatonin isn't regulated by the Food and Drug Administration because it is considered a dietary supplement and not a drug. So it is not labeled with personalized dosages, is not required to offer any official warning of side effects (which may be prolonged grogginess or a hangover effect, among other discomforts), and has no control for purity.

Staying in Gear

While crossing time zones can definitely bring on jet lag with a vengeance, the classic jet lag complaints can also occur within the same time zone, according to David Neubauer, M.D., associate director of the Johns Hopkins Sleep Disorder Center in Baltimore. "You might experience the same lousy feelings after flying from New York to South America as from New York to Cairo," he says. Even if you don't cross zones, many factors take a toll on your body, including low humidity, sitting for long hours, and of course, that stress that occurs after a flight of worrying if you remembered to lock the front door or pack rain gear. Here is how to fend off the post-flight turbulence.

PUT SOME SLEEP IN THE BANK. Try to maintain a regular sleeping schedule, ideally beginning two weeks before you leave, says Dr. Neubauer. Be especially strict about getting full nights of sleep the last few nights before you travel. If possible, give yourself an extra 15 minutes of shut-eye on those final days.

START OUT SMOOTH. Since stress can cause fatigue and deny you that all-important travel sleep, do everything you can to minimize tension. To keep organized, complete and cross off your checklist of "to do's" on the days before you take off. Avoid the stress of trying to pack the morning of your flight, Dr. Neubauer says.

LET THE LIGHT SHINE IN. If your flight is at night, be sure to get as much sunlight as possible during the day before you leave, says Dr. Ehret. If your flight is during the day, try to arrange for a window seat, ideally on the side of the plane that is exposed to the most amount of sunshine.

BEAT THE TIME. If you reset your watch to the time zone of your destination, you will start thinking in terms of the new environment, says James D. Frost, M.D., a jet lag specialist and professor of neurology at Baylor College of Medicine in Houston. Getting used to the new time helps you to psychologically adjust to the new place before you even arrive, he adds.

BE A CAMEL. If desert air is usually 20 to 25 percent humidity, it is no wonder you feel as if you are going to dry up and blow away after a six-hour flight in a typical airline cabin, which can plunge to levels between 20 percent and even zero humidity. Dehydration that occurs in flight is probably the main reason that airplane travelers often come to the ground feeling as though they were still up in the clouds, Dr. Ehret points out.

In addition to the zombie effect, dehydration can cause dry skin, dry and itchy eyes, headaches, and fatigue, adds Dr. Frost.

Be sure to drink like a camel and fill up on extra water (at least one glass) before boarding. Drink at least one glass an hour while you are in the air, says Dr. Neubauer.

BEWARE OF BUBBLES AND BOOZE. If you don't like water as much as the next humped desert mammal, you can drink juice and eat fruit like oranges, says Dr. Neubauer. Caffeinated and alcoholic beverages, however, only worsen dehydration, so don't overdo them. Don't substitute that whiskey sour for a Shirley Temple either. Carbonated beverages can cause gas pain and discomfort as the plane changes altitude, so stick with the flat stuff, he cautions.

KEEP YOUR ENGINE PURRING. A mini-workout as frequently as every 15 minutes can help ease the stiffness and fatigue from sitting long hours, says Dr. Neubauer. Stimulate your circulation by engaging your body parts from top to bottom. Inhale to the count of 10 as you clench, then exhale and deliberately release the just-tensed muscles. Clench and then release a few muscle groups at a time, starting with the facial muscles, working down through the neck and shoulders, back, stomach, buttocks, thighs, calves, feet, and hands. "Especially work the lower legs; when you sit for long hours, that is where fluid collects," he points out. You may also want to point and flex your toes and bring your knees to your chest if there is room.

DON'T CRASH EARLY. Even if you want nothing more than to hit the sheets for a few hours after your trip, taking a long nap when it is not bedtime is going to disturb your sleep later on, making it that much harder to adjust to your new time zone, says Dr. Frost. If you simply can't stay awake, limit your nap time to less than one hour, he advises.

RE-ESTABLISH YOUR EXERCISE ROUTINE. If you are used to exercising in the morning, do so when it is morning at your destination. If you normally work out at night, try to be as active as possible on the flight and when it is evening at your destination, says Dr. Ehret.

"Nothing beats a brisk walk in the sun as soon as you can," Dr. Neubauer adds. Not only will it refuel your jets and flush the fluid out of your seat-bound legs, but natural light is the most important thing that your body needs to readjust to the new time zone, he says.

JOCK ITCH
Block Locker Room Rash

Rest assured, this red, itchy rash around your groin *isn't* sexually transmitted. But that's about the only good thing you can say about it. Caused by the fungus *Tinea cruris*—the same denizen of locker rooms and hotel showers that causes athlete's foot—this infection can smell bad, cause a lot of discomfort, and take weeks to banish. So it makes sense to work in some regular measures to prevent the fungus from taking hold.

Secrets of an Itch-Free Groin

Doctors say that you can easily avoid getting jock itch in the first place. Here's how.

POWDER UP. "By covering the groin area with baby powder, you will help prevent the moisture that leads to jock itch," says James G. Garrick, M.D., director for the Center for Sports Medicine at Saint Francis Memorial Hospital in

San Francisco. Just sprinkle on a light dusting of powder whenever you change your underwear.

WEAR SHORTS UNDER YOUR JOCK. Athletic supporters can irritate the groin area, making it especially susceptible to the fungus. One of the best ways to escape this irritation is to wear a pair of all-cotton shorts under your jock. "The jock doesn't rub the skin nearly as much, and the cotton wicks some of the moisture and the perspiration away from the area by absorbing it," says Dr. Garrick.

STRIP DOWN. It is virtually impossible to keep the groin sweat-free while working out, but once you are finished, switch into dry clothes. "A lot of men sit around in their workout clothes after they exercise, but that is one of the surest ways to get jock itch," says Dr. Garrick. You need to peel off your workout clothes as soon as possible. And don't forget to launder them in between wearings, he adds.

KEEP YOUR TOWEL PERSONAL. When you go to the gym, bring your own clean towel from home for showering. The gym's towel may harbor the critters that cause the problem, cautions Dr. Garrick.

DRY FROM HEAD TO TOE. Dry yourself head to toe, literally. That damp towel you dried your feet with can spread the fungus, says Tobias Samo, M.D., an infectious disease specialist at Methodist Hospital in Houston. By drying your feet last, you avoid passing the germs from your toes to your groin. And wash that towel after every use.

GET YOUR AIR DRYER. If you have a hair dryer available, turn it on cool and blow-dry your privates. All that dry air helps to turn the dampness to desert, depriving the fungus of their moist hideaways. Use the dryer after every shower or bath when you are home, suggests Dr. Samo.

KIDNEY STONES
How to Stop Those Rocks from Rolling

Imagine a pea-size rock traveling ever so slowly through the small tube connecting your kidney to your bladder. Each time the pebble makes any progress, it gouges the tube (called the ureter), resulting in a sharp, excruciating pain. Whether you are a man or woman, that tiny rock has to push along through your pair of ureters.

In men, the rocky road to hell can cause a sharp pain that begins in the lower back. As the stone moves along, the pain seems to travel with it and strike with a vengeance in the abdomen, groin, and testicles. For women, the pain also begins in the lower back and can radiate to the abdominal and vaginal areas. It has been compared to giving birth. "It's one of the worst pains that a person can have," says Gary Curhan, M.D., Sc.D., director of the Partners Center for Kidney Stone Disease at Massachusetts General Hospital in Boston.

Fortunately, for most of us, kidney stones aren't inevi-

An Apple a Day Recipe

No-Stones Stuffed Potatoes

Potatoes are packed with potassium, which can help you sidestep kidney stones. These twice-baked potatoes are stuffed with a savory broccoli-cheese mixture.

4 large potatoes
½ cup skim milk, warmed
¼ teaspoon onion powder
¼ teaspoon garlic powder
⅛ teaspoon ground black pepper
1 package (10 ounces) frozen chopped broccoli, steamed

½ cup shredded reduced-fat Cheddar cheese
Paprika
1 teaspoon grated Parmesan cheese

Pierce the potatoes with a fork and place on a microwaveable plate. Microwave on high for 20 minutes, turning once, or until the potatoes are tender. Set aside to cool.

Meanwhile, in a large bowl, combine the milk, onion power, garlic powder, and pepper.

Preheat the oven to 400°F.

When the potatoes are cool, cut them in half lengthwise and scoop out the insides, reserving the skins. Add the potato insides to the milk mixture. Mash with a potato masher or hand mixer until smooth and creamy. Stir in the broccoli and Cheddar. Divide the mixture among the potato skins. Sprinkle with the paprika and Parmesan.

Place the stuffed potatoes on a baking sheet. Bake for 15 minutes, or until lightly browned.

Makes 4 servings. Per serving: 301 calories, 4 g. fat, 51% of Daily Value of potassium table. Here are a few simple dietary changes that can dramatically lower your odds of having a kidney stone. And if you have had attacks in the past, these tactics can help prevent a recurrence.

DRINK LOTS OF WATER. Your kidneys work as a sort of traffic cop for the body's waste products. They filter harmful substances out of the blood and redirect them out of the body via the ureters. In the presence of fluid, the waste dissolves and flows from the body without difficulty. But when the body is dehydrated, the waste products remain in crystalline form and can react with each other to form a stone made of either calcium oxalate or uric acid.

"Fluids are the single most important ingredient in the prevention of kidney stones," says John S. Rodman, M.D., associate clinical professor of medicine at Cornell University School of Medicine in New York City and co-author of *No More Kidney Stones*. "Theoretically, you could eat anything you wanted and never make a stone if you could drink enough."

The goal is to drink enough water to produce two quarts of urine a day. For most of us, eight eight-ounce glasses of water will do the trick.

If you exercise heavily, live in a hot and dry climate, or work in hot conditions, you will need to drink as much as 10 to 12 glasses a day.

You can tell how much waste is in your urine by checking the color: If it is dark yellow, the crystals are not dissolving, and you should increase your fluid intake.

EAT MORE POTASSIUM. In scientific studies, people who ate lots of fruits and vegetables rich in potassium cut their risk of developing kidney stones by roughly 50 percent. "We have found potassium to be more protective than any other dietary factor," says Dr. Curhan.

To increase your intake of potassium from food, you can easily get your daily minimum from bananas and potatoes.

Calcium to Prevent Kidney Stones

For many years, a low-calcium diet has been recommended to prevent kidney stones. But researchers at Harvard who studied the diets of 100,000 nurses for 12 years found that the more calcium there was in the foods they ate, the *less* likely the nurses were to develop kidney stones. Nurses getting more than 1,100 milligrams of calcium from food daily had one-third the risk that nurses getting less than 500 milligrams a day had. This confirmed an earlier study of men, showing a similar result.

These results, however, only applied to nurses who got extra calcium from food, like milk and yogurt. Those who took calcium supplements actually had a 20 percent higher risk of stones. Researchers think that the higher risk could be related to the fact that the nurses in the study took calcium supplements *between* meals rather than with meals.

Many women take calcium supplements to help prevent bone loss. There is a very low risk that women taking these supplements will develop kidney stones, says Gary Curhan, M.D., Sc.D., director of the Partners Center for Kidney Stone Disease at Massachusetts General Hospital in Boston. But if you have already had a stone, you are at high risk for another one. He recommends talking to your doctor about a diet that provides enough calcium without adding to your risk of getting stones in the future.

For people who have endured chronic stones, their doctors may recommend additional daily supplements, usually taken two or three times a day, to help prevent future attacks.

CUT BACK ON MEAT. Studies show that diets high in animal protein increase the chance of forming stones.

"Most people who develop stones eat too much meat," says Dr. Rodman.

How much meat is too much? Your daily total of meat should be no more than two three-ounce portions, or about 70 grams of protein. Measured by size, each portion should be no larger than a deck of playing cards.

KNEE PAIN
Put a Cap on It

From climbing stairs to kneeling in the garden, that critical hinge halfway down your leg gets a vigorous daily workout. So it's no wonder that knee injuries account for more than a quarter of all problems treated by orthopedic surgeons. And the way it is constructed—well, nothing's perfect.

"Essentially, it is like a round ball sitting on a flat surface, held in place by rubber bands. And the kneecap, it is like an ice cube on Formica," explains James M. Fox, M.D., an orthopedic surgeon and knee specialist with the Southern California Orthopedic Institute in Van Nuys and author of *Save Your Knees*.

No wonder many of us get kneecapped by Father Time. Osteoarthritis of the knee afflicts almost everyone to some degree by the age of 60, says Dr. Fox. This is the kind of inflammatory arthritis that is the result of wear and tear around and inside the joint.

You can, however, prevent knee problems. And the

first step you should take is out the door—to burn calories and to strengthen leg muscles.

LIGHTEN UP A BIT. "To prevent knee pain from osteoarthritis or injury, the first thing that you have to do is lose weight," says Dr. Fox. The reason, of course, is that more weight means increased pressure and stress on that weight-bearing joint. "If you throw a bag of sand in the trunk of your car for traction during the winter but then drive around with it all year, your tires will wear abnormally. If you weigh 10 extra pounds, you carry that extra weight around with you all the time, and your knees will wear abnormally. Those 10 additional pounds put 60 pounds per square inch of extra pressure on your knees every time you take a step."

Scientific studies support Dr. Fox's assertions. In a long-term study of 1,178 men, those who were 20 pounds overweight in early adulthood nearly doubled their chances of developing painful knee osteoarthritis later in life. In a study of 48 overweight women with knee osteoarthritis, who lost an average of 15$^{1}/_{2}$ pounds through treadmill walking and a reduced-calorie, low-fat diet, 40 percent of the women reported only half as much pain after losing the weight.

BUILD THE FATTED CALF. The second thing that you have to do is strengthen the muscles that support the knee joint—the calf muscle, the quadriceps on the front of the thigh, and the hamstrings on the back of the thigh. "Millions of Americans have experienced knee pain or knee injuries," says Dr. Fox. "Most of these pains, sprains, and strains could have been avoided with weight loss and proper muscular conditioning."

That is because the muscles guide the knee joint like reins guide a horse, says Dr. Fox. If the muscles aren't strong enough, the joint is wobbling all over the place and is more likely to be injured.

Walking Away from Knee Surgery

When osteoarthritis creates ever-escalating knee pain, some doctors will recommend surgery, but maybe there is a way around it. If you have osteoarthritis, you may be able to skirt the scalpel with a spin on an exercise bike or a walk in the park.

In one study, aerobic exercise was found to reduce pain and disability levels enough so that people with osteoarthritis considering knee replacement surgery "might be able to put it off for several years," says study leader Walter Ettinger, M.D. In some cases, exercise might be able to eliminate the need for surgery altogether.

The people who participated in the study worked out for 30 to 45 minutes, three times a week. Of the 439 people with osteoarthritis, the ones doing daily aerobic exercise reported a 12 percent reduction in knee pain as well as increased mobility when walking, climbing up and down stairs, and getting in and out of their cars. Those who lifted weights also reported significant pain reduction and mobility gains.

Exercise may unkink an arthritic joint because it strengthens muscles surrounding the knee, stabilizes the joint, and makes it less susceptible to pain, Dr. Ettinger notes. It may also increase production of pain-blocking substances called endorphins. And as exercisers noticed improvement, they developed an "I can do it" attitude that lessened their perception of pain.

Stronger leg muscles will also help prevent the pain of osteoarthritis of the knee, says Arthur Brownstein, M.D., clinical instructor of medicine at the University of Hawaii School of Medicine and director of the Princeville Medical Clinic in Princeville. "Ninety-eight percent of the pain in any arthritic joint is caused by weak muscles, tendons, and ligaments *around* the joint," he says. "Stronger muscles prevent pain by taking pressure off the joint."

Building the muscles in your legs doesn't mean that you have to hire Arnold Schwarzenegger as your personal trainer. "The best way to strengthen the hamstrings, quadriceps, and calf muscles is by walking," says Dr. Fox. He recommends doing it regularly for 30 to 40 minutes, three or four days a week, alternating with jogging or bike riding if you want to. It is a good idea to check with your doctor before starting any new exercise program.

WALK EVERY MOUNTAIN. Tired of walking a flat terrain all the time? Set your sights higher and try hill walking, suggests Dr. Brownstein. "You will really start to feel your quadriceps and hamstrings build in their strength and endurance once you start to walk up and down hills."

DON'T SHOOT YOURSELF IN THE FEET. If you exercise regularly but find that knee pain is starting to creep in, take a good look at your fitness shoes, says Dr. Fox. "The right fitness shoe keeps the knee stable and reduces impact, both of which are key to avoiding injury. Running shoes, for example, aren't meant for walking. They have a different tread and cushioning than is necessary for that activity."

To find the best fitness shoe, Dr. Fox recommends shopping at a shoe store that deals with many different types of fitness and sports activities and that carries lots of different brands. "Asking friends is a great way to get good advice about where to shop for fitness shoes," he adds. And if a friend has a favorite salesclerk at the store, get the name, too.

POSE FOR PREVENTION. While strengthening the muscles around your knees, you also have to keep those muscles flexible. The most effective technique to do this is "a simple yoga stretch called the pelvic pose," says Dr. Brownstein. In fact, the pelvic pose is so powerful a pain-stopper that it can also heal knee pain. "I've prescribed it for people with advanced osteoarthritis who were scheduled to have knee replacement surgery, and they have been able to regain full function with no pain."

To do the pelvic pose, kneel on a mat or carpeted floor with your heels beneath your buttocks. The tops of your toes should be flat on the floor, and your arms should hang freely from your sides. If you find that there is too much pressure on your ankles, roll up a towel and put it between the ankle joint and the mat or carpet. You can take this position anytime and hold it for as long as it is comfortable, Dr. Brownstein advises. "When you are going through your mail, instead of sitting at the couch and bending over a coffee table, do the pelvic pose and read the mail in that position. Do it when you are folding laundry, watching television, or reading. It is the best way to prevent knee pain."

DON'T POSE IN PAIN. If you already have some knee pain and you want to keep it from getting worse, you can still do the pelvic pose, but a modified version. When you start out, kneel upright near a sofa or bed, resting your arms on the mattress or sofa back for support. Put a stack of pillows or folded blankets on your calves behind your knees. "Slowly lower your body onto that stack," advises Dr. Brownstein. If the pain starts, just back off a little bit to a spot where it is no longer painful and rest in that position, supported by the stack. Now breathe deeply, slowly, and gently to bring oxygen into the muscle cells that you are stretching.

Repeat this modified pelvic pose and hold for as long as it is comfortable. Try to work up to 10 to 15 minutes, three to five times a day, suggests Dr. Brownstein. With each repetition, remove more and more of the stack so that you can put more weight on your legs. "Eventually, you will be able to come down all the way without pain so that you can take all of your upper-body weight on your lower legs," he says. "This will help your knees to heal."

GET SOME KICKS AT THE OFFICE. If you are sitting in an office chair all day, there is a good chance that your knee joints aren't being effectively lubricated, says Richard Braver, D.P.M., a sports podiatrist and director of the Active Foot and Ankle Care Center in Englewood and Fair Lawn, New Jersey. To prevent getting knee pain when you are in this plight, he recommends an easy 10-second exercise called the quad pump. This exercise tightens up the quadriceps, the front thigh muscles just above your knees. Here is how it is done.

You can do the quad pump while seated in your chair. Just extend your legs so that your heels are resting on the floor, then tighten your quadriceps. Hold the contraction for two seconds, then release. Repeat this five times, relax, then do a second set.

"Basically, these pumps cause the cartilage to secrete a fluid that bathes the joint in nutrients," says Dr. Braver. You can do this exercise whenever your knees feels stiff, he says, after sitting in a car, in a movie theater, or in a long meeting.

LARYNGITIS
You Needn't Get Husky

Angela loved that game last Saturday, even though she didn't want to go. After all, she started out with a cold. And she knew everyone was going to be rowdy. But as it turned out, the game was stupendous. Angela cheered loudly—along with everyone else—and afterward, she sang the alma mater at the top of her lungs. By Sunday morning, Angela's voice had diminished to the level of a very faint stage whisper. "I think I have laryngitis," she tried to tell her sleeping husband. He didn't even stop snoring.

Your vocal cords, high in your windpipe, are tight bands that vibrate as your breath passes over them. But if anything causes those cords to swell with inflammation, your speech will sound more breathy like a hissing cat than like human articulation. Too much enthusiasm, whether it is at the school game or the Saturday-night sing-along, can set you up for swollen vocal cords. More often, however, the laryngitis is caused by a viral infection. Here is how to keep your cords strumming.

How to Hold Your Hoarseness

Okay, you're hoarse, but you can still talk. Here is what you can do to help prevent your laryngitis from silencing you completely, says Blake Simpson, M.D., assistant professor of otolaryngology/head and neck surgery at the University of Texas Health Science Center at San Antonio.

DON'T WHISPER. "Whispering causes more trauma to the vocal cords than talking in a low volume with a normal voice," says Dr. Simpson.

DRINK PLENTY OF WATER. "When you replenish the water stores in your body, the mucus on your larynx will be thinner and more lubricating and more effective at stopping further damage." He recommends eight eight-ounce glasses a day. "And it has to be water, not herbal tea or juice."

REST YOUR VOICE. "Use your voice only when absolutely necessary for one to two weeks. Bring a pad of paper with you to communicate. Use e-mail," he advises.

AVOID SMOKY OR DRY ENVIRONMENTS. If you have to be in a dry environment—an airplane, for example—drink even more water, perhaps 10 to 12 glasses a day, he suggests.

IF YOU HAVE A COUGH, USE A COUGH SUPPRESSANT. "Coughing is very damaging to the vocal cords," adds Dr. Simpson.

STOP CLEARING YOUR THROAT. "Clearing your throat is very hard on the vocal cords," he says. "Instead of clearing your throat, take a sip of water or try to get rid of the sensation by swallowing."

DON'T USE A THROAT ANESTHETIC. "Using a throat anesthetic when you have laryngitis numbs the vocal cords so much that you are likely to traumatize them even more without knowing it," he says.

AVOID THE INFECTION. Most cases of laryngitis are what doctors call common viral laryngitis, a viral infection of the larynx that usually shows up along with a cold, bronchitis, or some other type of upper-respiratory tract infection. Frequently washing your hands and avoiding contact are the two best ways to prevent laryngitis, says Blake Simpson, M.D., assistant professor of otolaryngology/head and neck surgery at the University of Texas Health Science Center at San Antonio. "If someone has viral laryngitis, there is a reasonable chance that the virus could be passed by hand-to-hand contact, even when he uses a handkerchief," he says. So avoidance is the best prescription for prevention.

HALT THE HOLLERING. The second most common cause of laryngitis, says Dr. Simpson, is vocal abuse, traumatizing your vocal cords with hours of yelling or loud singing.

You are even more at risk for this type of laryngitis if you already have a cold or another kind of upper-respiratory infection, according to Dr. Simpson. So even if a cold doesn't keep you away from the game, clapping instead of yelling is the best way to root for the home team.

STOP THE BURN AND SPARE THE CORDS. Heartburn is a problem that afflicts just about everybody at some time or another. If you have had it, you may know that it is caused by stomach acid seeping up into the esophagus. The acid can also spill into the throat, which can damage the vocal cords so that the voice is husky and slightly lower in pitch, says Dr. Simpson.

One of the best ways to prevent this type of laryngitis is to either reduce or eliminate caffeine, according to Dr. Simpson. "Drinking caffeinated drinks really relaxes the lower esophageal sphincter," he says, which is the flexible valve that controls the stomach entrance. Cigarettes, alcohol, fried food, chocolates, and any candy, gum, or food that contains spearmint or peppermint also relax this valve and should be avoided.

GIVE UP WHEN IT GIVES OUT. To prevent laryngitis from going from bad to worse, give your voice a rest, but don't whisper, whenever your vocal cords start to hurt, Dr. Simpson advises. "If you experience vocal fatigue or pain in the throat when you are yelling, you should stop immediately and begin to rest your voice," he says.

DON'T SMOKE. There is a reason why constant smokers often have husky voices: Their vocal cords take a real beating when they are subjected to all that smoke rolling by. You will be less likely to get laryngitis if you swear off smoking, Dr. Simpson says.

LOW BLOOD PRESSURE
Keeping Your Cool

It is a hot and sunny August day—almost perfect weather, if it were just 10 degrees cooler. Not the kind of weather that's great for standing in line. But if that's what you are doing, you may find yourself beginning to feel thirsty, over-heated, and irritated. As more time passes, you may even feel light-headed, sweaty, and nauseated—almost as if you were going to faint.

Doctors call this a vagovagal reflex. Your brain sends an erroneous message to your heart to slow down, send blood to the arms and legs, and lower pressure. Heat, lack of water, and an excess of emotional stress can trigger this mind/body miscommunication, say doctors. Quite possibly, you are dealing with low blood pressure, medically known as hypotension. (Hypertension is the medical term for high blood pressure.)

If light-headedness is a frequent occurrence, the first thing to do is visit your doctor to find out whether your blood pressure is low. If so, your doctor can probably deter-

---

Are Your Medicines the Culprits?

Some medications can cause low blood pressure as a side effect, says David Robertson, M.D., professor of medicine, pharmacology, and neurology at Vanderbilt University in Nashville. The three biggest offenders are antidepressants (like Elavil or Norpramin), diuretics (like Diuril or Lasix), and high blood pressure medications (like Capoten or Catapres). If you feel light-headed, sweaty, or nauseated while taking any of these medications, consult your doctor about possibly lowering the dose or switching to a different drug, he advises.

---

mine what kind of low blood pressure you have, which is the first step in preventing it.

There are two major types of low blood pressure. The first is orthostatic intolerance, the most common type, when the blood pressure measurement drops less than 20 points on the top (systolic) and 10 points on the bottom (diastolic). The second and less common type is called orthostatic hypotension, when the drop is *greater* than 20 points systolic and 10 points diastolic.

At least 500,000 Americans, especially women under 35, are prone to frequent bouts of orthostatic intolerance, or OI. Symptoms include light-headedness, fatigue, nausea, headaches, confusion, muscle pain, palpitations, and sometimes fainting.

Orthostatic hypotension, or OH, seems more prevalent in people over 60. About 1 in 1,000 people in this age group have a weakened nervous system that causes low blood pressure almost immediately after they stand. They, too, may suddenly feel dizzy, faint, or confused from loss of blood pressure.

Unfortunately, medical science hasn't discovered how to prevent the onset of OI and OH. But if you have been diagnosed with either one, there are plenty of things that you can do to prevent the onset of dizziness or faintness that are so often associated with low blood pressure. Here is some advice from doctors.

Drink lots of water. Drinking eight eight-ounce glasses of water, and more if you know that you will be out in the hot sun, can help you if you have either type of low blood pressure, says Peter Rowe, M.D., associate professor of pediatrics at the Johns Hopkins University School of Medicine in Baltimore. Drink those glasses at regular intervals throughout the day.

Salt away. Doctors recommend eating as much salt as you can tolerate to treat low blood pressure.

When you have salt in your diet, you increase the amount of fluids in the bloodstream, raising the blood pressure. Unlike some people with high blood pressure who need to avoid salt, you can be liberal with the saltshaker and welcome the salted variety of pretzels, says Dr. Rowe. Also, people who have low blood pressure don't have to worry about the high sodium in many soups and canned foods.

Shop smart. People at risk for low blood pressure should try to avoid standing in line for a long time, particularly when it is hot, advises Dr. Rowe. Shop during off-hours, when the crowds have thinned. And if you are visiting an amusement park on a blazing hot day, ask someone else to hold your place in line.

Take stock in hosiery. For women, wearing support hose can create enough pressure on the legs to raise blood pressure, says David Robertson, M.D., professor of medicine, pharmacology, and neurology at Vanderbilt University in Nashville. You can get these stockings at some drugstores and medical supply stores, or your doctor can give you a prescription.

Keep moving. Whenever you do have to stand in line, keep your legs moving slightly, says Dr. Rowe. That will ensure that blood is pumped back to your heart to prevent low blood pressure. Crossing your legs while standing also helps.

SHIFT WHILE YOU SIT. A few minor adjustments while you are sitting can raise your blood pressure, says Dr. Rowe. Sit in a low chair to elevate your knees higher than your hips when you are lounging around at home. That position sends more blood to the heart and increases the blood pressure.

GET A LEG UP. Gravity causes blood pressure to increase in body parts that are far below the level of the heart. Your blood pressure is higher in your feet than your abdomen, says Dr. Robertson. Simply propping up one leg to a 45-degree angle (like on a chair rung) while you are standing can raise your blood pressure by 10 points, he says.

BE CAREFUL WHEN YOU EXERCISE. When people with OH exercise (except for exercises in water), their blood pressure drops, says Dr. Robertson. One reason is that the body heats up during exercise—and increased body heat causes a drop in blood pressure. So if you have OH, use caution if you work up a sweat, and sit down if you feel faint, he advises.

TAKE SHORTER SHOWERS. If you have OH, limit your showers to five minutes and keep the water slightly cool, says Dr. Rowe. Long showers in hot water tend to lower your blood pressure, and fainting away in the shower is a dangerous possibility.

BEWARE OF CARBOHYDRATES. For people with OH, a high-carbohydrate meal can cause blood pressure to fall. That is because your digestive system needs plenty of blood to work on processing those carbs, and it is drawn to its task from other blood-needy parts of the body. "If you are going to eat lots of carbohydrates—a big dessert, for example, or pizza—take it very easy for an hour or two afterward," says Dr. Robertson. Lounge around after your meal. And when you get up from your seat, rise slowly.

LUNG CANCER
No Smokes, More Salad

You won't find in this book any health problems more deadly than lung cancer. But at the same time, few conditions are more preventable. Since tobacco use causes almost 90 percent of all lung cancer, you have control of this beast.

Still, if 9 out of 10 lung cancers are linked to smoking, 1 out of 10 isn't. So to maximize your defenses, you can do more than shun cigarettes.

True, some of lung cancer's risk factors are out of your hands, such as a history of other lung diseases like pneumonia and asthma. And a variety of hormone-related reproductive factors can alter the risk for some women. But even if risk is written in your family history or your hormone-producing system, there are steps that you can take down the road toward prevention.

SHUN OTHER PEOPLE'S SMOKE. What used to be a hot debate is now a cold fact. "Environmental tobacco smoke is clearly a cause of lung cancer in nonsmokers," says Ross Brownson, Ph.D., professor of epidemiology at the

St. Louis University School of Public Health. "If your spouse smokes or you are around somebody who smokes, don't breathe their smoke." In fact, if you are right in the line of fire, you may be getting the worst of some of the noxious ingredients, according to Dr. Brownson, since the stuff is hotter at the public end than the puffing end.

A modern shift in your favor: "The social norms about smoking in public places have changed enough that you should be able to avoid environmental tobacco smoke," Dr. Brownson says. In other words, in these enlightened times, you can insist on smoke-free air without coming off as a pushy churl.

EAT YOUR FRUITS AND VEGETABLES. In addition to steering clear of tobacco smoke—your own or others'—probably the next best thing that you can do to prevent lung cancer is to eat more fruits and vegetables. "There have been hundreds of studies done all over the world on all kinds of people, and they all come to the same conclusion," says Jerry W. McLarty, Ph.D., chairman of the department of epidemiology and biomathematics at the University of Texas Health Center in Tyler. "Eat your fruits and vegetables. The connection is solid."

What's more, studies indicate that people who eat a variety of fruits and vegetables, including deep green vegetables, orange and yellow vegetables, cruciferous vegetables, citrus, and other fruits are at a lower risk of lung cancer. But, Dr. McLarty warns, that doesn't mean a good vegetable-and-fruit diet offsets the increased risk from smoking. "It is nowhere near being in the same league," he says.

JUST WASH THEM AND MUNCH THEM. There is some evidence that fruits and vegetables have a stronger protective effect when you eat them raw, according to Susan Taylor Mayne, Ph.D., associate professor of epidemiology and public health and director of cancer prevention and control research for the Yale Cancer Center at the Yale University School of Medicine. For one thing, researchers aren't sure

Stop in the Name of Your Lungs

The logic is simple enough: Smoking causes lung cancer, among a host of other evils. So don't smoke. And if you smoke, quit. But anyone who has tried in vain to do the right thing can tell you that it's not that easy.

It is no easier to stop smoking now than it ever was, but a lot more help is available. A veritable industry of smoking-cessation assistance is out there. And there is plenty of free information on quitting techniques, down to the smallest of helpful details, like what to do with the ashtrays. Here, though, are some of the big-picture ideas that can help you go into the battle better armed.

RESPECT THE ENEMY. Many a valiant soul has failed by underestimating the mission, thinking the task was simply to break the habit. "Smoking is much more than a habit," says Ellen Gritz, Ph.D., a clinical psychologist and chairman of the department of behavioral science at the University of Texas M. D. Anderson Cancer Center in Houston. "It is nicotine dependency."

And hardly a mild dependency. Consider this: You generally take about 10 puffs on each cigarette. If you smoke a pack a day, that's 200 puffs every 24 hours, or 73,000 puffs a year. "And each puff gets nicotine to your brain in under six seconds," Dr. Gritz says. "It is a phenomenally fast and efficient drug-delivery system."

REALLY MEAN IT. Given the might of your foe, you can't just dabble in quitting if you expect to get anywhere. "You have to make a commitment to stopping," Dr. Gritz says. "You have to set a quit date, and then you have to hold to it."

just what in fruits and vegetables fights lung cancer. Since cooking destroys some of the nutrients and other substances found in fruits and vegetables, you may be sautéing

MAKE A RESOLUTION. Dr. Gritz has done research indicating that a New Year's resolution may not be a bad way to make that commitment. "People who made up their minds and stopped for New Year's had a much higher rate of quitting than a random population," she says. Of course, there is nothing special about January 1. It is simply a way of solidifying the first prerequisite to stopping—setting a quit date.

WEAN YOURSELF. You don't have to give up nicotine suddenly. You can get chewing gum and skin patches over the counter that dose you with enough nicotine to ease the withdrawal process while you eschew cigarettes completely. And they help, according to Dr. Gritz, approximately doubling the quit rate of those in treatment programs. To derive maximum benefit, though, be sure to follow the instructions on the label.

GO TO THE PROS. There is no law forcing you to quit smoking on your own, especially these days when there are so many programs and aids available to help people stop. "Advice from a health-care practitioner doubles the quit rate compared to no advice at all," Dr. Gritz says. "And the more intense the treatment, the higher the quit rate."

HANG IN THERE. "Most relapses occur in the days or weeks immediately following quitting," Dr. Gritz says. "And that is very logical because you are experiencing withdrawal, and it can be quite severe." But somewhere between the third and six month, you will find that you have crossed a threshold and the hardest part is behind you.

away your allies. "Try to eat at least some fruits and vegetables raw," she says.

TEST YOUR HOME. Radon, by its own action and by its

interaction with cigarette smoking, is considered to be the second leading cause of lung cancer. Radon is a carcinogenic gas that, when geologic conditions are right, can seep into your home at dangerous levels. How can you tell if it has? "You can go to the hardware store and pick up an inexpensive test kit," Dr. Brownson says. "They are easy to use and give you a pretty good measure of the radon levels in your home."

If your home has a high level of radon, call a radon-control professional. He can both seal your home, especially the basement, to cut down how much radon can seep in and install a fan that helps ventilate radon safely.

OPEN YOUR KITCHEN WINDOW. Researchers have discovered an increase in lung cancer risk in Chinese and Taiwanese people who live in homes where excess vapors from canola oil (used in wok cooking) are allowed to accumulate. Though there is no indication yet that it is an important factor in the West, Dr. Brownson suggests that you make sure your kitchen is adequately ventilated if you do a lot of Chinese-style cooking. You should have a good vent hood over the cooking area, exhausting to the outside.

LYME DISEASE
Get Ticks Off

Lyme disease's function in this world is apparently to give us one more thing to worry about as we enjoy the great outdoors. But on the serious-o-meter, Lyme disease is light years ahead of, say, poison ivy. Left untreated, it can cause heart problems, nervous system problems, muscle pain, and many years of arthritis. "I've seen lives ruined and careers ended by this disease," says Dale Hamilton, Ph.D., a microbiologist and director of clinical microbiology at the Alvin C. York Veterans Administration Medical Center in Murfreesboro, Tennessee. "And I've seen it hit the young and old."

The guilty party is a corkscrew-shaped bacterium that sequesters itself in your nervous system after being deposited into your bloodstream, courtesy of a biting tick. The tiny little tick—usually a deer tick—isn't trying to make you sick. He is just hungry.

Gloomy as all this sounds, the odds aren't that bad. Ticks don't feed all year, and most deer ticks don't carry the Lyme disease bacteria anyway. Even if a germ-laden tick

Techniques of Tick Attack

You knew you were taking a chance when you rolled around in the bushes on a June afternoon in rural Connecticut. And sure enough, there is a little tick sucking on your skin like a baby at its bottle. What should you do?

RELAX. It may not be a disease-carrying tick. And it may not have had time to pass on the bacteria anyway. "Even most deer tick bites don't actually infect you," says Robert Schoen, M.D., clinical professor of medicine at the Yale University School of Medicine and co-director of the Lyme Disease Clinic in New Haven, Connecticut. If it does, there is time for early treatment.

GET IT OUT. Use narrow tweezers and pull from the head, which will be as close to your skin as possible. "Be careful not to squeeze its hind end," Dr. Schoen says. "You could actually inject the contents of the tick into you."

Your best effort may still leave the tick's barbed mouth clinging, according to Dr. Schoen. "That's okay," he says. "Keep the area clean, put some alcohol on it, and in a day or two, it will come out."

bites you, he doesn't always pass on the bug. But your preventive goal is simple: Keep those creatures off your skin.

KNOW THE TERRITORY. Lyme disease has occurred in most U.S. states and Canadian provinces, but the overwhelming majority of cases happen in the tick-friendly outdoors of the Eastern seaboard, from Massachusetts to Maryland. Another hard-hit region is in the upper Midwest, especially Minnesota and Wisconsin. Lyme disease is also a problem in northern California. "If you live in these places or visit them, you have to be careful to avoid tick bites," says Robert Schoen, M.D., clinical professor of medicine at the Yale University School of Medicine and co-director of the Lyme Disease Clinic in New Haven, Connecticut.

IF YOU ARE BITTEN, SAVE THAT TICK. "Put it in a bottle and stopper it up," says Dale Hamilton, Ph.D., a microbiologist and director of clinical microbiology at the Alvin C. York Veterans Administration Medical Center in Murfreesboro, Tennessee. "He will be all right for months, and it is possible to have that tick tested for the bacteria, should you develop symptoms of early Lyme disease."

WATCH FOR EARLY SYMPTOMS. "If you think that you have been bitten by a deer tick, you should consult a doctor," Dr. Schoen says. "But don't be surprised if he only recommends a watchful approach." What you are watching for are flulike symptoms and the telltale circular rash that rings out from the bite site like a bull's-eye.

GET EVALUATED. If your prevention efforts should fail and you do get Lyme disease symptoms, you are still better off if you get quick treatment. "If you jump on a Lyme disease case early enough and with sufficient antibiotics, you can knock it out," Dr. Hamilton says. Even if you don't have the rash, you should see a doctor if you know that you have been bitten by a tick and you are in an area where Lyme disease is known to occur.

CHECK THE CALENDAR. The offending ticks feed from about midspring through most of the summer, according to Dr. Schoen. So your risk is lower if you plan a camping or fishing trip for early spring or early autumn.

STAY ON THE TRAILS. Ticks hang out in the thicker woods or brushy areas. They don't fly, jump, or pounce. So as long as you are on the trail, you are much safer, says Nadu Tuakli, M.D., a preventive medicine specialist and a family practitioner in private practice in Columbia, Maryland.

TICK-CHECK OFTEN. When a tick bites you, it is usually after he has been piggybacking for a while. It can take a tick as long as 36 hours to transmit the bacteria to you, according to Dr. Hamilton. So if you get him out of your skin right away, there is a good chance that you are protected.

The problem is that you may not know he is there if you don't look for him. "The tick bite is often not painful, so frequent tick checks are a good idea," Dr. Schoen says. The tick is the size of a black peppercorn, and often there will be some redness around the bite. He can be anywhere on your body.

CHECK YOUR CHIHUAHUA. "While you are at it, check your dog for ticks," Dr. Tuakli says. "Pets like to run in and out of the woods, and that puts you at risk even if you don't go into the woods."

COVER UP. In the woods or brushy areas of the risky regions, says Dr. Tuakli, wear long sleeves and long pants tucked into your boots or socks. "You want your skin covered from the neck down," she says.

BE A GOOD GUY. In other words, wear white. "That makes it much easier to see ticks on your clothes," Dr. Tuakli says.

BE REPELLENT. Take out some anti-tick insurance by spraying your clothes with a promethrine-based repellent such as Permanone, suggests Dr. Hamilton. Treat your outerwear once or twice a season by spraying them until they are fully saturated and then allowing them to dry completely before wearing. Products such as Permanone are designed to be absorbed by material, so make sure you don't use them on bare skin. "Treat the clothes you use when you push the lawn mower or walk in the woods."

STRIP OUTSIDE. When you get home, tired and dirty from that weekend of backpacking, resist the temptation to stagger inside and flop down. You could be introducing a live tick to your down comforter. "It's better to take your clothes off outside or in the garage," Dr. Tuakli says.

DO SOME YARD WORK. If you live in a geographically high-risk area and especially if your property has woods,

Dr. Hamilton suggests keeping vegetation cut back away from the house and busy areas of your property.

And, Dr. Schoen says, place bird feeders well away from the house. "Feeders attract mice and mice attract ticks."

MEMORY LOSS
The Art of Cherishing Memories

You do indeed lose some short-term memory as you grow older. But that's natural. The natural decrease in memory function that may start at middle age is not a sign of senility or of serious dementia like Alzheimer's. "In fact, people between the ages of 65 and 75 are actually better at certain kinds of memory than young adults," says Carolyn Adams-Price, Ph.D., associate professor of psychology and chairman of the interdisciplinary gerontology program at Mississippi State University in Starkville. "Particularly in remembering to do things and keep appointments."

You are losing memory, not your mind. "Cognitive function is very complex, and memory is only one part of it," says Barbara Sherwin, Ph.D., professor of psychology and of obstetrics and gynecology at McGill University in Montreal. "No one is saying that your ability for abstract thinking or concept formation is compromised at midlife."

And, there are things that you can do to slow down

Remembering the Names Game

What is more common at social gatherings than exchanging business cards? Just this: The verbal dance you have to perform because you can't remember the name of the person you are supposed to be introducing to your spouse. "The number one memory complaint at any age is remembering names," says Forrest Scogin, Ph.D., professor of psychology at the University of Alabama in Tuscaloosa.

If you want to keep track of them, here are some guidelines that can help.

CONCENTRATE. Focus on the name when you are first introduced to somebody. "A lot of times, the reason you can't remember a name is that you never really got it to begin with," Dr. Scogin says. Deliberately store the name in your mental file.

REPEAT. "Ask the person right away if you have the name right," Dr. Scogin suggests. "Or use the name in the conversation that follows, like salespeople do when they talk you up." This will imprint the name in your memory.

ASSOCIATE. Immediately relating the name you hear to something else helps you lock it in. "How do you remember that a fellow is named George?" asks W. Scott Terry, Ph.D., professor of psychology at the University of North Carolina at Charlotte. "Think of five things you know about the name George." So, with the freshly introduced person now connected with George Washington, George III, *George* the magazine, Georgie Porgie, and George of the Jungle, it is easier to remember his name.

VISUALIZE. Mental imagery is a great name-remembering technique. The name of your new friend Ralph with the red hair will come back to you quickly if you form an initial image of, say, a red Irish setter whose bark comes out more like "Ralph!" than "Ruff!" Silly? Of course. That's the point. "If it is unusual, it stands out," Dr. Scogin says.

some of the loss, and plenty more that you can do to compensate for the rest.

GET SMART. "A pretty consistent line of research says that people of higher educational attainment tend to have less slippage in memory function as they age," says Forrest Scogin, Ph.D., professor of psychology at the University of Alabama in Tuscaloosa.

"But it is not too late to get more education," Dr. Adams-Price adds. "There are lots of people these days over age 60 getting advanced degrees."

FEED YOUR HEAD. Your brain doesn't know if it is learning in a classroom or in your living room. If you keep reading and keep learning new skills, the ongoing stimulation of your cognitive functions can minimize memory loss. "Anything that you can do to make yourself pay more attention helps," Dr. Adams-Price says. "There are lots of hobbies that require thinking—bridge, crossword puzzles, computer games, books, discussion groups."

READ RIGHT. One way to help prevent memory loss is by exercising your memory every chance you get—and that includes reading. While you are still in the middle of a good book that you are enjoying, imagine telling some one about what you are reading, says W. Scott Terry, Ph.D., professor of psychology at the University of North Carolina at Charlotte. "That helps you concentrate on it and remember more."

The way you read is also important in maintaining your memory. Don't try to just get through a book, cautions Dr. Terry. "Reflect on what you read," he suggests. "Repeat it. Rehearse it. Continually refresh your memory."

CONSIDER HORMONES. Research by Dr. Sherwin and others has found a solid link between menopause and memory loss in women. And like for many postmenopausal problems, hormone-replacement therapy (HRT) may help. "There is a decrease in certain aspects of memory with menopause," she says. "By giving estrogen to women, we can help bring them back to where they were." This could be an additional factor to consider if you are a woman making a choice about whether or not to use HRT.

SLOW DOWN. A memory lapse can be simple distraction; your mind just isn't on the ball. "Try not to operate on automatic pilot," Dr. Adams-Price says. "When you are not paying attention, that is when you make the mistakes."

A classic example: Without thinking, you turn left when you should turn right. Why? Because you usually turn left at that intersection. A classic solution: "Just slow down," says Dr. Terry. "Pause for a second and mentally form your intentions. Repeat to yourself what you are going to do."

GO FOR GINKGO. Many studies in Europe have shown that the herb ginkgo boosts the brain's ability to use oxygen and so improves the memory. It is available in convenient tablet form that is standardized to contain 24 percent ginkgo flavone glycosides. The standard dose is 120 to 240 milligrams a day, says Donald J. Brown, naturopathic doctor and author of *Herbal Prescriptions for Better Health* and editor of the *Quarterly Review of Natural Medicine*. Taking more than 240 milligrams per day may cause dermatitis, diarrhea, and vomiting. Also, be aware that this drug may increase the action of pharmaceutical MAO inhibitors, such as phenelzine sulfate (Nardil).

REMEMBER TO EXERCISE. There is compelling evidence that a habit of aerobic exercise can control memory loss. In one study, researchers found that volunteers who got an hour of aerobic exercise three times a week performed better on memory tests than those who didn't work out. Exercise, they speculate, keeps the blood flow to the brain peppy. Better blood flow means more oxygen and faster glucose metabolism. Exercise also reduces stress, which may interfere with your memory.

MENOPAUSE PROBLEMS
Managing the Midlife Move

No, you are not imagining things. Menopause problems really are more of an issue these days than they were a generation ago.

Not that symptoms have changed much, but women have. When menopause comes, typically around age 51, a woman is likely to be at the top of her career. She might have teenagers still living at home. Who has time for hot flashes?

"A generation ago, a woman's kids were usually gone by the time she turned 50, and she probably wasn't working," says Geoffrey P. Redmond, M.D., director of the Women's Hormone Center at the Center for Health Studies in Beachwood, Ohio. "If she didn't feel well, she could at least try to deal with it without the added stresses of outside work and small children."

Menopause, enlightened doctors will tell you, is not a disease. It is a natural phase of life when a woman stops menstruating and her production of hormones such as estrogen pretty much shuts down. "Menopause is not a single moment when periods stop," Dr. Redmond says. "It is an interval that may last for several years as the ovaries slow down and make less estrogen. Symptoms may emerge gradually over that time."

Some "symptoms" are subtle and long-term, such as an increased risk of heart disease, a significant loss of bone mass that can lead to osteoporosis, and a cumulative loss of short-term memory function.

Others are temporary and more immediate. These are the bothersome physical symptoms that come and go with annoying frequency during the several years of menopause transition (often beginning before a woman's last period). Here is a partial list.

Hot flashes. A natural periodic response to changing body-temperature regulation, they can make a woman feel as if she has been locked in a sauna, with the sensation of warmth usually starting in her chest and moving up to her face. They are also called hot flushes; *flash* carries a misleading sense of brevity.

Night sweats. Essentially, they are hot flashes that hit at night when a woman is sleeping.

Mood swings. It is a myth that menopause causes depression, but it sometimes brings pre-existing depression into focus. More often, the hormonal changes can result in a nonclinical kind of depression. It is also true that frequent bouts with other menopause-related symptoms, such as hot flashes or insomnia, aren't exactly what you would call mood boosters.

Sleep problems. Insomnia and other sleep-related difficulties are common and major menopause-related problems.

Dry skin. Cruelly, the cessation of ovarian function has the unwelcome effect of drying out skin, especially around the eyes. Some hair loss is also sometimes associated with menopause.

Bloating. There is much suspicion that the bloating

and weight gain that often accompany menopause are more of an age thing than a hormonal thing. But if either is a problem for you, you could probably care less about that distinction.

Bothersome sensations. A catchall category for some less-common but equally irking symptoms such as muscle pain, joint aches that mimic arthritis, and light sensitivity that can be very uncomfortable.

Doctors might argue that other health concerns should be more pressing in women's minds, such as the long-term risk of heart disease and osteoporosis. But for menopausal women, the symptoms of menopause take center stage. "Most women who come in for treatment are more concerned with being comfortable right now than with the long-term changes," says Donna Orofino Patno, R.N., a doctor of naturopathy and a certified nurse midwife with a clinical doctorate in nursing at the Women's Hormone Center at the Center for Health Studies in Beachwood, Ohio. "They will deal with the long-range problems, but they want to feel better first."

And that's the good part. There are ways that you can help prevent the night sweats, which sabotage sleep, as well as other menopause problems. And you can do most of these menopause strategies on your own. Here's how.

PULL THE TRIGGERS. Hot flashes are usually set off by something you did just before they started. So your first order of business is to identify those triggers so that you can avoid them. Do a little behavior survey on yourself, suggests Margery Gass, M.D., a gynecologist and director of the University Hospital Menopause and Osteoporosis Center at the University of Cincinnati. "Just note what was going on in the 10 minutes preceding the hot flush," she says.

WATCH THE SPICY FOOD. Certain foods can trigger hot flashes, and sizzling spices are a common culprit, according to Patno. "Be careful with hot, spicy foods," she says. Other usual suspects are hot beverages, caffeine, sweets, and alcohol.

SEE THINGS IN A NEW LIGHT. According to Dr. Gass, more than a few hot flashes are triggered by hot, bright lights. "Experiment with what kind of lights you are sitting under," she suggests. "You might want to consider fluorescent lighting or something that puts out a little less heat."

SHUN LATE COFFEE. Easing off on the java may sound like a no-brainer if you are having problems sleeping, but you can be fooled by your own history. "Your body changes, and a lot of women find that they can no longer tolerate caffeine in the evening like they used to," Dr. Gass says.

And there is another reason to watch how much coffee you drink: It might bother your bladder. "Whether it is decaf or regular, coffee can more easily provoke bladder irritation and cause a sense of urgency than when you were younger," says Dr. Gass.

CHUCK THE EVENING CHOCOLATE. Chocolate treats, as well, are sleep thieves. "People don't realize that chocolate can cause some insomnia," Dr. Gass says.

RELAX INTO SLEEP. For women making the menopause transition, a lot of things are conspiring against a good night's sleep. Good sleep habits help you turn things in your favor. The two most important of those habits, according to Dr. Gass, are regular sleeping hours and presleep relaxation.

"Be very consistent about your sleeping patterns," she says. "Try to do the same things every night before bedtime, and don't change your schedule a lot." Relaxing routines before bedtime can mean different things to different people. "For some, it is a warm bath," Dr. Gass says. "Find something that gets you in the frame of mind to sleep peacefully."

TAKE YOUR CALCIUM AT BEDTIME. Calcium is essential for osteoporosis prevention in postmenopausal women.

If you are a woman over 50 and you are using hormone-replacement therapy (HRT), you should aim for 1,200 milligrams a day, says Patno. For women who aren't on HRT or women who are over 65, Patno recommends 1,500 milligrams a day. But it has an added benefit for more immediate problems. "If you cap off your daily supply with a supplement or calcium-rich snack one to two hours before bedtime, it can help you sleep," she says.

UP YOUR VITAMIN E. Patno recommends "very liberal" use of vitamin E, assuming that you don't have diabetes or some other medical condition that would stop you from taking recommended doses in the high range. "Instead of taking that nice little 400 IU (international unit) capsule, talk with your doctor about taking 800 to 1,200 IU per day," she says. "That does wonderful things for hot flashes, night sweats, and problems with vaginal lubrication." If you are considering taking amounts above 200 IU, discuss this with your doctor first. One study using low-dose vitamin E supplements showed an increased risk of hemorrhagic stroke.

The vitamin E oil itself will help relieve the vaginal dryness that sometimes accompanies early menopause, according to Liliana Gaynor, M.D., clinical assistant professor in the department of obstetrics and gynecology at Northwestern University Medical School in Chicago. "Instead of taking your daily dose by mouth, just break open the capsule and apply the oil before intercourse," she says. You can use vitamin E like this two or three times a week.

GET YOUR B-COMPLEX. Low energy can be a problem when you are going through menopause, and supplementing the B vitamins can help prevent feelings of fatigue. "Vitamin B_6 is good not only for energy but also for mood swings and bloating," Patno says. "But don't go over 100 milligrams a day without talking to your doctor." Unstable gait and numb feet may occur when taking doses of vitamin B_6 at 50 milligrams to two grams daily over a prolonged time.

EAT SOY. Soy is an all-purpose health weapon that researchers now think fights short-term symptoms, such as hot flashes and vaginal dryness, and helps reduce the long-term risks of osteoporosis. That is probably because most soy products are rich in naturally occurring estrogens called isoflavones. "With moderate doses of anywhere from 30 milligrams to 70 milligrams of these isoflavones, you may see improvement in the severity of menopausal symptoms," says Gregory Burke, M.D., an epidemiologist and vice chairman of the department of public health sciences at the Bowman Gray School of Medicine of Wake Forest University in Winston-Salem, North Carolina.

You can get that amount of isoflavones in typical servings of tofu, soy powder, or soy milk—usually. "A problem you run into is finding a reliable source of isoflavones," Dr. Burke says. "You can eat two different types of tofu, and one may contain enough isoflavones, and the other, none." He predicts that the market will soon adjust to the rising demand for isoflavones in soy. "But until there is labeling that says how much isoflavones are in each soy product, you will probably have to call the manufacturer to find out," he says.

TREAT YOUR TOFU. Soft tofu is one of the best soy sources of symptom-relieving isoflavones, but let's check in with reality here. That bland blob isn't high on most people's list of favorite foods. Remember, though, that there is no rule saying that you have to take it straight. There are lots of things that you can mix it with in a blender. "Add anything to make it taste really good—bananas, strawberries, honey, vanilla, and some milk or soy milk," says Patno.

ADD SOME FLAXSEED. You get additional benefits when you add flaxseed to soft tofu. The flaxseed has its own weak estrogen-like micronutrients as well as lots of constipation-fighting fiber, according to Patno. She recommends adding about a teaspoon of flaxseed to one to two ounces of soft tofu.

SIP GARDEN SAGE TEA. "A cup of garden sage tea does

wonders for night sweats," Patno says. Make sure that it is *garden* sage, she cautions, and don't drink more than a cup every other night for two to four months while night sweats are at their worst, since this herb has been known to hurt the liver. Garden sage tea is available at many health food stores. Steep according to package directions.

WALK DOWN PRIMROSE LANE. Swallow 500 to 1,000 milligrams of primrose oil a day in capsule form to ward off dry cyc syndrome, a condition that often manifests itself in women at menopause, Dr. Gaynor suggests. You can find it at most health food stores.

EAT WELL NOW MORE THAN EVER. "Menopause can often be handled simply by good nutrition, adequate exercise, and a reduction in alcohol," Dr. Gaynor says. That means you might prevent uncomfortable symptoms if you cut down on sweets; eat as many unprocessed, whole foods as possible; and favor fruits and vegetables over fat.

"A good diet is incredibly important for menopausal women," Patno says. "Your basal metabolic rate is changing, so you will find that it is a lot easier to put on weight."

EXERCISE. "If you have never exercised before, now is the time to start," Patno says. Besides the proven array of physical benefits, vigorous activity sends mood up and stress down.

"Exercise certainly boosts endorphins," Dr. Gass says, referring to natural feel-good chemicals released by the brain. "And it is a good way to burn off extra anxiety." Shoot for at least 20 minutes of aerobic exercise, three times a week, with a focus on walking and other weight-bearing exercises. You should always check with your doctor before starting a new exercise program.

WEAR COTTON. When hot flashes do strike, ease the discomfort by being prepared. One way is by wearing loose cotton clothing. "Cotton fabrics breathe better than synthetics and allow your body to regulate its temperature better," Dr. Gass says.

LAYER YOUR CLOTHES. It is a time-honored technique for getting the best of hot flashes. "If you dress in layers, you can casually remove your jacket, then your vest, and so on," Patno says. "You don't have to feel as if your only choice to get cooler is to strip naked."

STAY OUT OF THE NOONDAY SUN. "Watch hot weather," Patno says. "Try not to do physical activity during the heat of the day in the summer. That's basic, but people don't think about it."

BEAT THE HEAT THE FUN WAY. Regular sex, two to four times a week, can reduce the number of hot-flash episodes, according to Christina Stemmler, M.D., director of the Center for Integrated Medicine in Houston. "That's because, depending on your age, you are stimulating the hormones you have left," she says. "Sex cranks them up."

TRY ST.-JOHN'S-WORT FOR MOOD. "As long as you are not on an antidepressant, St.-John's-wort is good for some of the mood swings that go along with menopause. It is very safe," Patno says. You can get this herbal tea or supplement in many drugstores and health food stores. To find out the right dose, just follow the instructions on the package. And if you are fair-skinned, avoid excessive exposure to sunlight when you are taking St.-John's-wort.

Preventing the Plummet of Sex Life

The only things about your sexuality that end at menopause are pregnancy, concerns about birth control, and menstruation hassles. You can put everything else into the "opportunity" category.

That doesn't mean that new sexual challenges don't arise. Dryness of the vaginal tissue is one common menopause-related problem, and there are others as well. Waning desire is common, and when you just don't feel much like having sex, it is unlikely that you will have a fulfilling sex life.

But for healthy and robust sexuality during and after menopause, the best defense is a good offense. There are things that you can do to keep the fires burning now and into old age.

THINK POSITIVE. "In a way, menopause is a built-in treatment for some of the conditions we suffered during our reproductive years," Dr. Stemmler says. Indeed, what's to complain about in saying goodbye to the fear of unwanted pregnancy? Or to birth control decisions? Or to romantically untimely menstruation? Or to premenstrual syndrome and menstrual cramps? "Focus on those positives," Patno says. "It can make a huge difference."

RETHINK YOUR SEXUAL PATTERNS. Sometimes decreased sexual desire is closely linked to your belief system. "Your expectations and beliefs can increase or decrease your desire," says Sheryl Kingsberg, Ph.D., a clinical psychologist and assistant professor of psychology in the departments of reproductive biology and psychiatry at Case Western Reserve University in Cleveland. "If a 50- or 60-year-old thinks that women of a grandmotherly age shouldn't be sexual, that may decrease her desire."

According to Dr. Kingsberg, we all have our comfortable and set ways of thinking about sexuality. We also have the option of changing them. "Every once in a while, just rethink the concept," she suggests. "Ask yourself where you got your beliefs. Rethinking your rules about what's okay and not okay creates the ability to be more sensual and have more fun."

GET CREATIVE. "Do things that you never dared to do when you were 30 or 40," Dr. Stemmler says. "Menopause is a great opportunity for that."

Besides opportunity, there is necessity. "There are physical changes with age," Dr. Kingsberg says. "Women notice differences in sensation in their breasts as well as in clitoral sensation. So you need to explore to see what works best now."

LUBRICATE. At menopause, lubricants will usually take care of vaginal dryness during intercourse. "Water-based lubricants work great," Dr. Kingsberg says. "Use them and use them liberally."

ASK ABOUT ESTROGEN CREAM. While lubricants can take care of vaginal dryness long enough for you to enjoy intercourse, they don't deal with the ongoing problem or with the thinning of the vaginal tissue that often accompanies menopause. Ask your doctor about a prescription for topical estrogen cream. "It treats the dryness and makes the vagina very moist," Dr. Stemmler says.

USE IT OR LOSE IT. "Sex is something you need to do in order to preserve the capability of doing it," Dr. Gass says. The longer you are sexually active, the longer your vaginal tissues will stay supple.

MENSTRUAL CRAMPS
Easing the Monthly Toll

Any woman who has ever experienced severe menstrual cramps knows that the word *cramps* doesn't sound quite bad enough to describe the pain.

Physiologically speaking, the term is accurate. Uterine muscle contractions naturally increase in intensity with the onset of menstruation. Sometimes they increase too much. Cramps are extreme contractions, explains Liliana Gaynor, M.D., clinical assistant professor in the department of obstetrics and gynecology at Northwestern University Medical School in Chicago. Fortunately, you can help prevent the pain.

TAKE AN NSAID. Nonsteroidal anti-inflammatory drugs (NSAIDs) are a class of over-the-counter drugs for menstrual cramps that is so far ahead of the pack that most doctors rarely recommend anything else. It is easy to take care of cramps with a drug like naproxen (Naprosyn), says Dr. Gaynor. It not only stops the present pain but also can help prevent upcoming discomfort. Just follow the label directions when you are taking it.

PREEMPT YOUR PAIN. Medical researchers are pretty sure that the uterine contraction problems that result in menstrual cramps are the work of an excess of contraction-inducing chemicals called prostaglandins. In addition to being pain relievers, NSAIDs help prevent prostaglandin production.

But for NSAIDs to work as a pain preventer, you have to time your doses. "The key is getting that anti-prostaglandin medication in there early," says Margery Gass, M.D., a gynecologist and director of the University Hospital Menopause and Osteoporosis Center at the University of Cincinnati. "If you're really regular, you can start taking it the day before your period. Otherwise, take NSAIDs according to label directions at the first hint of a symptom."

BRING OUT THE HEAT. Women have been using heat for relief from painful periods for centuries. There is no reason for you to stop that tradition if it can help prevent the pain. And it often does, says Donna Orofino Patno, R.N., a doctor of naturopathy and a certified nurse midwife with a clinical doctorate in nursing at the Women's Hormone Center at the Center for Health Studies in Beachwood, Ohio. "Get out the heating pad or the hot-water bottle and wrap it in a towel," she says. "Make yourself comfortable on the couch with a good book, put the pad on your belly, and cover yourself with a blanket." You may be able to prevent your cramps from getting worse.

CONSIDER THE PILL. If you choose to take oral contraceptives for birth control, you may find that they have another benefit; they help to prevent cramps. "Birth control pills help by suppressing ovulation," Dr. Gass says. "For most people, it can be a pretty benign way to manage cramps." Your doctor can help you decide if the Pill might be right for you.

Pricking Away the Pain

For an alternative therapy that might prevent many future episodes of monthly menstrual pain, some doctors are now recommending a treatment from the repertoire of Chinese medicine. "Acupuncture is extraordinary for menstrual cramps," says Christina Stemmler, M.D., director of the Center for Integrated Medicine in Houston. "For a very large percentage of women, menstrual cramps are either greatly improved or completely gone within a few cycles after acupuncture treatment."

Acupuncture is the ancient Chinese therapeutic technique that uses strategically inserted needles to unblock curative energy in the body. The traditional medical establishment has acknowledged that many of these treatments are effective. But if you are considering acupuncture for your cramps, Dr. Stemmler cautions that it must be done by skilled hands. Any doctor who recommends acupuncture can usually refer you to a qualified practitioner. Or look for a lay acupuncturist who is certified by the National Certification Commission for Acupuncture and Oriental Medicine.

MONONUCLEOSIS
How to Ban the Virus

With all those syllables and its Armageddon-like reso-
nance, mononucleosis sounds much worse than it is. Typically a low-grade infection brought to you courtesy of the
Epstein-Barr virus, mono generally resolves itself without
treatment in a matter of weeks.

But it is no fun to have, as a cursory glance of the symptoms makes clear: weakness, fever, loss of appetite, malaise,
headache, muscle pain, nausea, and sore throat. What's
more, those who are most likely to have these symptoms—
young people from adolescence through college-age—are
probably the least likely to welcome the uninterrupted bed
rest that mono demands.

Preventing mononucleosis is fairly simple. Here is
some doctors' advice for you or for the highly susceptible
teenagers in your home who might need to know.

MISS THE BUSS. No one has ever launched a "safe kissing" campaign to help prevent mononucleosis, but maybe

someone should. "Saliva-sharing is mono's transmission mode of choice, and also why it was called the kissing disease; so it makes sense to keep your lips away from danger," says Joseph Marzouk, M.D., an infectious disease specialist at the Infectious Disease Medical Group in Oakland, California.

STICK TO YOUR OWN EATS. You might not want to think about it, but a little saliva can transfer the virus to food if you happen to be sharing a plate with someone who has mono. "If you know somebody who has mononucleosis, it is probably best not to share food or utensils with that person," says Dr. Marzouk.

PREVENT ANYTHING WORSE, TOO. Mono may do more harm when you don't have it than when you do. Uh . . . how's that again? "There are other illnesses like strep throat, hepatitis, or even HIV infection that can mimic mononucleosis," Dr. Marzouk says. "You may assume that you have mononucleosis when you really have a more serious illness that can be difficult to treat if not discovered early." To prevent another health problem from rapidly getting worse, he advises, make sure that you get a diagnosis from a physician as soon as you feel the symptoms.

STAY AWAY FROM THE ROUGH STUFF. Your spleen often enlarges with mono, which means that you need to prevent a rupture. If you have had mono, reduce the danger of rupturing your spleen by steering clear of any jarring physical activity, even if you are feeling better. "Take it easy until your doctor has told you that your spleen has gone down," says Paul Ellner, Ph.D., professor emeritus of microbiology at Columbia University in New York City. "Avoid contact sports and heavy lifting."

Giving Mono an Early Kiss-Off

You may have taken your best step toward preventing mononucleosis without even knowing it. That is because people who have had the virus once are unlikely to have a second run-in. "You are unlikely to get it twice," says Margaret Lytton, M.D., a family practitioner in private practice in Narberth, Pennsylvania. "Once you've had it, you are immune."

What's more, your first mono experience may already be out of the way, and you may not even realize it. "Almost everybody gets this disease and recovers from it," Dr. Lytton says. "A majority of people, actually, probably get the disease in infancy when there are usually very mild symptoms. So you might have had a sore throat as a kid, and that was your mono."

Although chances are that you've already had mono, you will want to follow basic guidelines for prevention. In developed countries such as the United States, the infection develops more often in the teenage years or older than it does elsewhere. "And that is when you get more severe manifestations," Dr. Lytton says.

MOTION SICKNESS
Stop Those Unsettling Experiences

Sometimes the worst thing about motion sickness isn't the dizziness. Or the nausea. Or even the vomiting. No, the worst thing about motion sickness is that while you are feeling miserable, everybody else in the car or on the boat is enjoying the view and feeling fine. What's going on here?

"Motion sensitivity varies with the individual, and we don't know why," says Craig Buchman, M.D., an otologist in private practice in Miami.

You get sick when the balance system in your inner ear senses motion that contradicts what your eyes perceive. Seasickness may be the most common variety—just think of how many different ways a ship can move at once. But many a Sunday drive has been ruined by unwelcome queasiness. "The fact is that almost any kind of moving conveyance can produce motion sickness, whether it is a boat, a car, a plane, a horse, an elephant, or a camel," says Millard Reschke, Ph.D., a senior scientist for neuroscience at NASA's Johnson Space Center in Houston.

But there are almost as many ways to prevent motion sickness as there are vehicles to cause it. Here are some doctors' recommendations for moving without moaning.

TAKE THE WHEEL. Even the most nausea-prone road worrier seldom gets sick while driving. "If you are controlling the vehicle, you are controlling the motion," Dr. Reschke points out. "That reduces the conflict in your brain."

RIDE SHOTGUN. If you are not driving, sit in the front seat. The backseat is the worst because you are exposed to more motion than you are in the front, Dr. Reschke says.

There is another plus to being nearer the windshield. "You can maximize the visual input there," says Brian Blakley, M.D., an otolaryngologist in private practice in Winnipeg. "The movements your inner ear senses are confirmed by vision in the world outside the car." When you are getting information from two sources, your eyes as well as your ears, you are less likely to be dizzy, he explains.

DEVELOP A DISTANT STARE. Watching the telephone poles zip by only increases your brain's perception of the motion and your stomach's rebellion. "You are better off focusing on a landmark far down the road," Dr. Reschke says. "A mountain in the distance will work fine."

HOLD STILL. Keeping your head movement to a minimum helps fight motion sickness, Dr. Blakley says. "If you want to look at something, try to keep your head still and move your eyes instead."

TAKE A NAP. "Sleep is an excellent way of preventing motion sickness," Dr. Reschke says. Not everyone can sleep in a moving vehicle, of course, but nature tends to care for many who are prone to motion sickness by making them sleepy. Perception of motion isn't sent to the brain, so queasiness doesn't trouble those who are sleeping soundly.

READ SOME OTHER TIME. Even though you vowed to finish that Stephen King novel, save your reading for when you are not moving. "You get ill much faster when you read because you are effectively putting yourself into a 'room' that moves with you," Dr. Reschke says. This increases the conflict between what you see and what motion you feel, he explains.

TAKE A PILL. Over-the-counter motion sickness medicine such as Dramamine as well as stronger prescription versions work by reducing your brain's awareness of the sensory conflict, says Dr. Blakley.

Take them at least a half-hour before your trip. "If you wait until motion-sickness symptoms start, they are not going to work," Dr. Reschke says. And remember, this stuff makes you drowsy, so don't take Dramamine when you are the driver.

LEAN WITH THE TURNS. If curvy highways trigger your motion sickness, don't fight the turns. "You may notice that a bus driver always moves into the turn, but passengers tend to do the opposite," Dr. Reschke says. "It's better to do what the driver does."

DON'T LOOK DOWN. Advice for shipboard travelers: "The worst thing that you can do is bend your head over and watch the waves go by in the water," Dr. Buchman says. Instead, keep an eye on the horizon.

As long as you are on deck with the wind in your face and an eye on the horizon, you help to reduce motion sickness, Dr. Blakley explains.

SHUN THE CABIN. It is best to spend as much time as you can up on deck while at sea, Dr. Buchman says. "Seasickness is usually worse if you are below."

STAY ACTIVE. You may be able to keep seasickness at bay simply by not giving yourself time to think about it. "A lot of balance-system problems depend on how aware you are of them," Dr. Buchman says. "If you stay very active on a big cruise ship, for example, your brain can basically override what's going on in your stomach."

BE AWARE. Motion sickness doesn't usually hit all at once. Before you get sick, you often become "aware" of your stomach or throat. "Take that as a warning," suggests Dr.

Getting Over the Queasies at Sea

Here's a thought to cheer you as the rolling sea churns your stomach into a nauseated liability: Things get better.

"It is very common for seasickness to resolve itself after the first few days," says Craig Buchman, M.D., an otologist in private practice in Miami. "So hang in there."

In fact, even your car sickness can fade if you take those motor trips more often. "As you continue to experience these kinds of motion environments, your brain stores the memories," says Millard Reschke, Ph.D., a senior scientist for neuroscience at NASA's Johnson Space Center in Houston. "And that can protect you tomorrow in the same situations that are making you sick today."

One catch: The very medicine you take to get through the rough times inhibits the learning that your brain needs to do. "So if motion sickness is not too horrific for you, try to ride it out rather than taking a lot of suppressants like Dramamine," advises Dr. Buchman.

Reschke. "If you are on a boat, get up on deck and find a landmark."

If you are in a car, be sure to stop and get out. "It always makes you feel better to get some fresh air," Dr. Buchman says.

MUSCLE CRAMPS AND SPASMS
No More Knots

Sore muscles hurt, but it is sometimes a nice kind of pain, isn't it? It is like a reminder that you exercised too hard or hiked that trail where lesser mortals fear to venture.

But muscle cramps? There is nothing good about them. The pain is intense, sudden, and often inconveniently timed, striking as it does in the midst of physical activity or at night when you are trying to sleep. Usually, your muscles are masters of movement, expanding and contracting with mind-boggling efficiency. But sometimes, one will contract against your will, knot itself up, and stay there. That hurts.

Researchers have identified a lot of cramp causes, but doctors aren't 100 percent sure just how and why cramps happen, especially the nocturnal version. In fact, there is some confusion about what they are supposed to be called. With muscle spasms, you can actually see and touch the knotting muscles, and the spasm is usually injury-related. Muscle cramps, on the other hand (or usually on the other leg), can just happen, says Joel Press, M.D., medical director

An Apple a Day Recipe

Magnesium-Max Salad

Cramping up? The magnesium in spinach may help ease those muscles. This simple spinach salad is also a smart way to use leftover fish. Almost any white fish will do. Try cod, flounder, haddock, halibut, or even canned tuna.

⅔ cup low-fat plain yogurt
2 tablespoons lemon juice
1 tablespoon chopped fresh parsley
1 clove garlic, minced
5 cups torn spinach

12 ounces cooked white fish, cut into 1" chunks
1 carrot, cut into matchsticks
3 scallions, sliced

In a large bowl, stir together the yogurt, lemon juice, parsley, and garlic. Add the spinach, fish, carrot, and scallions. Toss to coat. Divide among 4 salad plates.

Makes 4 servings. Per serving: 129 calories, 2 g. fat, 33% of Daily Value of magnesium

at the Rehabilitation Institute of Chicago. Despite the difference between the two problems, Dr. Press believes that both may be caused by similar mechanisms. "There may be a lot of overlap between the two," he says.

So it makes sense that there is a lot of overlap in your prevention strategy for both.

MEET YOUR MINERAL NEEDS. When you lose water, you lose vital minerals along with it. And some people aren't getting enough of those minerals in the first place. Either way, mineral deficiency can cause cramps. Make sure that you are getting adequate calcium, potassium, and magnesium in your diet. Dairy products such as milk, yogurt, and cheese are good sources of calcium. Magnesium is abundant in tofu, beans, seeds, and leafy green vegetables. And you can get your potassium in vegetables and fruit, especially bananas, Dr. Ullis says. "Usually, you can get what you need if you are conscientious about your diet and if you take in enough water and other fluids," he says.

DRINK UP. "Dehydration is probably the number one cause of muscle cramps," says Edward R. Laskowski, M.D., co-director of the Sports Medicine Center at the Mayo Clinic in Rochester, Minnesota. "When you sweat or exercise for long periods, what you lose is water. That is what you should replace."

DRINK WHEN IT IS COLD. Guzzling water is a good anti-cramp strategy for all seasons, according to Dr. Laskowski. "A lot of people think that they don't need to drink water if it is cold," he says. "But winter air is very dry and easily dehydrates you. So drinking water is very important for skiers and wintertime cyclists, for example."

LAP IT UP EARLY. Don't wait until you are panting to get yourself hydrated during exercise. "Usually, by the time you are thirsty, you may be significantly down on your water content," Dr. Laskowski says. "So it is a good idea to drink going into an exercise. Then keep drinking throughout it."

GUZZLE ON TILL DUSK. It is not just heavy exercisers who need to get enough water to avoid cramps. "A lot of times just being in a state of relatively low water volume can trigger cramps at night," Dr. Laskowski says.

The solution is simple. "Increase your fluids," says Karlis Ullis, M.D., assistant clinical professor of sports medicine at the University of California, Los Angeles, School of Medicine. "And make sure that you are drinking enough fluids throughout the day."

STRETCH IT OUT. Tight muscles are more likely to

cramp up, so a good stretch is good protection, especially before and after you exercise. "Stretching is really important," Dr. Ullis says. "Before you go to bed, stretch all the major muscle groups, especially the areas that tend to irritate you. Hold each stretch for 30 to 40 seconds to get at the deep tissues."

SOAK IN SOME EPSOM. Dr. Ullis suggests adding Epsom salts to your post-exercise tub soak. "Epsom salts is basically magnesium," he says, "so you get more muscle relaxation."

USE THE SALTSHAKER. "If you have lost liquid after exercise, add a little more salt to your food," suggests Dr. Ullis. Sodium chloride helps you retain water. You need to be careful about using excess salt if you have been diagnosed with high blood pressure, but otherwise, let your tastebuds dictate your salt needs, he says.

NAIL PROBLEMS
Have Never-Fail Nails

It hardly seems fair, does it? How can little things like fingernails cause such big problems? Broken nails are ugly. Hangnails are ugly and painful. Ingrown nails are ugly and painful and potentially harmful. And nail fungus is ugly and painful and potentially harmful and disgusting.

It is also unfair that some of us are born with brittle, problem-prone nails. Others find that their nails start acting up when they get older. But all of us can avoid problems if we do right by our nails. Here's how.

FIND SOME REAL TOOLS. "Your nails aren't screwdrivers, and they aren't scrapers," says Richard K. Scher, M.D., a nail specialist and professor of dermatology at Columbia-Presbyterian Medical Center in New York City. "A lot of the problems I see are from people abusing their nails by using them as tools."

GET CREAM ON THE NAIL. Dry nails crack. And dry skin around the nails forms hangnails. "Using moisturizing lotions on a regular basis keeps the nail hydrated and prevents tearing while also keeping the cuticle softer so that it cracks less," says Paul Kechijian, M.D., clinical associate professor of dermatology at New York University Medical Center in New York City and a dermatologist in Great Neck, New York. "Apply the moisturizer to your palms," he says. "Then rub the nails of your right hand on your left palm and vice versa. This gets the moisturizer into your nails."

GO NATURAL. Eschew nail polish altogether because the process of removing the polish dries out and damages the nail, suggests Dr. Kechijian. "Just leave them alone, buffing them lightly for a slight sheen and a more finished look."

But if you can't do without nail polish, read the label. Make sure that your polish doesn't contain formaldehyde or toluol (sometimes called toluene), says Dr. Scher, and don't use removers that contain acetone, he advises.

DOUBLE UP ON GLOVES. When you put your hands in water, the nails absorb water and expand. When you remove them from water, the water evaporates and the nails contract. All that expansion and contraction makes your nails more brittle. So the less your hands are in and out of water, the better off your nails will be, says Dr. Kechijian.

But somebody has to do the dishes. Rubber gloves keep the water away but make your hands sweat, creating the same problem. The solution is to "get an inexpensive pair of cotton gloves and put them on under the rubber gloves," Dr. Kechijian says. "The cotton gloves absorb the sweat and keep the hands dry."

KEEP THEM SHORT. "The longer the nail, the more likely it is to become traumatized," Dr. Kechijian says. But don't go overboard. "It is a mistake to try to cut down into the corners of the nails because they tend to become ingrown fingernails or toenails," he says. "It's better to cut straight across." And while you are at it, make sure that you use good, sharp scissors or clippers and try to clip when the nails are soft.

CLIP AFTER A BATH. Cut your nails as soon as you get out of the tub, says Dr. Kechijian. Your nails are softest right after they have soaked and before all the water has evaporated out of them.

GET SUPPLEMENT SUPPORT. Strong nails require adequate vitamin intake, Dr. Scher says. Be sure that your vitamin supplements include minerals, especially zinc and iron. "And make sure that there is biotin in the supplement," he says. "Biotin is very helpful for brittle nails." Your multivitamin should contain the Daily Value of these three nutrients.

INVEST IN YOUR CUTICLES. Nail damage is often self-inflicted. "Nail biting is a big problem," Dr. Scher says. "Besides causing infection, it can cause permanent injury." His tip for keeping yourself from snacking on your fingernails is to treat yourself to a manicure, with all the extras. "If you spend good money getting your nails done, you are less likely to chew them up," he says.

HAVE BAD TASTE. Sabotage the taste of your fingernails, says Dr. Kechijian. How? Try one of those bitter-tasting nail products that are designed to discourage nail biting. They are available at any drugstore. Trying to bite your nails after putting this stuff on your nails will inspire an instant "yecch."

IF THE SHOE FITS, WEAR IT. There are ways to be kind to your toenails, too. "Make sure that your footwear fits properly," Dr. Scher says. If your shoes are too tight, it can lead to nail fungus and to ingrown toenails to boot. If you are a runner, buy new running shoes every several months, he advises. "Those cruddy old shoes can harbor fungus over time."

KICK YOUR SHOES OFF. "I don't care what kind of shoes you wear, they are going to make your feet sweat," Dr.

Kechijian says. He advises going around as much as you can in stocking feet in your home.

USE SOME SANDALS. Wear sandals at the poolside or in the gym shower, says Dr. Kechijian. They diminish your chances of picking up or spreading a fungus that may damage your nails and feet. And wear sandals in the summer. "The more you keep your feet cool and dry, the less likely the fungus will have a chance to grow."

NECK AND SHOULDER PAIN
New Tricks to Prevent Old Cricks

A house painter spends several hours painting a ceiling. His neck is bent backward, and his arms are stretched overhead.

A grocery clerk raises boxes of sugar onto a high shelf. He bends and reaches without the aid of a stepladder.

A writer on deadline cradles a phone while typing frantically on an awkwardly angled computer keyboard.

If you have neck pain, you may need to make some important changes in your routine. You can help prevent neck pain—and often-related shoulder pain—by changing a few bad habits and adding a few beneficial ones.

TAKE A BRIEF BREAK. Don't spend too long doing any one repetitive activity. It is always smart to break up your routine, says Karl B. Fields, M.D., professor of family medicine at the University of North Carolina and director of the Family Practice Residency and Sports Medicine Fellowship at Moses H. Cone Memorial Hospital in Greensboro.

Often, this is easy to do. If, for example, you have three hours of computer work and an hour of photocopying to do, Dr. Fields suggests breaking up the tasks into smaller chunks of time to vary your muscle movements and to prevent neck and shoulder cramps. After working at the computer for an hour, why not stand up, stretch, and do some photocopying? Alternating the tasks will help.

LIMBER UP YOUR LIMBS. "Muscles can get stiff if the neck is in one position too long, and then pain can set in," says Douglas Einstadter, M.D., assistant professor of medicine at Case Western Reserve University in Cleveland. To avoid the tightness leading to pain, he advocates taking a break every hour or two to stretch and relax.

Even a couple of minutes of stretching can help. If you can move around a bit throughout the day, he says, it often helps prevent neck problems.

DESTRESS TO STOP SPASMS. Tightness and muscle spasms are often brought on by anxiety and stress. "If you are under a lot of stress, just a twist, a bend, or a sudden head or arm movement can trigger a spasm," says Andrew Barkin, D.C., a certified chiropractic sports physician in private practice in Valley Stream, New York.

Muscles also fatigue faster in people who are stressed. "If you find that you are stressed a good deal of the time, then you need to look at relaxation as a part of prevention," says Dr. Fields.

"For some, relaxation may be blowing off steam at the gym," he observes. "But if you already exercise enough, a hot bath, shower, or whirlpool may be a good relaxer."

COUNT AS YOU BREATHE. Breathing techniques also help people relax and may help prevent painful muscle spasms, according to Dr. Barkin. "Inhale deeply through your nose, exhale deeply through your nose, count to three and repeat," he says. Try it for several minutes. You can do it anywhere, and it will help prevent neck pain. (This also helps assuage the pain if you already have a crick.)

FIND KEYBOARD COMFORT. Quite often, neck and shoulder pain is traceable to a workstation that is poorly

Work It Out

Simple exercises for the neck and shoulders can provide the muscle stretching that keeps you loose and limber. Try these neck stretches to keep good muscle tone and prevent aches and pains in your neck, shoulders, and other upper-body areas, suggests Ira Schneider, D.C., a chiropractor in private practice in Santa Monica and Thousand Oaks, California. Here are the four types of stretches that he recommends.

1. Lateral bending. Gently lower your ear to one of your shoulders, and hold for 15 seconds. Slowly return your head to the starting position, then lower it to the other shoulder. Do these stretches in the morning and in the evening, suggests Dr. Schneider.
2. Gentle rotation. Turn your head to one side, hold that position for three to six seconds, and then rotate your head very slowly and back to the other side.

arranged. Be sure that you have a chair that supports the small of your back so that you don't have to lean or slouch to get comfortable. When typing at a computer, make sure that you sit up straight in a comfortable, nonstraining posture.

Your keyboard should be at the proper height so that your forearms are perfectly horizontal when your fingers rest on the keys. If it isn't the correct height, all your muscles get put in an awkward position, and it can lead to neck ache, says John McShane, M.D., director of primary care sports medicine at Thomas Jefferson University in Philadelphia.

EYEBALL THAT MONITOR POSITION. Keeping the computer monitor at the proper height can help you avoid muscle strain. "Be sure that your monitor is set at eye level.

Repeat. Do these stretches in the morning and again in the evening.

3. Shrugging. First, shrug your shoulders up and down. Roll your shoulders forward and then backward. Then lower your chin toward your chest to flex your neck forward. Finally, place your hands on either side of your neck and slowly tip your head back, extending the neck only until it reaches the shoulders, says Dr. Schneider.

4. Turtling. Lying on your back, lift your head three to four inches, hold for an instant, and then lower your head to the floor. Repeat 15 times, advises Dr. Schneider.

When doing any of these exercises, beware of bouncy, jerking, or fast movements, warns Dr. Schneider. He advises against a very common neck stress reliever, head rolls—rotating your head in a circle. "This exercise can cause wear and tear on the small joints of the cervical spine," he warns.

For proper positioning, the top of the monitor screen should be at or just below eye level," says Dr. Einstadter. If it is, your head will automatically be in a comfortable position.

If you find that you are moving your head forward to look down at the monitor, that changes your center of gravity, says Ira Schneider, D.C., a chiropractor in private practice in Santa Monica and Thousand Oaks, California.

BEWARE PHONE FOLLIES. "Cradling a telephone between your head and shoulder is a common cause of neck and shoulder pain," says Dr. Schneider.

Instead, try a headset. "It's great for people who tend to cradle the phone," says Dr. McShane. A headset allows you to keep your head, neck, and shoulders in a normal, comfortable posture.

When to Worry

If neck pain radiates down your arm, it could be a sign of a disk problem in the neck. "You should seek medical attention," says John McShane, M.D., director of primary care sports medicine at Thomas Jefferson University in Philadelphia.

Also, take note if the pain goes down through your arm and into your fingers. It could mean a degenerative or herniated disk. "See a physician if you have any numbness, tingling, or weakness in the arm, because it may be a sign of nerve compression," says Douglas Einstadter, M.D., assistant professor of medicine at Case Western Reserve University in Cleveland. Your doctor may recommend treatment that focuses on taking the pressure off the disk so that it doesn't irritate the nerve.

HAVE A FLOOD OF FLUIDS. "Well-hydrated muscles fatigue less quickly than muscles that are poorly hydrated," says Dr. Fields. He encourages good fluid intake. "Water is used to transport minerals and electrolytes, which help with muscle contractions," he says. But remember that fluids with caffeine, like coffee and soda, are not helpful because they don't hydrate you very well. Choose water, sports drinks, or juices instead.

BALANCE YOUR ELECTROLYTES. Calcium, magnesium, potassium, and sodium are known as electrolytes, and they play a role in muscle contraction. "Muscle cramping is sometimes due to not having enough electrolytes in your system," says Dr. Schneider. For example, "magnesium is good in relieving muscle spasms and can help to increase the integrity of ligaments and muscles," says Dr. Barkin.

You can help avoid cramping by making sure to get enough foods that introduce these valuable minerals into your system. If you consume sports drinks such as Gatorade, you help replace all the electrolytes that are lost when you exercise hard, says Dr. Barkin. In addition, he suggests eating lots of leafy green vegetables, wheat germ, and cereal grains that are rich in magnesium. "Calcium can help to relieve muscle irritability," he adds, noting that dairy products, fish, cereal, and leafy green vegetables are all good sources.

BE A BACKPACKER. Lots of people get neck and shoulder pain from carrying a heavy pocketbook or briefcase because the weight is most often only on one side of their bodies. "A knapsack is a good alternative to a shoulder bag as long as it is lightweight," says Dr. Barkin. It divides the weight evenly between the two sides of your body.

"It's best to use a knapsack," agrees Dr. McShane. "But if you do carry a shoulder bag, alternate it from side to side on a regular basis."

AVOID PILLOW FIGHTS. Bad pillow habits can lead to neck pain. "Using too many pillows stacked too high overflexes the neck. While you are asleep, the neck should be maintained at a normal curvature," says Dr. Einstadter.

To avoid morning neck aches, use a pillow that supports your head and keeps your neck straight. Your head should neither droop back nor tip forward.

GO BELLY UP. Sleeping on your stomach means that your neck is twisted to the side. This position is detrimental to the neck and shoulders because it puts your neck in an abnormal position, says Dr. Einstadter. To avoid waking up with neck pain, try sleeping on your back.

BUY A WIDE STRAP. Larger-breasted women experience more bra-strap-induced neck pain because their straps support extra weight. The closer to your neck your bra strap lies, the more it impinges on the muscle that runs from the shoulder to the neck, causing pain in that area. "To prevent neck and shoulder pain, a bra should have good support in back as well as in front," says Dr. McShane.

"Larger-breasted women should make sure that they wear a bra with good support and shop in a store that carries larger-size bras so that they can be fitted properly," adds Dr. Barkin. Look for bras with comfort straps that are wider than the average bra strap and have extra cushioning. Wider straps spread out the pressure over a wider area.

TAKE CLASS ACTION. The Hindu discipline known as yoga is often cited for its benefits to the musculoskeletal system of the neck, shoulders, and back. Yoga classes can teach people how to benefit from concentration, meditation, and breathing exercises. To relieve neck tension, sit in a chair and grip the side of the seat with your left hand to stabilize your shoulders. Place your right hand on top of your head, drop your head toward your right shoulder and gently resist your hand with your head. Hold this pose for 10 seconds. Repeat on the other side.

"Yoga achieves muscular relaxation with the idea that all parts of the body should be in harmony," says Dr. Fields.

Yoga offers many strategies for preventing pain throughout the body, including in the neck and shoulders, explains Dr. Barkin.

DO SAFE SITUPS. If situps are part of your fitness regimen, be sure that you are not putting extra strain on your neck. Sometimes, people yank their heads with their hands to help pull themselves up. This action can cause neck pain.

"Cradle your head gently during situps," says Dr. Schneider. "Do not force it up, but allow it to come up at its own speed." Many experts suggest that instead of putting your hands behind your head when you are doing situps, just cup your ears with your fingers. This will keep you from straining your neck.

NIGHTMARES
Keeping the Beasties at Bay

It may be hard to accept right after you wake up screaming and sweating from a particularly ghastly dream, but nightmares often serve a productive purpose. "They can be a message from within that something is going on in your life that you are not coping with consciously," says Alan Siegel, Ph.D., president-elect of the Association for the Study of Dreams, an international organization based in Vienna, Virginia; a clinical psychologist in Berkeley and San Francisco; and co-author of *Dream Catching*.

While an occasional nightmare is not uncommon in adults, it is the recurring, unchanging, and disturbing ones that you need to do something about, according to Dr. Siegel. It is often best to take the lead from your local garage mechanic: "Open up the hood" of your mind. Find out what the problem is. Then fix it.

And, just like fixing a balky engine, this approach can prevent future problems. Here are some things that experts suggest you do to help stop nightmares from haunting your sleeping hours.

NEUTRALIZE IT. "Accept the nightmare," says Larry J. Feldman, Ph.D., director of the Pain and Stress Rehabilitation Center in New Castle, Delaware. "When you resist it, you give it power." The best route to acceptance is to seek the possibility that the nightmare is there for a purpose. "Making that assumption takes away a lot of the nightmare's sting," he says.

REASSURE YOURSELF. You are probably not proud of the way you behave in your nightmares, but a key step to leaving the nightly rut is to rid yourself of shame. "We all have nightmares, and it is okay to have them," Dr. Siegel says. "Reassuring yourself about that breaks the spell that the nightmare has over you."

A good shame-busting tactic is to speak up. "Tell a friend, tell a counselor, or just write it down," Dr. Siegel says. "Getting it out reduces the stigma." And make dream-talk a habit. "If you make discussion of dreams more of a regular feature of your conversation, then nightmares are less intimidating if they come," he says.

RELAX. "As long as your tension is running out of control, you will never make any sense out of your nightmare," Dr. Feldman says. He recommends this simple relaxation technique: "When you repeat the word *relax* to yourself a few times a day, your brain starts sending out chemicals that trigger the relaxation response," he says. "Then when a nightmare wakes you up, you can trigger those chemicals again by reminding yourself to relax."

EASE INTO SLEEP. An hour of stress-free relaxation before going to bed is always good sleep hygiene, but it also can help prevent nightmares, according to Dr. Feldman. "The best way to prevent a nightmare is to be in a relaxed state when you go to sleep," he says.

Dr. Feldman recommends two relaxation methods for

helping you get into this relaxed state. Your goal with these techniques is to increase serotonin production, which helps you sleep, and decrease your body's levels of cortisol (a stress hormone). You can set this physical process in motion through thinking and breathing in a relaxing manner when you are already in bed and lying awake in the dark, he says.

For the first technique, simply breathe in and out slowly, focusing on the air as it passes through your nose, the back of your throat, and into your lungs. Each time you exhale, repeat the word *sleep* or *relax*. Paying attention to your breathing also loosens your diaphragm and takes your mind off problems, he says.

Another technique that you can try involves counting backward from 100 to 1, but with a twist. Each time you inhale, think of the number, and then think of the word *sleep* as you exhale, Dr. Feldman says. This is another way to take your mind away from stressful thoughts.

START A DIALOGUE. "Talk to your nightmare," suggests Dr. Feldman. "Ask the characters or symbols in it what they are telling you." Will they answer? Probably not. "But just by asking, you enter a mind state in which you are more open to your own intuitive responses," he says. "You are more likely to hear that wee voice inside you, your wiser side, your higher self."

DO A REWRITE. Take control of your nightmare by re-scripting it, Dr. Siegel advises. "Create a new ending or put a new twist on the story," he suggests. Of course, your dream demons may not stick to their lines in their next appearance, but don't let that discourage you. "Keep rehearsing it," he says. "Or try it different ways. Consider it a kind of assertiveness training of the imagination."

RESOLVE IT. The dagger in the heart of your nightmare is to decode its message. "The dream is a metaphoric statement about something that is unresolved in your life," Dr. Siegel says.

Your Child's Nightmares

Young children are more vulnerable to nightmares because they have less control over their world, says Alan Siegel, Ph.D., president-elect of the Association for the Study of Dreams, an international organization based in Vienna, Virginia; a clinical psychologist in Berkeley and San Francisco; and co-author of *Dream Catching*. You know it is up to you as a parent to help them make it through the night, and a few parental strategies just may help them keep their childhood demons at bay. The question is, how can you help? Here are some ideas.

USE A PLAYFUL APPROACH. "If your child is dreaming of a spider, tell him that you are going to sweep that spider away with a broom," says Dr. Siegel. "Then literally sweep a broom. That's very effective."

WELCOME THE NIGHTMARE. Kids need to be reassured that bad dreams don't mean that they are bad little boys or girls, Dr. Siegel says. Soothe their fear and reassure them. One way to do that is to welcome the nightmare by offering to talk about it or draw a picture of it, so it won't be so scary.

EMPHASIZE CREATIVITY. "Dreams are a way for kids to express their feelings," Dr. Siegel says. "Try to connect on that dream level through dream-talk. It is a wonderful source of creativity."

START EARLY. "Talk to your two-year-old about his dreams," Dr. Siegel says. "As soon as he can start putting a few words together, he can tell you a little about what he is seeing in his sleep."

"When you play out the dream through rescripting, you eventually get some insight about how that metaphor relates to what is out of kilter in your life," Dr. Siegel observes. "Then take action to resolve the problem."

CHECK YOUR MEDICATIONS. Medications, prescription or over-the-counter, can sometimes induce nightmares, according to Quentin Regestein, M.D., director of the Sleep Clinic at Brigham and Women's Hospital in Boston. "Take stock of what drugs you are taking and what drugs you are withdrawing from," he advises. Medications that alter your nervous system are particular pharmacological villains, he says, but that doesn't mean you should simply stop taking prescribed medicine. Examples of drugs that may cause nightmares include beta-blocking antihypertensive medications like propanolol (Inderal) or metoprolol (Lopressor). And some antidepressants may also be associated with nightmares if they are taken at bedtime, Dr. Regestein says. If taking a new prescription is followed by particularly florid and unpleasant dreams, discuss it with your doctor.

OILY HAIR
Time for an Oil Change

A brief history of hair: The wethead was dead, then reborn. The dry look reigned, until it was overthrown by mousse. Hair fads come and hair fads go, but one thing stays: Nobody wants oily locks.

So why do a lot of us have them? "People come in all types," says Victor Newcomer, M.D., clinical professor of dermatology at the University of California, Los Angeles, School of Medicine. "There are some people who produce a lot of excess oil at one extreme, and then there are those—usually blondes and redheads—who produce very little oil. Most of us fall somewhere in between."

In other words, if you have oily hair, it is almost certainly because you were born that way. Consider it a trait rather than a condition, dermatologists say. But however you categorize it, you don't have to go through life with your hair looking like a wet cocker spaniel's. Here is what doctors say you can do to ebb the flow.

DO A DAILY DE-OILING. The best way to get rid of

Baby and Flakes

The perfect shampoo for your oily hair problems may be as close as your two-year-old's tub. "Baby shampoo is actually the best detergent shampoo there is," says Dorian Gravenese, M.D., a dermatologist in private practice in New York City. "Even though its alkaline nature makes it mild, it is still a great degreasing agent."

Chances are, there is another possible savior in one of your bathroom cabinets. "If you have a really oily scalp and baby shampoo doesn't seem to help it, try upgrading to one of the dandruff shampoos," Dr. Gravenese says. "They usually have drying agents such as zinc pyrithione or sulfides."

hair oil is also the most obvious one—wash it away. And then keep washing it away because that oil comes back like a pesky relative. "If you have oily hair, get used to washing it daily," says Alan S. Boyd, M.D., assistant professor of dermatology and pathology at Vanderbilt University in Nashville.

TAKE IT TO THE LIMIT. If once a day is good, is twice a day better? Try it, suggests Dorian Gravenese, M.D., a dermatologist in private practice in New York City. "The idea is to shampoo often," she says. "And while shampooing twice a day is not a good idea if you have a dry scalp, it is usually not a problem if you have oily hair."

There are limits, of course. "Too much repeated wetting and drying can aggravate any kind of hair," says Thomas Helm, M.D., assistant clinical professor of dermatology and pathology at the State University of New York at Buffalo and director of the Buffalo Medical Group Dermatopathology Laboratory in Williamsville. If you are washing your hair too frequently, it will become brittle and dry with an increase in split ends. Also, your scalp may become itchy and inflamed, he says.

USE AN OIL-STRIPPER. Take a little extra time to find a shampoo that gets the job done. The best ones (surprise) are those specifically formulated for oily hair. "They mean it when they say that on the label," Dr. Boyd says. "Those shampoos generally have more detergent, and that is what strips the hair of built-up oil."

There is another reason to choose your weapon wisely. "There are a lot of shampoos out there that are specifically trying to add moisture back into hair, and that is exactly what you want to avoid," Dr. Gravenese says. "So look for the words 'for oily scalp' or 'for oily hair.'"

DOUBLE UP. If oil is in your locks, you really can't settle for the lather-up-and-get-out shampoo routine. "Lathering twice each time you shampoo is never a bad idea," Dr. Boyd says. "Leave it on at least five minutes the second time before rinsing it off."

KEEP YOUR CONDITIONER OIL-FREE. Conditioners aren't obligatory for oily hair, but a lot of people still prefer to use one. That calls for more label reading. "If you need some kind of conditioner, put one on that is oil-free or at least has fewer oily properties," Dr. Boyd says.

DO A HORMONE CHECK. It is rare that excess oil production in the scalp is due to anything besides genes, but for some women, there might be another factor. If your formerly normal scalp turns oily, birth control pills may occasionally be a culprit, according to Dr. Boyd. "The hormonal manipulation can sometimes increase the glands' oil production, and that can give you an oily sensation in your scalp. If that is the case, you can consider stopping birth control pills."

On the male side, there is a similar hormonal connection, but with a much easier decision to make. "We all know the pitfalls of androgenic hormones that some men use who want to bulk themselves up," Dr. Boyd says. "They will also increase oil on the skin and hair as a side effect, which gives you one more reason to steer clear of these drugs."

OILY SKIN
For That Drier Look

Teenage skin, you no doubt remember, can drip enough oil to send OPEC prices plummeting. Mother Nature, bless her heart, usually caps the gushers as we mature, but sometimes she forgets. So a lot of us glow our way through life in a way we would rather not.

Bad luck in the gene-pool sweepstakes is to blame, so there is no real cure for oily skin. "Sorry, only one body per person," says Victor Newcomer, M.D., clinical professor of dermatology at the University of California, Los Angeles, School of Medicine. "But if you produce a lot of oil, you can do things to take care of it."

SCRUB UP. "Washing often with a lot of soap and water removes oil," Dr. Newcomer says.

What kind of soap should you use? "Look for one with more detergent and less fatty substances," says Dorian Gravenese, M.D., a dermatologist in private practice in New York City. "The heavier the fat—like in a bar of Dove soap—the more you want to avoid it." Find soaps that are

---

Oil-Free Makeup

You want to use makeup, but the last thing you need on your face is more oil. Fortunately, you are living in face-friendly times. "Look for products with the word *noncomedogenic* somewhere on the label," advises Dorian Gravenese, M.D., a dermatologist in private practice in New York City. "That means they are safe to use and are essentially oil-free."

Still, dermatologists recommend that you take any makeup for a test drive before buying, no matter what the label says. "Even oil-free products might create oil or just look heavy," she says. "Ask for samples, put one on each side of your face, and see how they work."

Moisturizers also come oil-free. Do you need them? Not really. "With oily skin, you have nature's moisturizer," Dr. Gravenese says.

---

formulated for oily or acne-prone skin, like Neutrogena, she suggests.

WARM YOUR HIDE. Water temperature makes a difference, too. "Hot water works on the oil on your face as it does with the grease on your plates," says Alan S. Boyd, M.D., assistant professor of dermatology and pathology at Vanderbilt University in Nashville. "It is better than cold water at stripping off the oil." Use water that is comfortably hot, he advises.

FIND AN EXFOLIANT. The best soaps for washing oily skin are often sold as anti-acne washes or bars, dermatologists say. They can be detergent- or sulfur-based (both enemies of oil), but the key ingredient is benzoyl peroxide. "These soaps are good at stripping off oil," Dr. Boyd says. "And benzoyl peroxide is a mild exfoliant, which gives you a dry sensation." Oxy 10 Balance Maximum Medicated Face

Wash and Fostex Medicated Bar are two products containing benzoyl peroxide.

TAKE SOME ACID. There are other cleansing options. "Salicylic acid–based washes are very effective for oily skin," Dr. Gravenese says. "And glycolic acid is a natural oil remover." All can be found in drugstore products; just check product labels for ingredients. Clear Logix and Neutrogena are two salicylic acid acne washes. Glycolic acid facial cleansers include Alpha Hydrox and Aqua Glycolic.

GET ROUGH. If that sheen comes back too soon after washing, Dr. Gravenese recommends a mild astringent. Most of the available astringents, such as Sea Breeze, use alcohol, which is a strong degreaser, according to Thomas Helm, M.D., assistant clinical professor of dermatology and pathology at the State University of New York at Buffalo and director of the Buffalo Medical Group Dermatopathology Laboratory in Williamsville. "Occasional use is okay, but it can get irritating if you use it regularly."

The more upscale department-store astringents blend witch hazel with other ingredients to reduce irritation, so they may be an attractive alternative if you have very oily skin, says Dr. Gravenese.

RAID YOUR TEENAGER'S MEDICINE CHEST. If anti-acne washes help, anti-acne creams help even more. "It is the benzoyl peroxide agent that keeps the oil at bay," Dr. Gravenese says. "And with creams or gels, that agent stays on your skin longer." Two brands with benzoyl peroxide are Johnson's Clean and Clear Persa-Gel and Clearasil.

DON'T OVERDO IT. In your ongoing oil war, there is a point of diminishing returns, Dr. Gravenese warns. "If you overwash or use astringents excessively, your body will react by actually producing more oil," she says. "So you have to monitor yourself."

BYPASS THE POWDER ROOM. Unlike most oily skin treatments, retinoids actually reduce your oil production.

The most well-known is Retin-A, although its cousin, marketed as Differin gel, is making inroads. You will need a prescription for these medications.

While the idea of a prescription medication may not appeal to you, there may be practical considerations that come into play. "For a lot of business people with oily skin, it is just not practical to stop during the day to wash your face," Dr. Gravenese says. "And men aren't socialized for powder-room trips. So for a lot of people, moving up to retinoids is a good way to get oil production down."

OSTEOPOROSIS
Planning Zero Fractures

The hip fractures and other broken bones that often haunt older adults are by no means a predetermined price for living long. In fact, the condition that weakens your bones enough for them to break easily, osteoporosis, can be fought against in youth. And some experts say that it is never too late to take measures that help prevent bone loss.

"Osteoporosis results from loss of bone tissue," says Michael Kleerekoper, M.D., an endocrinologist and professor in the departments of internal medicine, obstetrics and gynecology, and pathology at Wayne State University in Detroit.

"The more bone tissue you start with," says Dr. Kleerekoper, "the more you can afford to lose. So during childhood and adolescence, you want to optimize what you get."

But prevention doesn't stop when you reach voting age. Doctors say that it is just as crucial into and beyond middle age, when you lose bone mass instead of accumulate it. With men, the loss is gradual, but women can lose as much as 3 percent per year for the first 10 years of menopause. No wonder, then, that osteoporosis is more common in women than in men.

"In maturity, your goal is to slow or stop the loss of bone," says Kendra Kaye Zuckerman, M.D., assistant professor of medicine at Allegheny University of the Health Sciences and director of the osteoporosis program at Allegheny University Hospital in Philadelphia. "You can prevent it from ever reaching the point where the bone is fragile enough to break."

Here are the strategies that have helped the strong-of-bone to stay fracture-free throughout their lives.

GET YOUR MIRACLE MINERAL. "It is really important to get adequate calcium all throughout life," Dr. Zuckerman says. "Calcium during the growing years helps increase peak bone mineral density and later in life helps slow bone loss."

But how much is adequate? "That's somewhat of a fluid target," says Steven T. Harris, M.D., clinical professor of medicine and radiology and chief of the osteoporosis clinic at the University of California, San Francisco. "The general recommendation is to aim for somewhere between 1,000 and 1,500 milligrams per day, whether through diet or supplements or a combination of the two."

You should keep it toward the high end of that range if you are under age 24, over age 65, or postmenopausal and not taking estrogen, Dr. Zuckerman notes.

MAKE DAIRY A DAILY THING. Unlike a lot of vital minerals, calcium isn't typically plentiful in the American diet. You have to make a conscious effort to get enough. "The only reasonable way to do that in the diet is through dairy products," Dr. Kleerekoper says.

A tall glass of milk, a thick slice of cheese, a cup of yogurt, or a good-size serving of cottage cheese will each provide you with about 300 milligrams of calcium. And that is as much calcium as you are likely to get from all the rest of the food you eat that day, according to Dr. Zuckerman.

Other good, but less-rich, sources of dietary calcium include broccoli, sardines (especially canned with bones intact), and tofu. "When you buy juice or cereal or bread, buy it fortified with calcium," she adds.

GO NONFAT. Don't let fear of fat keep you from getting calcium from dairy products. The nonfat versions are just fine. "People tend to think that there is less nourishment in them, but it is not so," Dr. Kleerekoper says. "If you take the fat out of dairy products, you are not taking the calcium out."

TAKE VITAMIN D. "Vitamin D helps you metabolize calcium and use it effectively in building bone," says Dennis Black, Ph.D., associate professor of epidemiology and biostatistics at the University of California, San Francisco. "The recommendation is 400 IU (international units) a day, but there is data to suggest that something around 600 IU can be more beneficial, especially for older people." Your body converts sunlight to vitamin D, but often that is not enough. You also need fortified foods like milk and cereal. Also, make sure that vitamin D is included in your multivitamin.

SPRINKLE IT ON. You can boost the calcium content of just about any dish without changing the taste much. "Just add nonfat powdered milk to soups or drinks or casseroles," Dr. Zuckerman suggests.

SWALLOW CALCIUM SUPPLEMENTS. The surest and easiest way to get enough calcium to retard osteoporosis is to take calcium supplements," Dr. Black says. And to help your body absorb and use that calcium, look for supplements that also contain vitamin D.

The carbonate versions are the most popular, not to mention the cheapest. They can be pills or chewable; even Tums doubles as a calcium supplement. "Take them with food and a full glass of water for better absorption," Dr. Zuckerman says.

"If you are taking most of your calcium as supplements,

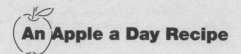

An Apple a Day Recipe

Bone-Building Stuffed Shells

Increased calcium intake is the number one way to improve bone health. Broccoli and ricotta cheese are both packed with calcium. And they are delicious together in these quick stuffed shells.

16 jumbo pasta shells
 1 carrot, finely chopped
 3 scallions, finely chopped
 1 teaspoon canola oil
1½ cups finely chopped broccoli florets
 1 tablespoon chopped fresh basil or
 1 teaspoon dried

 1 clove garlic, minced
 1 container (15 ounces) fat-free ricotta cheese
½ cup grated Parmesan cheese
1½ cups tomato sauce

Cook the pasta in a large pot of boiling water according to the package directions. Drain and cool slightly.

Meanwhile, combine the carrot, scallions, and oil in a microwaveable bowl. Cover with vented plastic wrap and microwave on high for 2 minutes. Stir in the broccoli, basil, and garlic. Cover and microwave for 3 minutes. Add the ricotta and all but 2 tablespoons of the Parmesan. Stir until well-blended.

Spoon the stuffing into the shells. Place the shells in an 8" square microwaveable baking dish. Top with the tomato sauce. Microwave on medium for 7 minutes, or until the shells are heated through. Rotate the dish once during cooking. Sprinkle with the remaining 2 tablespoons of Parmesan.

Makes 4 servings. Per serving: 274 calories, 6 g. fat, 26% of Daily Value of calcium

don't take it all with one meal," Dr. Zuckerman adds. If the carbonates give you constipation, calcium citrates such as Citracal are another option, according to Dr. Zuckerman. These can be taken between meals.

THROW IN SOME TRACE ELEMENTS. Zinc, copper, and manganese may be bit players on the bone-building scene, but there is some evidence that they may help your skeletal health, according to Dr. Harris. "If you are going to be taking a multivitamin, it makes sense to hedge the bet and include a multimineral element in what you take," he says.

DON'T SALT IT AWAY. One element that your bones don't want much of is sodium. "When your body gets rid of that sodium, it takes the calcium with it," Dr. Kleerekoper says. Sodium is added to many canned goods and processed foods, so if you lean toward fresh foods in your diet, you will automatically dodge more salt. After that, just go easy with the saltshaker.

GO EASY ON THE SOFT DRINKS. They contain phosphorus, which has to stay in proper balance with your calcium. "Soft drink consumption probably has some impact on bone health," Dr. Harris says. "The negative effects of low calcium consumption seem to be magnified by a high phosphorus consumption."

CARRY THAT WEIGHT. So-called load-bearing or weight-bearing exercise, in which you work out while supporting your own body weight, helps build bone, experts say. Running, aerobic dancing, or walking are recommended

Dose Up on Estrogen

Calcium, vitamin D, weight-bearing exercise—those are all great for keeping as much bone mass as possible. But menopause-related bone loss can often be so rapid that your best prevention efforts might not be able to keep up with it. That's why doctors often recommend going straight to the source of the problem—that is, replacing the lost estrogen.

"Estrogen replacement is the first recommended treatment of osteoporosis in postmenopausal women," says Kendra Kaye Zuckerman, M.D., assistant professor of medicine at Allegheny University of the Health Sciences and director of the osteoporosis program at Allegheny University Hospital in Philadelphia. "Taking estrogen in supplemental form prevents the rapid loss of bone."

The best known procedure is hormone-replacement therapy (HRT), which provides at least one other hormone besides estrogen to help balance out some of estrogen's side effects.

But for postmenopausal women who forgo estrogen-replacement therapy, there are alternative bone-saving prescription medications available. Here are some that you can ask your doctor about now.

Alendronate. Sold under the commercial name Fosamax, it has been approved by the Food and Drug

anti-osteoporosis exercises. "Also, using weights can help bones in different parts of your body," Dr. Zuckerman says. Note well: The benefits last only as long as you exercise regularly.

But the specific "pro-bone" benefits of load-bearing exercise are small compared to the tremendous overall health advantages of exercise in general. "I prefer to encourage people to just be active," Dr. Harris says. "If you love to

Administration (FDA) as a drug that helps reduce osteoporosis. "It is a really good inhibitor of bone breakdown. And it decreases fractures in older people with osteoporosis," says Steven T. Harris, M.D., clinical professor of medicine and radiology and chief of the osteoporosis clinic at the University of California, San Francisco.

Alendronate is not the simplest medication to take, however. "You have to swallow the pill first thing in the morning with six to eight ounces of water every day," Dr. Zuckerman says. "Then you can't eat or drink anything, take any other pills, or lie down for 30 minutes."

Raloxifene. This is the first of the so-called SERMs (selective estrogen receptor modulators) to get FDA approval for the prevention of osteoporosis. The trade name is Evista. "What's interesting about SERMs is that they have some of the properties of estrogen but not some of the negative effects," Dr. Zuckerman says. "Raloxifene builds a small amount of bone, but it doesn't cause the breast tenderness or menstrual bleeding that estrogen sometimes does."

Calcitonin. This is a hormone approved for treatment, not prevention, and it is usually prescribed as a nasal spray (one brand is Miacalcin). "The improvements in bone density are smaller with calcitonin than with other treatments, and the fracture protection is likely to be correspondingly less," Dr. Harris says.

swim, swim. There is not much evidence that swimming is good for you from a skeletal perspective, but it is far better to faithfully do something you like to do than not do the 'right' exercise."

GET PROTEIN FROM SOY. Not only is it a good source of calcium but soy may also contribute in other ways to building bone mass. Soy contains isoflavones, which are plant estrogen-like compounds, or phytoestrogens, that

Avoiding Falls

Osteoporosis doesn't hurt. That's what's so sneaky about it. You don't think there is really anything going on until a silly little fall results in a not-so-silly fractured hip.

The risk of that skyrockets in your older years. So while you still want to do all you can to keep as much bone strength as possible, there is another item on your prevention agenda.

"The prevention strategy is different in your sixties, seventies, and beyond," says Michael Kleerekoper, M.D., an endocrinologist and professor in the departments of internal medicine, obstetrics and gynecology, and pathology at Wayne State University in Detroit. "Now you have to think about the complications of bone loss, which are fractures. And there are many things you can do to prevent fractures."

KEEP EXERCISING. Exercise is more important when you are older, not less, because it does more than help save bone. "Exercise reduces your risk of falling," says Dennis Black, Ph.D., associate professor of epidemiology and biostatistics at the University of California, San Francisco. "And it helps your reaction time if you do fall." So all activities are beneficial, whether weight-bearing or not, when it comes to preventing falls. "Activities that help your balance, like tai chi, and anything that keeps you vigorous are helpful," he says.

may behave like the body's natural estrogens in preventing bone loss after menopause. According to Bahram Arjmandi, R.D., Ph.D., associate professor in the department of nutritional sciences at Oklahoma State University in Stillwater, soy isoflavones may behave in both an estrogenic and antiestrogenic manner. "Soy isoflavones may exert the beneficial effects of estrogens on bone but without any ad-

FALL-PROOF YOUR HOME. Get rid of loose cords, small stools, and other assorted stumbling blocks. "It sounds trite, but you need to move these things out of the way to prevent falls," Dr. Kleerekoper says.

STAY IN SIGHT. "Make sure that you wear your prescription glasses properly," Dr. Kleerekoper says. "For example, don't go outside with reading glasses." The distortion of images—or blurriness—could alter your depth perception and your ability to react.

LIGHTEN YOUR BURDEN. You are more likely to fall when you are struggling with heavy, awkward things. "When you go to the supermarket, tell the clerk to put fewer groceries in each bag," Dr. Kleerekoper suggests.

TEAM UP. Winter is no friend of weak bones. "Don't walk outside when the ground is slippery without some sort of support," Dr. Kleerekoper says. "Take a walking stick or a friend or a spouse."

ILLUMINATE THINGS. Those nocturnal sojourns to the bathroom aren't much different than a walk through a dangerous dark alley, as far as your bones are concerned.

"Without some lighting, the likelihood of tripping is quite high," Dr. Kleerekoper warns. "Leave a night-light on." Concerned about the small increase in your electric bill? "It is not too expensive compared to the cost of a fracture."

verse effects on your breasts and uterus, where high levels of estrogens can promote cancer," he says.

Research has not yet proven which form of soy isoflavones is best in terms of potential skeletal health benefits, Dr. Arjmandi cautions, but he says that consuming 50 milligrams of total soy isoflavones a day has shown benefits you can enjoy with modest consumption of soy products. For instance, 30 to 50 milligrams of total iso-flavones can be obtained by consuming a half-cup of textured soy protein, one ounce of roasted soy nuts, one cup of soy milk, or a half-cup of tofu. All of these should be available at your local health food store.

CHEAT THE MEAT. Dr. Arjmandi emphasizes that Americans have to be careful not to add to already sufficient protein and energy intakes, no matter how beneficial these food sources may be. Use soy as a substitute for, not a supplement to, your protein intake, he says. In other words, when you eat more soy, eat less meat.

In fact, there is evidence that cutting down on animal protein is good for your bones. "There are actually a number of reasons why you ought to avoid excessive animal protein," Dr. Harris says. "One is that in older people it probably aggravates the normal rate of bone loss."

EAT FLAXSEED. Flaxseed is a rich source of polyunsaturated fatty acid, especially alpha-linolenic acid, which has been shown to decrease the rate of bone loss. A clinical study by Dr. Arjmandi and his colleagues has shown that daily consumption of 40 grams of flaxseed has positive effects on bone. When a group of postmenopausal women ate this amount of flaxseed every day, cooked into breads and muffins, the added ingredient helped reduce the rate of bone loss. In this study, the flaxseed also helped reduce urinary loss of calcium.

LEAVE YOUR CIGARETTES AT THE BAR. The link between smoking and osteoporosis is weak, but it is there. "Tobacco use is associated with an earlier menopause, lower body weight, and probably enhanced breakdown of estrogen," Dr. Harris says. "Consequently, it is associated with a tendency toward osteoporosis."

Alcohol abuse is also a risk factor for osteoporosis, according to Dr. Zuckerman. "It looks like heavy alcohol use suppresses the osteoblasts, which are the cells that lay down bone tissue," she says.

OVERWEIGHT
You Don't Have to Go Over

Eat right, keep moving.

You have just read all that you need to know about how to prevent being overweight. That simple set of instructions should be easy to follow, but not for 35 percent of Americans who are unable to prevent being overweight.

Of course, once we are overweight, we usually want to trim down for a whole lot of reasons, some related to health, others having to do with looks. And it is never too late to lose weight. But the fact is, it's a whole lot easier to prevent putting on pounds than to try losing them later on. And if there is one thing we all know, it's that weight gain is likely to happen if we don't take forward-looking steps to stop it.

"People stray," notes G. Kenneth Goodrick, Ph.D., a psychologist, assistant professor of medicine at the Baylor College of Medicine in Houston, and author of *Living Without Dieting*. "We tend to go back to our old eating habits even after we learn to enjoy low-fat eating. We tend to return to sedentary ways even though we enjoy exercising."

But despite the momentum toward weight gain, you can stop it from happening, experts say. And there are plenty of good reasons to avoid excess pounds, reasons that go beyond vanity or social acceptance. "The significance of excess weight is more than cosmetic," says Patrick M. O'Neil, Ph.D., a clinical psychologist and director of the Weight Management Center at the Medical University of South Carolina in Charleston. It takes a huge toll on your physical health, hc points out.

Preventing the Health Risks

Controlling your weight and avoiding weight gain as you get older are important ways to prevent a host of weight-related health problems.

Indeed, if you are more than 20 pounds over your ideal weight, you are at greater risk for a rogues' gallery of potentially deadly conditions, including diabetes, high blood pressure, coronary heart disease, endometrial cancer, obstructive sleep apnea, and breast cancer. What's more, most people who are overweight tend to avoid exercise, and that avoidance just adds to the toll paid for extra pounds. "If you have a sedentary lifestyle and are overweight, you are at higher risk of cardiovascular disease and other health problems," says Lawrence J. Cheskin, M.D., a gastroenterologist, associate professor of medicine at Johns Hopkins University, director of the Johns Hopkins Weight Management Center in Baltimore, and author of *Losing Weight for Good*. And if you already have a medical condition such as high cholesterol, being overweight puts you at higher risk for complications.

"The good news is that even modest amounts of weight loss can improve your health significantly," says Dr. Cheskin. Loss of 10 percent of body weight can reduce blood pressure, high cholesterol, triglyceride, and high blood sugar levels.

If you have just put on a few extra pounds and want to avoid gaining more, these arguments for better health may seem convincing. But in addition to being convinced, you may also have to take some action to ensure that your weight doesn't creep ever upward.

"It isn't just a question of deciding to be strong-willed and determined or upbeat and positive," Dr. O'Neil says. "Lifestyle changes are where it's at for long-term success with your weight."

A lot of us tend to cringe at the phrase "lifestyle changes." Sounds like someone is trying to tinker with our identity. But all it means is taking control of what you eat, how often you eat, and how much and often you move around. "Despite everything you hear about recent discoveries linking genetics and obesity, when you get right down to it, we humans have had these same genes for thousands of years," Dr. O'Neil says. "The problem is of more recent origins. It is in our lifestyle."

Some Ways to Stop the Weighting

Genetics does play a role in obesity, of course, but not as big a role as you do. "It is a myth that genes compel you to be heavy," says Stephen Gullo, Ph.D., president of the Institute of Health and Weight Sciences in New York City and author of *Thin Tastes Better*. "For the vast majority of us, genes may set the lower limits of our weight, but we set the upper limits by our food choices."

Nonetheless, we all know that most of us tend to put on weight as we age. And if there is one thing we can't prevent, it is the aging process. But we can prevent eating more and exercising less as we get older. And first of all, "you have to have strategies for food control in your life, strategies that work," Dr. Gullo says.

To make those strategies work, you will need some co-operation, particularly from your spouse. Of course, it is ideal if you and your spouse, as a team, can avoid overeating and work together as a sort of built-in social-support group. But it is probably not wise to push the matter. "You can't change your spouse," Dr. Goodrick says. "You can only set an example." You can also arrange things so that the love of your life doesn't inadvertently (or intentionally) sabotage your efforts. If your spouse continues to whip up chicken-fried steaks with biscuits and gravy when you are in the mood for a fresh salad, it is time for a talk.

When you talk, tell it straight and clear, Dr. O'Neil says. "Only you know what you want from the significant people in your life when it comes to support for your weight-controlling efforts," he says. "You may want a cheer-leader, you may want a cop, you may want to be left alone. It is your job to communicate."

Weighing In with Lower Fat

The nuts and bolts of eating right for maintaining a healthy weight aren't all that complicated. In fact, it is a good bet that most people know pretty well what is best. As Dr. Cheskin summarizes it, "A reasonable approach for main-taining your weight is a diet that is high in complex carbo-hydrates, high in fiber, moderate in protein, and low in fat."

A complex carbohydrate is a baked potato. Fat is the sour cream and butter you shouldn't put on it. Fiber is vege-tables. Fat is the oil you shouldn't fry them in. Protein is a lean cut of meat. Fat is the gravy you shouldn't pour over it.

"Dietary fat promotes weight gain because it is a very dense source of calories," Dr. O'Neil says. "Also, when you consume excess calories from dietary fat, you store those calories as body fat more efficiently than excess calories from other sources. And fat in food makes it taste good, so it encourages you to eat more."

But fat isn't the only food that makes you fat. All food has calories, although some foods have much more than others.

A calorie is a convenient unit of measurement for the amount of energy in food. Eat more energy than your body expends, and it is stored for future use. That's excess weight, which is exactly what you are trying to avoid. Thirty-five hundred unused, stored calories turns into one pound of fat on your body, says Dr. O'Neil.

Your mission for preventing weight gain, should you decide to accept it, is to eat fewer calories when you are not involved in activities that burn up those calories. In the long run, your schedule of cutbacks doesn't have to be anything drastic, but consistency matters. And experts have many strategies to help you reduce your consumption of high-calorie foods.

BE CONSCIOUS OF CALORIES. "It is important to educate yourself about the foods that you are likely to eat," Dr. O'Neil says. "Spend some time up front learning their relative calorie content. That will help you make better choices."

To get a better idea of foods that are high in calories, begin by reading labels on packaged foods to help increase your awareness, Dr. O'Neil suggests. If you want even more information, you can get a calorie-counter paperback book that lists thousands of different foods.

THINK DENSITY. "Go for foods that are lower in calorie density," Dr. O'Neil says. "Instead of a cup of grape juice, for example, you can have two full cups of fresh grapes. You get more volume for the same calories."

Most types of cheese, for instance, are high in calories. Even a sliver of cheese has more calories than a plateful of salad.

The Diet Debate

If you have been watching your weight go up and you are worried about the rising pounds, you may be wondering whether popular diets really work. Is it possible to prevent future weight gain by putting yourself on a popular diet plan? "All diets work because they are all designed to get you to eat fewer calories," says Marion Nestle, Ph.D., professor of nutrition and food studies at New York University in New York City. But, she points out, what good is a diet if you start gaining weight again as soon as you stray from the program?

If you want to live the rest of your life at your best weight, diets alone don't work. "You will also need to stay physically active," says Dr. Nestle. There are lots of reasons why.

Diets miss the point. "Thin is a process, not a destination point," says Stephen Gullo, Ph.D., president of the Institute of Health and Weight Sciences in New York City and author of *Thin Tastes Better*. "Your goal is to live your life in control of food."

They are often not healthful. Crash diets, in particular, often neglect good nutrition practices. "Ask yourself if the diet would be healthy if you followed it in the long run," says Patrick M. O'Neil, Ph.D., a clinical

---

"You can eat a lot more food if it is lower in calorie density," Dr. Goodrick says. "That way, you and your body don't feel deprived as you eat fewer calories."

DON'T FALL INTO THE FAT-FREE TRAP. Here is a telling conundrum: Manufacturers keep coming out with low-fat or fat-free versions of their best-selling foods, but Americans keep getting fatter anyway. "One of the great delusions of the 1990s is that 'no-fat' means 'non-fattening,'" Dr. Gullo says. The truth is, you are often getting just as many

psychologist and director of the Weight Management
Center at the Medical University of South Carolina in
Charleston.

They sap energy instead of boosting it. "People on
traditional restrictive diets are drinking a lot of coffee and
caffeinated and sugar-free soft drinks all day," says G.
Kenneth Goodrick, Ph.D., a psychologist, assistant
professor of medicine at the Baylor College of Medicine in
Houston, and author of *Living Without Dieting*. The caffeine
and sweet drinks may provide bursts of energy, but they
can't make up for a deficiency of nutritious foods. These
people are not getting enough energy, he says.

They lead to obsession. "When you eat less than you
should, you become obsessed about food, which is the
exact opposite of what you want for weight management,"
Dr. Goodrick says.

They require willpower. "Eating properly is enjoyable,
and it doesn't take much willpower if you do it right," Dr.
Goodrick says. "But it takes a lot of willpower to stick to
restrictive diets."

They make you fatter. "When you lose weight on a
diet, you lose fat and muscle," Dr. Goodrick says. When
you gain weight back, which usually happens when you go
off a diet, the fat comes back first, he says. "So you end up
with more fat than when you started."

calories from the no-fat version, even if the calories aren't
coming from fat.

The term *fat-free* can be a trap if you start to believe that you can eat any amount of the foods that are ad-
vertised that way. "Be aware that if you overeat fat-free
foods, you could sabotage your weight-maintenance plan,"
says Dr. Gullo.

RESPOND TO HUNGER WITH HEALTHFUL SNACKS. Dr.
Gullo recommends trying to eat every three to four hours,

which may mean a nutritious low-fat snack between lunch and dinner. When you feel the urge for food coming on, he suggests snacking on something healthy such as a fat-free waffle with jelly or a slice of whole-grain toasted bread topped with a piece of melted nonfat cheese. Just be sure not to overdo it. Never skip a meal and eat snacks instead because that's the worst thing you can do if you are trying to control your eating habits and weight, he says.

REPLACE A FEW THINGS. Just modify the foods you eat in your favorite meals, and you may find it a lot easier to prevent gaining weight. If you like chicken, for instance, trade legs and thighs for low-fat skinless chicken breasts—and bake the chicken instead of frying it.

GIVE IT TIME. Changing your eating lifestyle can be like going to the opera or watching golf on television—a lot of people assume they hate the idea before they have given it a chance. Those who do stick with a lower-fat nutrient-dense lifestyle, however, rather than going on a crash diet, almost always prefer it, according to Dr. Goodrick. "Gradually, you learn to adapt to new foods and new cooking techniques that help you eat healthful meals."

SHUN THE FOODS THAT MAKE YOU EAT MORE. "Certain foods create their own compulsion for more and more," Dr. Gullo says. "Trying to just have a little bit doesn't work. I've never met anyone who could eat one peanut and stop."

Interestingly, the intensity of the compulsion varies according to sex. "Women seem to have the most problems with cookies and chocolate and things like that," Dr. Gullo says. "With men, it is more often chips, peanuts, and bread. If you start negotiating with those foods, the negotiations can last a lifetime."

BAN THE FOOD BOMBS. "Do not bring into your home any food that you have a history of overeating," Dr. Gullo says. "If it is one of your 'trigger' foods, just don't put it in the shopping cart." You don't need to be challenged by having those foods on your shelf at home. "Protect yourself," he says. "That's the essence of weight control."

DON'T CONCEDE TO FAMILY DEMANDS. If you are buying for your children, spouse, or both, that shouldn't be a reason to bring trouble foods into the house. "Every single person who loves potato chips says that they have to buy them for the children, husband, or wife," Dr. Gullo says. Don't let that happen, he cautions. Bring home fruit or individual-size bags of pretzels for family members to snack on instead.

THINK SMALL. Buying the large economy size saves money, but giant-size purchases ring up numerous calories. "Some people who buy the large boxes eat much more of the product than if they had bought the small box," Dr. Gullo says.

THROW OUT THE LEFTOVERS. If you perpetually snack on leftovers, just remember that they have just as many calories as they did the first time they were served. If you serve a special meal for guests and you have high-fat, high-calorie leftovers, let your guests take them home or throw them away, Dr. Gullo advises. "Calories cost more than money if you have to wear them."

SNACK ON THE RIGHT STUFF. Many women crave sweets or just get hungrier during the days just before their periods. Dr. Gullo recommends mellowing out with a healthful snack. Have it at whatever time of day you feel hungry, he suggests. "Make sure that it is strong on fiber, such as a bean salad. Or have some fresh vegetables with a little bit of protein in the form of an egg-white omelet, a can of tuna, or two ounces of turkey."

PUT AWAY THE SERVING BOWLS. "Don't serve meals family-style, with the serving bowl on the table," Dr. O'Neil advises. "Each individual plate should be prepared in the kitchen and then brought to the table. That way, you are not inclined to have seconds if you shouldn't."

The Goal to Go For

Since excess weight puts you at risk for many health problems, you may need to set some weight-loss goals to help avoid those risks and prevent disease. But what should be your long-term weight goal? And what short-term goals should you set to help you get there? You have a better chance of attaining your goals if you make sure that they are sensible and reasonable right at the beginning. Here are some guidelines from experts.

BE REALISTIC. "Most people's long-term weight-loss goals are more ambitious than they have to be," says Patrick M. O'Neil, Ph.D., a clinical psychologist and director of the Weight Management Center at the Medical University of South Carolina in Charleston. "If you weigh 170 pounds and your long-term goal is to weigh 120, even though you haven't weighed 120 since you were 16 and now you are 45, that is not a realistic goal."

Your body mass index (BMI) is a good indicator of whether or not you need to shed pounds. The ideal BMI range, according to the National Institutes of Health, is between 19 and 24.9. If your BMI is between 25 and 29.9, you are considered overweight. Any number above 30 is in the obesity range.

To calculate your BMI, take your height (in inches) and multiply it by itself. (So if you are 5 feet 4 inches tall, you would multiply 64 by 64 to get 4,096.) Next, divide your weight in pounds by that number. Finally, take that result and multiply it by 705.

For instance, if you are 5 feet 4 inches tall and you weigh 150 pounds, you'd divide 150 by 4,096 and multiply by 705 to get a BMI of about 26.

"From a health standpoint, if your BMI is at 31, getting

down to 24 might be an unrealistic goal," says Dr. O'Neil. Just try to lose 10 percent of your body weight, and you will be decreasing your risk of disease, he says.

SET APPROPRIATE OBJECTIVES. "Losing weight for vanity is psychologically less helpful than losing weight to improve health," says G. Kenneth Goodrick, Ph.D., a psychologist, assistant professor of medicine at Baylor College of Medicine in Houston, and author of *Living Without Dieting*. "You have made a big step forward if you decide to exercise and eat right so that you will feel better and have more energy to do something positive with your life."

FOCUS ON DOING, NOT LOSING. "Rather than saying that you are going to lose a pound this week, say how much you are going to exercise this week," Dr. O'Neil says. "Your weight within a span of a week is not completely in your control, but your behavior is."

USE MEASURABLE MEASURES. "Saying that you are going to be 'more positive' this week or that you are going 'to really get serious' this week is not a goal that you can actually measure," Dr. O'Neil says. This is another reason to focus on the amount of exercise you are getting. You should be able to count up the minutes of exercise and say, "I met my goal" or "I didn't."

BUILD BIT BY BIT. "Short-term goals should not be pie-in-the-sky," Dr. O'Neil says. "For example, if you have never exercised at all, your best goal this week might be to find three different one-mile routes that you can walk next week."

KEEP UP THE SELF-ENCOURAGEMENT. "An all-or-nothing attitude only sets you up to fail," Dr. O'Neil says. "Learn to evaluate your efforts fairly and objectively." If you fall short of some goals, just look ahead to next week. You don't need to have a perfect record, he points out.

SERVE ON SMALLER PLATES. Let the fancy restaurants serve those little dollops of expensive delicacies that look like a bull's-eye on a huge white plate. "Using smaller plates can help your attitude," Dr. O'Neil says. "It looks like there is more food."

SLOW DOWN. Eating too quickly is a common mistake. The trouble is that it takes 15 to 20 minutes for your brain to get the message that your belly has had enough. In other words, you can still be eating when you don't really want to.

"When you get to the end of the meal and you are thinking that you are still hungry, give yourself 15 minutes," Dr. O'Neil advises. That gives your stomach time to catch up to your brain and let you know you are satisfied.

EAT BEFORE YOU EAT OUT. "Never go to a restaurant hungry," Dr. Gullo advises. Research shows that people eat more when they eat in a social setting, especially where they know people, than when they eat alone. And if you are going out to dinner with friends or relatives, make sure that you are not ravenous when you arrive.

DROWN THE TEMPTATION. "If you do arrive at the restaurant hungry, a carbonated beverage or any cold liquid kills appetite," Dr. Gullo says. "Or order a tomato juice, which is a very powerful appetite suppressant."

BE BLIND TO THE BREAD. Breadbaskets are insidious enemies of a weight-conscious lifestyle, especially if you are a man. "If you know that you can't have half a roll without having three, don't have any," Dr. Gullo says. "It doesn't make any difference if you use butter or not. I've never known one male who has kept his weight off after going back to the breadbasket."

ORDER WITHOUT THE MENU. Many of us enter a restaurant with every intention of choosing foods that are healthful, nutritious, and low in fat. But for some people, a tempting menu can be too much to resist. "It is written to stimulate your desire to buy food," Dr. Gullo points out.

If you find that alluring descriptions undercut your

best intentions, don't even ask for the menu, Dr. Gullo advises. Instead, just ask the waiter questions about what you want. "Ask what kind of grilled fish they recommend today," Dr. Gullo suggests. "Or just order a specific item, like grilled chicken breast. You don't need the menu for that."

Taking such a puritanical approach to dining, however, isn't something that you have to do every single day, according to Dr. Gullo. He says that he allows his patients to have a featured menu meal two or three times per week.

SAVE YOUR SALAD. You probably know that pouring on high-fat dressing adds fat and calories to an otherwise innocent salad. But do you know how much? "If you use the wrong kind of dressing, a salad can have more grams of fat than a cheeseburger," Dr. Gullo says. "Use balsamic vinegar or mustard," he suggests. "If you are at a restaurant, ask for a vinaigrette on the side."

TREAT YOURSELF TO DESSERT. At restaurants, you can enjoy dessert without sacrificing your weight at the altar of the dessert tray. "Go with berries," Dr. Gullo says. "Or if you must have something sweet, order a sorbet instead of ice cream. Tell them not to bring the little cookie with it." Or, if you would just like to try a bite or two of a scrumptious-looking dessert, share it with others at the table.

STIFLE THE FEELING. Cravings have killed many weight-management efforts because too many people give in to them too easily, according to Dr. Gullo. "Remind yourself that a craving is just a feeling, not a command," he says. "Studies indicate that the average craving passes in 4 to 12 minutes."

Making Moves That Matter

A lot of us live our lives like penned animals. Built to move, too often we put ourselves in a cage. We have bodies designed for racing across the savannas, but we live a lifestyle

---

Watch Your Medications

It would be a shame to have your weight-control efforts undermined by medicine you have to take, but it happens. Weight gain can be a side effect of many kinds of medications, such as antidepressants like amitriptyline (Elevil) or phenelzine (Nardil), some birth control pills, and steroids like prednisone. To find out if a medication that you are taking lists weight gain as a side effect, read the fine print on the label or package insert or get a printout from your pharmacist.

"If you notice weight gain and think it is tied to a medication, tell your doctor," advises Patrick M. O'Neil, Ph.D., a clinical psychologist and director of the Weight Management Center at the Medical University of South Carolina in Charleston. "There may be an alternative medication that doesn't have weight gain as a side effect."

---

designed for migrating from the bed to the breakfast table to the car seat to the office chair to the restaurant booth to the living room couch and back to the bed.

It wasn't always this way. "Not that long ago in the United States, a man who worked on a farm did the equivalent of 15 miles of jogging every day," Dr. Goodrick says. "And his wife did the equivalent of 7 miles of jogging."

Today, our daily obligations of work and home keep us tied to our chairs, and if we want exercise, we have to seek it out. "The obesity problem is probably caused at least as much by lack of physical activity as by eating too much," Dr. Goodrick says. "People need to move around."

That does not mean that a lap or two around the old high school track will offset a daily dose of donuts. "Exercise alone is not very efficient," Dr. Cheskin says. If you just exercise and don't change your diet, he points out, you may be able to prevent weight gain or even lose a few pounds for a while. But it is not something that you are likely to sustain unless exercise is part of an overall program. The more regularly you exercise, the easier it is to maintain your weight. Here's what to do every day to make sure that you get the exercise you need.

GET QUALITY ZZZS. "Make sure that you get adequate sleep," says Dr. Goodrick. Good sleep habits are conducive to exercise, he points out. If you feel worn out during the day, you are less likely to get much physical activity during the day. Also, there is evidence that people who are tired tend to eat more, using food as a substitute for the rest they need.

WALK THE WALK. It is probably the easiest exercise program of all. In fact, it may be all you ever have to do, according to Dr. Goodrick. "Gradually build up to at least 30 minutes of brisk walking five times a week," he says. "Brisk walks themselves have health and psychological benefits that are well worth the while."

WALK THE TREADMILL. When the weather is bad, you might not feel like going outdoors. But if you have a treadmill in the television room, you can catch up on your favorite shows while you are doing your daily good turn for your weight-maintenance plan, Dr. Goodrick suggests. Most of us watch television anyway, and indoor exercise equipment enables anyone to turn a sedentary activity into a healthy walk.

SEIZE THE TIME. Excuses aside, lack of time is certainly a limiting factor in most lifestyles. Dr. Goodrick suggests a basic guideline for incorporating exercise into your schedule. "Get as much exercise as you can that feels good without letting it interfere with your work or family life," he says. If you need to, remind yourself that you are preventing many health problems when you prevent weight gain—and keeping your health is a gift to your family as well as yourself.

Can You Rub Your Cellulite Risk Away?

Every time you turn around, a new cellulite-fighting potion hits the market. The only thing that these formulas will reduce is the size of your bank account, says Donald Robertson, M.D., medical director of the Southwest Bariatric Nutrition Center in Scottsdale, Arizona.

But even though the potions won't work, there is some evidence that anti-cellulite massage can help. Elliot Greene, past president of the American Massage Therapy Association and a massage therapist for 25 years in Silver Spring, Maryland, explains that a study published in the *Massage Therapy Journal* revealed that "a Swedish massage stroke called vibration actually contributes to the beakdown of body fat."

"A deep massage using the knuckles or elbows may also help break up the dimples that come with cellulite," says Dr. Robertson. For the best results, he suggests receiving a deep massage targeting the troubled areas at least two or three times per week.

PANIC ATTACKS
Free Yourself from This Savage Emotion

They can happen to the smartest among us. When he wasn't contemplating the origins of man, Charles Darwin was frequently overwhelmed by panic attacks that left him crying hysterically and feeling as if he were about to die. Ironically, the condition kept the celebrated naturalist so socially isolated that it probably helped him focus on his concept of natural selection, a theory that took him 22 years to write.

"Had it not been for this illness, his theory of evolution might not have become the all-consuming passion that produced *On the Origin of Species*," says Thomas Barloon, M.D., associate professor of radiology at the University of Iowa College of Medicine in Iowa City, who has written about Darwin's medical history.

But Darwin, who spent a lifetime seeking a cure, probably wouldn't have been comforted by that thought. And certainly, few of the estimated 3.3 million Americans who get panic attacks would consider them a blessing in disguise. These surges of unexplainable fear and anxiety can have a crippling effect on a person's life, says David A. Spiegel, M.D., medical director of the Center for Anxiety and Related Disorders at Boston University. The attacks usually occur suddenly, either without cause or in situations where a person feels at risk although no apparent danger exists. Symptoms include shortness of breath, hot and cold flashes, dizziness, chest pain, racing heart or palpitations, sweating, and nausea. The symptoms are sometimes so intense that people suspect they are having a heart attack.

Although the attack itself may only last for a few minutes, fear of another attack can cause a person to avoid situations believed to trigger panic, such as driving a car or being alone, says Albert Carlin, Ph.D., professor of psychiatry at the University of Washington School of Medicine in Seattle. In severe instances, like Darwin's, some people become so fearful that they don't venture outside of their homes for months or even years.

But if Darwin exemplifies someone with panic disorder, he is also a symbol of hope for others who have this problem. Eventually, Darwin traveled the world, sufficiently confident in his power to deal with his attacks.

The cause of panic attacks isn't fully understood, but researchers believe that heredity or childhood trauma plays a role, says Edmund Bourne, Ph.D., author of *The Anxiety and Phobia Workbook*. Often, before a panic attack becomes disabling, there are early signs that one is coming. Here are some simple self-help techniques that doctors offer to fend off panic attacks before they get a good grip.

BREATHE SLOWLY, BREATHE DEEPLY. Slow, deep breathing from your abdomen is your best defense against panic attacks, Dr. Bourne says. Slow breathing can relieve muscle tension, dizziness, and many other early symptoms before they blossom into high panic.

So when you feel a panic attack coming on, place a hand on your abdomen and inhale slowly and deeply through your nose to a count of four. As you breathe in, your hand should rise, a sign that you are breathing correctly. When you have taken a full breath, pause for a moment and then exhale slowly through your nose or mouth to a count of four. Allow your whole body to relax and become as limp as a rag doll. Do 10 repetitions or more, if necessary.

ACKNOWLEDGE IT. Fighting panic will only make your symptoms worse, Dr. Bourne says. When you sense panic on the horizon, try to let the early symptoms flow through you without fighting them—beyond breathing deeply and slowly. If you feel dizzy, don't try to escape it, sit down and allow it to happen. If you can do that, the dizziness may subside within three to five minutes without escalating into a full-fledged panic attack.

YAK TO RELAX. Chatting with someone nearby will help get your mind off your anxious thoughts, Dr. Bourne says. This works well whether you are driving a car, flying on a plane, or standing in line at the grocery store. If you have to give a speech, let your audience know that you feel anxious about it. When you tell people how you feel, instead of trying to hide your fear, you can help lessen the feeling.

SAY THE SECRET WORDS. Some people find that repeating a single reassuring phrase for the first minute or two after they begin to feel panicky can stop an attack, Dr. Bourne says. Try using statements like "This is just anxiety. . . . I'm not going to let it get to me" or "These are just thoughts, not reality." Experiment with different mantras, then pick three or four phrases that seem to work best for you and jot them down on an index card. Carry the card with you in your purse or wallet. Pull it out and read it when you feel symptoms coming on, Dr. Bourne suggests.

TEND YOUR GARDEN, BREAK A SWEAT. Regular physical exercise can help prevent panic. Get in the habit of doing a gentle daily workout. Even walking outdoors for 10 minutes can help dissipate panic, Dr. Bourne says. Physical activity such as housecleaning or gardening is also an excellent way of fending off an attack.

COUNT SHEEP. Simple repetitive tasks such as counting backward from 100 by threes or adding up numbers on license plates can help distract your attention and subdue early panic symptoms, Dr. Bourne says.

If you are prone to panic, avoid coffee, colas, and other caffeinated drinks. They can heighten anxiety and make you more vulnerable to an attack, Dr. Carlin says.

JUMP-START YOUR LIFE. If you are experiencing panic attacks, it may be because there is psychological stress somewhere in your life. Perhaps you feel trapped in a bad marriage, a lousy job, or another dead-end situation. See if you can figure out if there is something that needs to be addressed, and if so, consider counseling—marital or individual. Some lifestyle adjustments may be enough to short-circuit panic attacks for good, Dr. Bourne says.

PELVIC INFLAMMATORY DISEASE
Safe Sex Is Your Best Defense

Each year, more than one million American women develop pelvic inflammatory disease (PID), a bacterial infection of the upper reproductive tract that can lead to infertility, ectopic pregnancy, and chronic pelvic pain.

"It is one of the 10 most common diseases among women and certainly ranks high as a cause for hospitalization," says Gary Newkirk, M.D., clinical professor of family medicine at the University of Washington School of Medicine in Seattle and director of the Family Medicine Residency Program in Spokane.

The disease usually develops after a woman has been infected with a sexually transmitted disease (STD) such as gonorrhea or chlamydia. These STDs cause swelling and scarring in the fallopian tubes, which weaken the body's defenses and allow bacteria that are normally safely confined to the vagina to move deeper into the reproductive system. These bacteria invade the fallopian tubes, where they can form painful abscesses, Dr. Newkirk says. Without treatment, these abscesses can also block the fallopian tubes, resulting in infertility, or can spread to the abdominal cavity.

Like most infections of the reproductive system, nearly all pelvic inflammatory disease is preventable if you know your partner and take some simple sexual hygiene precautions.

GO STEADY. PID is most common among women who have multiple sexual partners, Dr. Newkirk says. So try to maintain a mutually monogamous relationship.

CREATE A ROADBLOCK. If you have more than one partner or you know that your partner is not monogamous, use condoms, diaphragms, and other barrier forms of contraception—even if you have gone through menopause. They form an essential line of defense against PID and other infections of the reproductive organs, Dr. Newkirk says.

MAKE IT GOOD, CLEAN FUN. If you use sex toys, you can contract vaginitis and even pelvic inflammatory disease, in some cases, unless these devices are properly cleaned, says Jill Maura Rabin, M.D., chief of urogynecology and of the division of ambulatory care at Long Island Jewish Medical Center in New Hyde Park, New York. Wash them thoroughly with soap and hot water before each use.

POSTPONE SEX AFTER CHILDBIRTH. After childbirth, the reproductive tract needs time to recover and is especially vulnerable to infections like PID. So forgo sex for at least six weeks after giving birth, advises Dr. Maura Rabin. "If you have sex too soon after giving birth," she says, "you can get PID from unprotected intercourse if the penis pushes bacteria into the unhealed upper reproductive tract."

DECLINE TO DOUCHE. Women who douche have a 73 percent higher risk of developing PID than those who don't, according to researchers at the Mount Sinai School of Medicine in New York. Douching may flush bacteria deep into the reproductive tract where they can cause infection and pain, Dr. Newkirk says.

PNEUMONIA
Keep This Beast Caged

Thanks to modern science, many of the diseases that cursed the ancient world have been subdued. Smallpox has been eradicated, measles is an endangered species, and polio is on the wane. But pneumonia still thrives.

Historically, pneumonia has been one of the world's great killers, claiming hundreds of millions of lives in the centuries prior to the development of antibiotics. As recently as the 1930s, pneumonia was the leading cause of death in the United States. The disease still strikes about 4.2 million Americans and kills nearly 82,000 annually, according to the National Center for Health Statistics. Only heart disease, cancer, stroke, chronic respiratory ailments, and accidents cause more deaths.

Particularly susceptible are smokers, people over age 60, and those with chronic health problems, such as asthma, heart disease, diabetes, alcoholism, kidney ailments, emphysema, and AIDS, says Harry Steinberg, M.D., chief of pulmonary medicine at Long Island Jewish Medical Center in New Hyde Park, New York.

Often, the disease is preceded by a cold or flu. But occasionally, it can develop rapidly without any preceding symptoms, Dr. Steinberg says. That is what happened to Muppet creator Jim Henson, who contracted an aggressive form of bacterial pneumonia in 1990 and was dead within hours.

Pneumonia causes phlegm, fluid, and debris to build up in the lungs, clogging your airways. This buildup disrupts the lungs' ability to remove carbon dioxide from your body and deliver life-giving oxygen to your blood and vital organs, Dr. Steinberg says.

Although in rare cases pneumonia is caused by fungi or parasites, it is usually caused by a virus or bacteria. Most of us are exposed to these organisms every day.

"The problem with pneumonia is that, unlike other diseases, no single organism causes it," says Steven A. Green, M.D., chairman of the department of family practice and a family-practice physician at Sharp Rees-Stealy Medical Group in San Diego. "So it is unlikely that we will ever find a way to eradicate it."

You can, however, lower your risk of getting pneumonia. Your best defense against the disease is a strong immune system, Dr. Steinberg says. Here are a few ways you can prevent pneumonia from sneaking up on you.

SAY *SAYONARA* TO SMOKING. People who smoke are more susceptible to pneumonia, Dr. Green says. Smoking kills hairlike structures in your airways called cilia that help keep your lungs clear of bacteria and other pneumonia-causing organisms.

Smoking also lowers your immunity, so you are less capable of fighting off the infection.

SEEK SLEEP. Get at least six to eight hours of sleep a night, Dr. Green says. It will help keep your immune system in tip-top form so that it can fend off pneumonia, particularly during the cold and flu season.

SEEK SERENITY, TOO. Stress hampers your immunity and may make you more susceptible to pneumonia and other respiratory ailments, Dr. Steinberg says. Taking a few moments each day to practice meditation, deep breathing, and other forms of relaxation may help keep the disease at bay.

BUILD A DEFENSIVE DIET. Eating a balanced diet will help keep your immune system alert so that it can clobber any organism that might cause pneumonia, Dr. Green says. Try following the recommendations of the U.S. Department of Agriculture Food Pyramid: Eat at least five servings of fruits and vegetables, six servings of grains, and a variety of proteins including dairy products, fish, poultry, beans, or meat each day.

RUN FOR YOUR LIFE. Regular exercise such as running or walking 20 minutes a day, three times a week, can help keep your lungs strong and pneumonia-free, Dr. Steinberg says.

SCRUB, SCRUB, SCRUB. One of the best ways to prevent respiratory infections including pneumonia is thoroughly washing your hands, says Dr. Green. So during the cold and flu season, be sure to cleanse your hands frequently with soap and warm water, particularly after personal contact like shaking hands.

GET A FLU SHOT FIRST. The flu doesn't directly cause pneumonia, but it can weaken your immune system so that pneumonia-causing microbes can infiltrate your lungs. An annual flu shot in susceptible or at-risk people can prevent that, Dr. Steinberg says.

ASK ABOUT THE OTHER NEEDLE. Men and women over 60, people who have respiratory diseases like emphysema or asthma, and others particularly susceptible to pneumonia might consider getting a pneumococcal vaccine. The vaccine can help prevent the most common strain of bacterial pneumonia, Dr. Steinberg says. Ask your doctor if the vaccine is right for you.

POSTNASAL DRIP
Turn Off the Tap

When he died, Edward Lawton, an English physician, was remembered not so much for his accomplishments, but for his nose.

"[He] was a tall man with a long and distinguished nose whom people sometimes mistook for General de Gaulle," his obituary in the *British Medical Journal* began. "Not surprisingly, he was called 'The General' by friends and patients."

Unlike Dr. Lawton, few of us have noses that are worthy of immortality. In fact, you probably seldom notice your snout unless you have a nagging case of postnasal drip.

Everybody has some postnasal drainage going on all of the time, however, says Jack B. Anon, M.D., chairman of the nasal and sinus committee of the American Academy of Otolaryngology/Head and Neck Surgery and an otolaryngologist in Erie, Pennsylvania. Healthy noses and sinuses produce about a quart of clear, thin mucus each day. This sticky mucus humidifies and heats the air as it is sucked into the lungs. It also traps dust and helps destroy bacteria before it enters the lower respiratory system. Normally, you swallow the mucus without even being conscious of it.

"You only become aware of postnasal drip if the mucus thickens, as it does when you have allergies, colds, or another disease," says Thomas Kidder, M.D., associate professor of otolaryngology and human communications at the Medical College of Wisconsin in Milwaukee. Literally hundreds of airborne irritants can trigger excessive postnasal drip, he says. Some of the more likely culprits include molds, pollen, dust, dust mites, cigarette smoke, and dry air often caused by heating or air-conditioning.

Food allergies also can increase annoying nasal secretions, Dr. Anon says. Here is how to prevent postnasal drip.

IDENTIFY THE TROUBLEMAKER. If you suspect an allergy is causing your postnasal drip, the first thing to do is to identify it, says Thomas Platts-Mills, M.D., Ph.D., head of the division of allergy and clinical immunology at the University of Virginia Medical Center in Charlottesville. A skin test is your best bet. Using a needle, your doctor or allergist pricks different allergens into your skin. If an itchy welt appears, you have found your culprit.

If it turns out that you are allergic to dust or dust mites, Dr. Anon suggests these dust-busting ways to protect yourself from them in your bedroom, throughout your house, and in the great outdoors.

MAKE YOUR BED MITE-FREE. If you cover your mattress and box spring in zippered vinyl coverings, the allergens will be trapped inside. Also, make sure that you have polyester pillows, which are made from foam, a material that gathers less dust than feathers and can be washed frequently. And wash your sheets once a week to make sure that you drown the microscopic critters.

BECOME A HOUSE-ROVING VACUUM VIRTUOSO. To help eliminate the mighty mites around the house, Dr. Platts-Mills says that you should dust and vacuum your house at least once a week. Since curtains and heavy drapes can be contaminant-catchers, be sure to vacuum them, too. Just slap on the attachment and give them a once-over, he advises.

REFURBISH THE FURNITURE. Couches and chairs can be dustbins, too—especially items with heavily textured fabrics, says Dr. Anon. Vacuum the Victorian love seat that your Aunt Flo left you in her will.

IN POLLEN SEASON, GUARD THE ENTRY POINTS. Spring and summer are the peak seasons for pollen, a prime cause of allergies and postnasal drip, Dr. Platts-Mills says. Air-conditioning can help slash your exposure to these pollens. Be sure to follow the manufacturer's directions and regularly change the filter.

If you don't have air-conditioning, use fans, but not the type that fits into your window since they blow pollen into the room. Also, keep your windows closed as much as possible during the pollen season, Dr. Platts-Mills suggests.

WIPE OUT THE MOLDY OLDIES. Molds are yet another problem that can cause postnasal drip, Dr. Platts-Mills says. At least once a week, scrub mold-prone areas like the bathroom and kitchen with diluted bleach or use a product that kills mold and fungus, such as Lysol.

SCRUTINIZE YOUR MENU. Postnasal drip can be aggravated by a food allergy. If you suspect that a certain kind of food might be the cause, just eliminate it from your diet and see if the nasal blockage eases. Or get a skin test, which can help to determine if you are allergic to a particular food.

WATER YOURSELF. Six to eight eight-ounce glasses of water a day will help dilute mucus and prevent postnasal drip, according to Dr. Kidder. "You lose a lot of moisture from your lungs and nasal passages during the course of a day. So the mucus in your nose tends to be thicker if you don't keep yourself well-hydrated," he says.

You can also use over-the-counter nasal saline sprays

as needed. The saline spray will help keep mucus from thickening, he says.

WATER THE AIR, TOO. Crank up your humidifier in the winter months, Dr. Anon suggests. Furnaces tend to dry out household air, which can thicken mucous secretions and lead to postnasal drip. Be sure to clean and dry the humidifier well between uses to prevent mold.

SNUFF THE PUFFS. Smoke damages hairlike structures in the nose called cilia that help flush mucus into the throat. If the cilia aren't working properly, the mucous layer in the throat will thicken, creating the sensation of postnasal drip, Dr. Anon says. Avoid all forms of smoking, including secondhand smoke that is common in many bars and restaurants, he urges.

PREMATURE EJACULATION
Take Control of the Flow

Speedy sex used to be good sex. "From an evolutionary standpoint, rapid or premature ejaculation makes a great deal of sense. Two million years ago, if you took 10 minutes to have intercourse, you probably would have been eaten by a saber-toothed tiger before you ejaculated. So if you took just 10 seconds to ejaculate, your chances of surviving and producing lots of offspring would be greatly enhanced," says Roger Crenshaw, M.D., a sex therapist and psychiatrist in private practice in La Jolla, California.

But life no longer boils down to the survival of the fastest. For most of us, lovemaking has evolved into a lingering pleasure. Yet for some men, that experience is frustratingly elusive. In fact, premature ejaculation is by far the most common male sexual problem.

Despite its prevalence, premature ejaculation is surprisingly hard to define. A wide range of men—some of whom last less than 30 seconds and others who hold out for

15 minutes or more—complain about the problem, Dr. Crenshaw says.

Here are some simple ways to prevent premature ejaculation from disrupting your sex life.

TALK IT OUT. Discussing the problem with your partner will take some of the edge off and possibly help you resolve the problem, according to Barbara Bartlik, M.D., a psychiatrist and sex therapist at the New York Hospital/Cornell Medical Center in New York City.

If your partner is willing to help you overcome the problem, you can discuss whether there are ways that you can satisfy her sexually without intercourse. With more sex play in your repertoire, there is less attention on ejaculation.

"If people can talk about these things and work them out together, then there isn't a sexual problem. It is when communication breaks down that people get into trouble," Dr. Bartlik says.

EMBARGO EROTICA. Abstain from erotic books, magazines, and videos. Viewing or reading these materials makes it harder for you to concentrate on physical sensations in the penis. And learning to focus on those physical sensations that occur just prior to orgasm is the key to the treatment of premature ejaculation, Dr. Bartlik says.

BUNDLE UP. Try using three layers of condoms when you have sex. It will reduce penile stimulation and can help delay ejaculation, Dr. Bartlik says. As you become more confident during your sexual encounters, you can gradually peel down to one condom—or none at all if you are in a monogamous relationship with a woman who is using another form of birth control.

GET BACK TO BASICS. Ask your partner to agree to a moratorium on foreplay and intercourse, suggests Robert W. Birch, Ph.D., a sex therapist in Columbus, Ohio, and author of *Male Sexual Endurance*. Instead, schedule an hour twice a week when you can lie naked together and just cuddle and caress. It will help you relax in a sexual environment without worrying about performance. Given the role anxiety plays in rapid ejaculation, the couple must learn to relax. Massage your partner's back, the backs of her legs, her shoulders, and her arms. If this stimulates you to the point that you feel as if you are about to ejaculate, stop, get up, and walk around the room. Don't return to your partner until you feel the urge pass. The point of this exercise is to find a balance where you can relax and feel pleasure in giving and receiving, yet remain in control, he says.

DO YOUR HOMEWORK. Once you learn to relax, you might want to try the stop/start technique, a classic method for preventing premature ejaculation that will require practice, patience, and some cooperation from your partner, Dr. Birch says.

Ask your partner to caress your penis with a dry hand. As she is doing this, imagine that you are at the foot of a ladder, Dr. Birch says. Keep close track, and as your excitement surges, imagine that you are beginning to climb up that ladder, a rung at a time. It is your job to keep yourself from falling over the top, so you must anticipate the point of no return. As your partner strokes your penis, you will begin climbing the ladder faster and faster.

Now shift your focus from the sensation of her hand stroking your penis to your location on the imaginary ladder. Lie perfectly still. Keep your eyes closed and avoid any sexual thoughts or images. When you feel close to the point of no return, tell your partner to stop. At this point, she should let go and sit back. Allow yourself to level off and visualize yourself descending back down to the foot of the ladder. When you are absolutely sure that you are back under control, ask her to begin again. Do this five or six times a session before allowing yourself to ejaculate. Practice this technique as often as you are comfortable for at least two weeks, Dr. Birch recommends.

BOTTOM OUT. Avoid the traditional man-on-top position, Dr. Crenshaw advises. In that position, the nerves in your penis will be more aroused, you will thrust harder, and the muscles in your back, legs, and arms will be more tense—a perfect setup for premature ejaculation. You will last longer if the woman is on top, he says, because your whole body will be more relaxed. Relaxation of large body muscles is the key.

PREMENSTRUAL SYNDROME
It's Not Just in Your Head

Premenstrual syndrome is a riddle wrapped in a mystery inside an enigma. In fact, it has baffled doctors dating back to Hippocrates, the father of modern medicine, who noted premenstrual-syndrome-like symptoms among ancient Greek women nearly 2,500 years ago.

Premenstrual syndrome (PMS) actually isn't a disease, but rather an eclectic mix of more than 150 physical and emotional symptoms, according to Andrea Kielich, M.D., clinical professor of internal medicine specializing in women's health at the Portland Clinic in Oregon. These symptoms commonly include irritability, depression, mood swings, bloating, tender breasts, fatigue, forgetfulness, headaches, and food cravings.

Although estimates vary, some researchers believe that up to 40 percent of menstruating women have PMS to some degree. Many of them experience just a few symptoms beginning 3 to 14 days prior to their periods. Although bothersome, the symptoms are usually mild and disappear once menstruation begins, says Jean Endicott, Ph.D., director of the Premenstrual Evaluation Unit at Columbia-Presbyterian Medical Center in New York City.

But for many others, perhaps as many as 15 percent of all menstruating women, PMS is a much bigger problem. They have severe multiple symptoms that often disrupt relationships, cripple job performance, and in the most extreme cases, have been blamed for child abuse, suicides, and violent crimes.

Although there is no surefire prevention plan, there are some lifestyle steps that you can take to minimize the impact of PMS.

Food Fighters: Less Fat, Lotsa Pasta

The first line of defense is nutritional. Follow these food and drink rules to get less stress from PMS.

Squash fat. Eating too much fat can ignite biochemical changes in the body that may worsen your symptoms, says Glenn O. Bair, M.D., director of the Bair PMS Center in Topeka, Kansas. He suggests limiting the amount of fat in your diet to less than 20 percent of calories. Here is how to figure out your fat.

Divide the average number of calories you eat daily by 5 (that's 20 percent of your calories). Then divide the result by 9 (there are 9 calories in 1 gram of fat). The result will tell you how many grams of fat you are allowed. Once you know this, carefully reading food labels, which list fat in grams, should help you keep your dietary fat under control.

Nosh on noodles and nectarines. Pastas like spaghetti and linguine and other foods like fresh fruits and vegetables, whole-grain cereals, and whole-grain bread may help relieve food cravings and mood swings, Dr. Kielich says. These foods are loaded with complex carbohydrates, which have a vital role in the production of mood-enhancing chemicals in the brain.

Eat at least 100 calories of complex carbohydrates every three hours, Dr. Bair suggests. Plain popcorn, pretzels, rice cakes, or a baked potato are good choices for between-meal snacks.

CURTAIL CAFFEINE. Coffee, cola, chocolate, and anything else that contains caffeine can give an unwanted jolt to breast pain, anxiety, and other PMS symptoms, Dr. Endicott says. Switch to decaffeinated coffee or herbal teas. It is best to avoid caffeine all month, but especially in the days prior to your period, she suggests.

STAY AWAY FROM THE BOTTLE. Resist the temptation to numb PMS with beer, wine, or other alcoholic beverages, Dr. Endicott says. Although you may feel better while you are drinking, in the long run alcohol actually will worsen your symptoms because a hangover on top of PMS will make you feel really rotten.

SOCK IT WITH SUPPLEMENTS. Daily supplements of 400 IU (international units) of vitamin E, 50 to 100 milligrams of vitamin B_6, 1,000 milligrams of calcium citrate, and 300 to 500 milligrams of magnesium citrate or aspartate may relieve breast tenderness, backaches, irritability, and other PMS symptoms, says Vickie Lovin, M.D., a gynecologist in private practice in Hickory, North Carolina.

If you are considering taking vitamin E in amounts above 200 IU, discuss this with your doctor first. One study using low-dose vitamin E supplements showed an increased risk of hemorrhagic stroke. Supplemental magnesium may cause diarrhea in some people, and people with heart or kidney problems should check with their doctors before taking supplemental magnesium. Over a prolonged time, unstable gait and numb feet may occur while taking vitamin B_6 in doses above 50 milligrams.

Ease On down the Road

Tension can aggravate the symptoms of PMS, Dr. Kielich says. She recommends activities that cut down on stress. Practicing yoga; listening to soothing music; taking a long, hot bath; and other pleasurable activities can help knock down stress.

TREK AROUND A LOT. Increasing exercise during PMS can help relieve symptoms, Dr. Kielich says. In particular, aerobic exercise like walking, running, or swimming stimulates the production of endorphins, brain chemicals that can improve mood. Exercise also improves blood flow to your reproductive organs and may prevent cramping, swelling, bloating, and other painful symptoms of PMS. So if you normally walk for 20 minutes, three times a week, try taking daily walks the week before your period, she suggests.

TAKE BACK THE NIGHT. If you have PMS, avoid working at night or doing routine tasks that require staying up past your normal bedtime, says Katharina Dalton, M.D., author of *PMS: The Essential Guide to Treatment Options*. The area of the brain called the hypothalamus that controls day/night rhythms is located next to the part of the brain that regulates menstrual hormones. Dr. Dalton's theory is that any disturbance in the day/night rhythm can interfere with your menstrual cycle and aggravate symptoms like irritability and fatigue.

Dr. Bair adds that hormones are at their lowest at night, all the more reason to snooze or lose.

PROSTATE CANCER
Eating Well Is the Best Defense

No other human organ is as susceptible to cancer as the prostate. Each year, an estimated 209,900 American men are diagnosed with the disease, making it the most prevalent form of cancer in the United States. Although lung cancer claims more than twice as many men's lives each year, prostate cancer is the second most lethal male cancer, killing 41,800 men annually.

In fact, the disease is so common that by age 65, nearly two of every three men may have microscopic cancers growing in their prostates, the walnut-size gland that is wrapped around the urethra, the tube that drains the bladder. And some doctors believe that if men lived long enough, every man would develop the disease.

Curiously, the vast majority of men who have the disease will never know it. That's because prostate cancer is normally a very slow growing tumor, often taking 20 to 30 years to become large enough to be detected by any currently available tests or to cause serious health problems. By then, many older men who had these small tumors will have long since died of other causes such as heart disease and stroke, says William R. Fair, M.D., professor of urologic oncology at Memorial Sloan-Kettering Cancer Center and director of the Prostate Diagnostic Center, both in New York City.

"Clearly, many more men die *with* prostate cancer than from it," Dr. Fair says. "So if we could just slow the growth of the tumor so that it takes 40 to 60 years to progress instead of 20 to 30, that would amount to a cure for many men."

Doctors suspect that dietary changes may help men stall the progress of disease and prevent it from becoming life-threatening. Here are a few prostate protectors.

GO LEAN ON FAT. Lowering your fat intake to 20 percent of your total calories (that's about 44 grams of fat if you eat 2,000 calories a day) is one of the best things that you can do to slash your risk of developing aggressive prostate cancer, Dr. Fair says.

American men, who on average eat about 34 percent of calories from fat, are about eight times more likely to develop advanced prostate cancer than men in Japan and China, where people traditionally get only 10 to 15 percent of their calories from fat. In addition, the disease develops much more slowly and is far less deadly among men in these countries than it is with men in the United States.

Some researchers theorize that excess fat drives up levels of testosterone, a male hormone that promotes cancer growth. In animal studies, Dr. Fair has found that low-fat eating—that is, getting less than 20 percent of calories from fat—can virtually halt the progression of tiny tumors.

"The tumors almost disappear," Dr. Fair says. "They grow so slowly that they will probably never be life-threatening. And that, to me, is tantamount to prevention."

TURN AWAY FROM RED MEAT. Beef and other red meats are loaded with saturated fat, a type of fat linked to development of several cancers including prostate cancer. In one study of 51,000 American men, those who ate the most red meat were 2.6 times more likely to develop advanced prostate cancer than men who avoided meat consumption.

One theory, reports Dr. Fair, is that the fat in red meats triggers the production of hormonelike substances called prostaglandins that stimulate prostate cancer growth.

"Personally, I eat no red meat, and I think that's the best way to go given the apparent link between red meat consumption and prostate cancer," Dr. Fair says. "If you can't bear to live without it, make it a once-a-month treat and choose a well-trimmed cut like filet mignon that has less fat than T-bone steak."

CATCH SOME FISH. One reason why advanced prostate cancer is rare in China may be the quantity of fish in the diet. One study compared cancer rates of American men to men living in Shanghai, China, where people consume three times as much fish in their daily diet. The rate of prostate cancer for the American men was a dramatic 25.9 times higher than for the Chinese.

In a laboratory study, animals fed a diet supplemented with omega-3 oils, the "healthy" oils that are present in many fish, developed prostate tumors one-quarter the size of the tumors in animals that lacked omega-3's, according to Dr. Fair.

Try eating at least two servings a week of fish rich in omega-3's like salmon or tuna, suggests David Rose, M.D., associate director and chief of the division of nutrition and endocrinology at the American Health Foundation in Valhalla, New York.

An Apple a Day Recipe

Lycopene Soup

This creamy tomato soup packs in the lycopene that can help prevent prostate cancer. It has plenty of flavor without a lot of fat.

½ cup nonfat sour cream

2 scallions, minced

1 teaspoon prepared horseradish

1 tablespoon olive oil

1 large onion, chopped

3 cloves garlic, minced

1 teaspoon dried basil

6 cups seeded and chopped tomatoes

2 cups fat-free milk

2 cups low-sodium vegetable juice

1 tablespoon balsamic vinegar

In a small bowl, combine the sour cream, scallions, and horseradish. Set aside.

Warm the oil in a medium saucepan over medium heat. Add the onion and garlic. Cook for 4 minutes, or until soft. Add the basil and tomatoes. Cook, stirring often, for 5 minutes, or until the tomatoes begin to release their juices. Puree the mixture in a food processor or with a handheld blender.

Return the mixture to the pan. Stir in the milk, vegetable juice, and vinegar. Simmer over low heat, stirring often, for 10 minutes. Do not boil.

Divide the soup among 4 bowls. Swirl 2 tablespoons of the sour cream mixture into each bowl.

Makes 4 servings. Per serving: 194 calories, 4 g. fat

Discover the joy of soy. Instead of meat, try substituting tofu, miso, and other soy foods in salads, casseroles, and soups, Dr. Fair suggests. Men in Japan eat lots of soy-based foods, benefiting from significantly high levels of genistein and genistin, two substances found in soy that may help clamp down on the disease, a study shows.

Researchers suspect that the phytoestrogens in soy foods may reduce the production of testosterone, a male sex hormone believed to fuel prostate cancer growth. Phytoestrogens also may prevent the growth of blood capillaries that normally form around prostate tumors. Without these capillaries to nourish it, a tumor has difficulty growing.

Learn to like lycopene. A study at the Harvard School of Public Health tracked the eating habits of almost 50,000 health-care professionals for more than six years. The researchers came to the conclusion that lycopene, an antioxidant compound that gives tomatoes their distinctive red color, helps fight cancer.

As little as two servings a week of foods made with cooked tomato sauce can help men halve their risk of developing aggressive prostate cancer, says Edward Giovannucci, M.D., assistant professor of medicine and nutrition at Harvard Medical School and Harvard School of Public Health.

Lycopene also is found in raw tomatoes and other fruits and vegetables like pink grapefruit and watermelon. But cooked tomato sauce seems to provide the greatest benefit. Researchers have found that using olive oil when you're making tomato sauce makes it easier for the body to absorb larger amounts of the antioxidant.

So make spaghetti and other foods made with tomato sauce a centerpiece of your meals two or three times a week, Dr. Fair says. But avoid the high-fat extras that so often come with the sauce such as pepperoni and cheese or fat-laden meatballs. (When you place an order at the local pizzeria, ask them to go light on the cheese and hold the meat toppings.)

PSORIASIS
Relieving the Itch

Psoriasis is an unsightly, chronic condition in which skin cells develop faster than normal and cluster on the surface of the skin. They often form swollen lesions, topped with silvery white scales.

The ancient Greeks considered it the curse of the gods and sometimes forced psoriasis sufferers to ring a bell to warn of their approach—in part because the disease was thought to be contagious. It isn't, but for the more than six million afflicted Americans, psoriasis is often painful. It causes the skin to itch, burn, sting, and bleed easily.

Although doctors aren't sure what leads to psoriasis, some researchers suspect that it is an inherited disorder in which the body's immune system attacks its own skin.

When someone has psoriasis, his skin cells grow abnormally, and the rate of cell growth is much faster than normal, says Ross Bright, M.D., medical director of the Psoriasis Medical Center in Palo Alto, California. Doctors and researchers have not been able to explain what sets this process off, but there is evidence that it may be triggered by emotional stress, illness, or injury to the skin.

There is no surefire way to prevent psoriasis. Once an itchy patch appears, it tends to spread—for a very simple reason: Scratching the itch can cause tiny wounds in the skin that lead to the development of new patches. It is pretty tough not to scratch an itch. Still, psoriasis can be controlled with drugs and intensive ultraviolet therapy. And if you use these self-help techniques, you may be able to prevent it from spreading and minimize its impact on your life.

SLICK UP YOUR SKIN. Moisturize all of your skin, not just the affected part, twice a day, says Gerald Krueger, M.D., professor of dermatology at the University of Utah School of Medicine in Salt Lake City. He recommends using about an ounce of thinly applied petroleum jelly or other greasy over-the-counter skin lubricants like Cetaphil or Eucerin cream. The moisturizer will help soothe the itch and prevent psoriasis from spreading, he says.

OIL UP YOUR BATH. Besides using commercial lotions and creams, try adding baby oil or olive oil to your bath, says Jerome Z. Litt, M.D., assistant clinical professor of dermatology at Case Western Reserve University School of Medicine in Cleveland and author of *Your Skin: From Acne to Zits*. A couple of capfuls may be enough to prevent new outbreaks and control existing ones, he says. But use extra care getting in and out of the tub and be sure to clean it well afterward because these oils can be extremely slippery, he cautions.

BE DELICATE WITH YOUR DERMA. Your skin isn't an old cowhide, so don't treat it that way, advises Dr. Krueger. Resist the temptation to vigorously scrub with brushes and washcloths, which can damage your skin and aggravate psoriasis. Instead, use your bare hands to gently wash with warm water and a moisturizing soap. Then pat yourself dry or leave your skin slightly damp and apply moisturizer.

UNCOIL YOUR SPRING. Sometimes stress can make you scratch or pick at your wounds, and, of course, that only aggravates the psoriasis. To help avoid some of these nervous habits, Dr. Krueger suggests reaching into the stress-buster tool chest for something to help you relax. Here are a number of possibilities.

- Meditation
- Deep breathing
- Yoga
- Tai chi
- Aromatherapy
- Any hobby you can lose yourself in—from gardening to collecting antiques

CHECK YOUR MEDICINE CHEST. A few frequently prescribed drugs for conditions such as arthritis, high blood pressure, and migraines can worsen psoriasis, Dr. Krueger says. If your psoriasis is flaring, ask your doctor if one of your medications could be behind it. Then ask your doctor about switching prescriptions.

ELECTRIFY YOUR LIFE. To avoid nicks and cuts that can spread psoriasis lesions on areas of the body where you shave, use an electric razor, suggests John Romano, M.D., professor of dermatology at the New York Hospital/Cornell Medical Center and Saint Vincent's Hospital in New York City.

GET SOME SUPPORT. The National Psoriasis Foundation offers telephone counseling and support groups and publishes newsletters updating members on medications, research, and social services. The yearly membership fee is a donation in any amount. For more information, write to the National Psoriasis Foundation at 6600 SW 92nd Avenue, Suite 300, Portland, OR 97223.

RASHES
Steer Clear of Certain Substances

Most rashes are warnings, our immune system's way of telling us that there is an intruder in the neighborhood. They are allergic reactions to either something we ate or some environmental irritant—a chemical, a fabric, your sister's cat. Unlike hives, which are distinct, red bumps with whitish centers, rashes are usually just red and itchy. But they are similar to hives in that *something* is triggering the problem. The best way to prevent the return of the redness is to try these precautions.

INVOLVE YOUR DOCTOR. The best defense against round two with a rash is to find out what caused the outbreak in the first place. When you get a rash, it is always a good idea to consult a dermatologist. If you are allergic to a particular food, he can do some sensitivity tests to figure out whether it is strawberries or peanuts, for instance, that your body doesn't care for, says Jerome Z. Litt, M.D., assistant clinical professor of dermatology at Case Western Reserve University School of Medicine in Cleveland and author of *Your Skin: From Acne to Zits*.

BE A DETECTIVE. Ask yourself some sleuthing questions. Have you recently eaten anything that is not a normal part of your diet? If the rash is on your face, have you changed your makeup recently? Or your soap? Or your perfume? Or hair spray?

"If you suddenly get a rash, figure out what you have done differently in the last 24 to 36 hours," says Dr. Litt. "If the rash is on your body, were you wearing a new article of clothing? Have you changed your laundry detergent or fabric softener? By noting this information, you can help your doctor determine the cause of the rash." And once you have determined what's causing the rash, the simplest preventive is to stay away from whatever provokes it, he adds.

INTERVIEW WAITERS. If you are allergic to a food, it is important that you avoid it. If you are allergic to peanuts, for instance, don't be timid about asking the waiter if the tandoori chicken is cooked in peanut oil.

BECOME FOOD FINICKY. Sometimes an offending food can be a minor ingredient of processed frozen or canned foods. Read labels carefully. Dr. Litt says to look for dyes like FD&C red and FD&C yellow or preservatives like sulfates.

READ BEFORE YOU TOUCH. The same advice applies for any products that you are in contact with regularly, such as paints, lotion, and detergents. If you are trying out a new soap, for instance, read the label carefully to make sure that it doesn't have the chemical that sets your skin screaming. It may be acetone, fragrances, lanolin, deodorants, vitamin E, turpentine, dye—and other things, says Dr. Litt.

GET FUSSY ABOUT CONTAMINATION. Our immune systems are finely tuned, so it is important to avoid even incidental contact with an allergen. Avoid cutting boards or counters that could be tainted with rash-causing allergens contained in the soaps or detergents you used to clean it.

GLOVE UP. If you are prone to rashes on your hands, wearing gloves while doing household cleaning or home improvements is wise. Dr. Litt recommends cotton liners inside rubber, plastic, or vinyl gloves. If you don't wear the cotton liners, sometimes the rubber or vinyl itself can cause a rash. Gloves that come with built-in liners don't offer enough protection, he says.

COAT YOUR JEWELRY. Some people find that they have allergic reactions to jewelry, especially if it contains nickel. Try this trick, offered by Wilma F. Bergfeld, M.D., head of clinical research in the department of dermatology at the Cleveland Clinic. "You can coat your jewelry with clear nail polish or polyethylene sprays so that the metal doesn't touch your skin." Though it wears off eventually and needs to be renewed, the coating won't harm the metal, and it won't hurt gemstones either, if some of the polish or spray happens to get on them.

DUCK RAZOR RASH. Razor burn isn't caused by an allergic reaction, but just by irritation of the skin. There are ways to train your hair to grow properly so that you can avoid razor chafing, says Dr. Litt. "Men should shave down on the face only once and up on the neck only once," he says. "This will help to train the hair to grow out straight, preventing razor bump rash."

His advice for women who shave their legs? "Always shave down to prevent nicks and irritations."

SCRATCH NOT. Rashes can be very itchy, so sometimes it's tough not to scratch. But do your best not to. Scratching can spread a rash and prevent it from healing. In some cases, scratching can lead to infection, cautions Lenore Kakita, M.D., assistant clinical professor in the department of medicine, division of dermatology, at the University of California, Los Angeles.

SLATHER YOUR SKIN. Keeping your skin healthy means keeping it clean and moisturized. If your skin is damaged, red, or scaly, it is more prone to be injured or infected, according to Dr. Bergfeld.

Use "bland" lubricants—ones that have no dyes, fragrances, or other additives that can irritate the skin. The lu-

When It's Rash to Ignore a Rash

Sometimes rashes are more than a discomfort that you would like to prevent. The onset of a rash could signal a threat to your health or even your life. Call your doctor right away if a rash covers more than 20 percent of your body and comes with other systemic symptoms like fatigue, headache, and flulike symptoms, says Wilma F. Bergfeld, M.D., head of clinical research in the department of dermatology at the Cleveland Clinic.

There are rashes that can be signs of potentially life-threatening illnesses. For example, purple spots on the skin and a temperature of over 100°F may be signs of meningitis. If you have these symptoms, call a doctor right away.

Hives that rapidly cover a large area of the body are usually triggered by an allergy to drugs, food chemicals, or an insect sting. This violent allergic reaction can lead to unconsciousness. And some people are susceptible to anaphylactic shock, when areas around the throat and lungs swell up, leading to asphyxiation.

Of course, not all rashes call for immediate emergency care. If your only symptom is a rash, you can just call your doctor and ask what to do. But if you are also having difficulty breathing, get to the emergency room immediately.

bricants will keep skin moist and supple, says Dr. Kakita. "Frequent lubrication is helpful for dry skin. It is good to leave a little water on the skin after bathing, then lubricate. You can buy bland lubricants over the counter," she says. Many lotions and creams don't contain dyes, fragrances, and other elements that can irritate skin, she says.

REPETITIVE STRAIN INJURY
Prevention, Hands Down

A secretary entering endless data at the keyboard. An Internet enthusiast surfing the Web for hours every night, clicking the mouse again and again. A clerk at the supermarket checkout, waving item after item over the bar-code scanner. A carpenter hammering nails all day. A musician practicing a piece until it is perfect.

All those folks—and anybody else who performs a specific task with his hands and arms over and over again, day after day—are candidates for a painful condition called repetitive strain injury, or RSI. The most common RSI is carpal tunnel syndrome, in which the nerve that runs through a small tunnel of bone in the wrist is pressed and pained by the swelling of nearby tendons, causing tingling and numbness in the hand. More than 800,000 Americans per year visit a doctor for this problem. But there are plenty of other spots for RSI: the elbow, the forearm, the thumb, the shoulder, the top side of the hand, the palm side of the

Strength Training: Will It Overpower Your Hands and Arms?

For people involved in repetitive hand and arm actions at work, strength training the upper limbs, using the type of weight-lifting machines found in fitness centers and gyms, will aggravate or even cause repetitive strain injury, says Robert E. Markison, M.D., associate clinical professor of surgery at the University of California, San Francisco, School of Medicine, and a hand surgeon in San Francisco.

Despite the many benefits of upper-body workout machines, they are not helpful for people who are already doing repetitive upper-body motion all day long. "They add wear and tear to the muscles of the upper limbs," says Dr. Markison. "And they add a mantle of muscle to the neck, back, and chest that can crowd nerves in those regions, which can contribute to repetitive strain injury."

Instead of working out with weight machines, Dr. Markison says to walk. "It is the most natural thing you can do, and there is a swing of the upper limbs that creates tone and fitness."

fingers—almost any spot where the muscles of the hands and arms are used again and again.

Most of that damage is preventable, says Robert E. Markison, M.D., associate clinical professor of surgery at the University of California, San Francisco, School of Medicine, and a hand surgeon in San Francisco. And he should know. Not only has Dr. Markison been counseling and treating people with RSI for 15 years in his surgical practice, he is also a musician who took it upon himself to redesign various types of musical instruments so that those who play them would be less likely to develop RSI.

Full-blown RSI doesn't happen overnight. Dr. Markison advises to stay alert for the warning sign: temporary pain. "If you have discomfort that lingers for more than half an hour after the task, you are probably doing too much," he says. If you take preventive measures early, you can head off RSI before it becomes a serious problem. Here is advice on sidestepping repetitive strain.

TAKE 15 AND STRETCH. Experts agree that breaks are a must, especially if you are doing data entry on a keyboard for hours a day, says Karen Allen, a senior physical therapist in the office of environmental health and safety at the University of Virginia in Charlottesville. Try every 15 minutes to take 1-minute mini-breaks, she says. You can do these while still seated at your desk.

During those mini-breaks, Allen recommends doing two easy stretches to help prevent RSI.

Stretch #1: Make a fist, then span or spread your fingers as far as possible. Relax. Repeat this three or four times.

Stretch #2: Hold your arms straight out in front of your body with your palms facing down. Bend your hands up, so that your palms face away from you. Hold that stretch for five seconds. Then bend your hands down, so that your palms are facing toward you. Hold that stretch for five seconds. Repeat three or four times.

Be sure to leave your work space after every two hours of continuous computer use, says Allen. "For those breaks, give yourself 15 minutes to get away from your desk and move. Walk around a little bit and shake out your hands," she advises.

CUT THE CAFFEINE. Avoid caffeinated drinks—coffee, tea, or soda, recommends Dr. Markison. Because caffeine is a diuretic, you will need to urinate more frequently. And when there is less fluid in your body, there is a loss of blood volume. This means that you get less circulation to the hands, he explains.

PRACTICE POSTURE PREVENTIVES. Awkward posi-tioning while you work can be a major factor in causing RSI, says Dr. Markison. The key to good posture, he says, is to bring the work to you rather than wrapping yourself around the work. If you are a computer operator, for exam-ple, sit upright, with limbs that are relaxed and flexible rather than strained and rigid.

To avoid postural errors, Dr. Markison says, watch out for these clues.

The tipped-forward head. This can triple the force running through your spine and the muscles of your neck, compressing nerves and vessels in those areas, which can lead to problems in the arms and hands.

The extended arms. Don't put your limbs forward any farther than you have to. The farther away they are from your body, the more your circulation is reduced. Avoid the elbow extended, palm-down position when using a mouse.

BREATHE AWAY STRESS. Stress is another contribut-ing factor to RSI, says Dr. Markison. To counter stress while at work, breathe more deeply. Just take a couple of deep breaths every now and then, he says. It is the simplest way to deal with stress in the workplace, and it helps restore blood flow to the hands.

He also suggests that people who must sit at key-boards entering written data speak the words in a whisper as they are typing. "If you look at people in high-speed, data-entry situations, their breathing is often shallow or halted. But when typists whisper the words as they are typed, they force themselves to breathe more deeply," he says.

SCARRING
How to Save Your Skin

Our skin and tissues have remarkable powers to heal themselves. Given enough time and the proper conditions, all the different tissues in skin, even the blood vessels and nerves, can grow back, creeping in from the edges and slowly growing up from the bottom of a wound. But sometimes, if the wound is deep or becomes infected or keeps tearing open as it heals, there is likely to be a noticeable scar.

A scar is simply an abnormal arrangement of skin cells. It may be shiny and thin, hard and rough-textured, white or dark. It can be a reminder of where the wound was "stitched up." Sometimes a scar can be so tough and fibrous that it interferes with your ability to move a joint.

"It is easier to take measures to minimize a scar early on than to have to correct one later," says David H. McDaniel, M.D., assistant professor of clinical dermatology and plastic surgery at Eastern Virginia Medical School of the Medical College of Hampton Roads in Norfolk and director of the Laser Center of Virginia in Virginia Beach. Here is what experts recommend.

DON'T SCRATCH A RASH, ESPECIALLY THE CHICKEN-POX. Lots of scars are remnants of childhood chickenpox. Scars are a result of scratching. If your child has chickenpox, start giving an oral antihistamine as soon as you see him begin to scratch. Simply use an over-the-counter brand of diphenhydramine hydrochloride, such as Benadryl Allergy Liquid, at the dosage recommended for children, Dr. McDaniel says.

For poison ivy or other itchy skin patches, apply a topical hydrocortisone cream, such as Cortaid, to subdue the itch and short-circuit scratching, adds Dr. McDaniel. If an over-the-counter hydrocortisone cream doesn't relieve your itching, your doctor can prescribe a stronger-concentration cream.

USE BUTTERFLY BANDAGES TO CLOSE SMALL CUTS. These very narrow adhesive bandages, which are available at drugstores, can be used to keep a small wound closed until it heals, which will minimize scarring, says Dennis J. Lynch, M.D., chairman of the department of surgery at the Scott and White Clinic, chairman of surgery for the Texas A&M School of Medicine, both in Temple, and president of the American Society of Plastic and Reconstructive Surgeons.

"For very superficial cuts, they can be used instead of stitches," he says. "For many cuts, however, they are not adequate. They are likely to work best on areas of your body where tension on your skin is minimal, such as your forehead."

To use them, pinch the cut closed with your fingers and apply as many of the small strips as you need to keep it closed, he says. Usually, these strips stick to your skin even when you shower—and you can leave them in place until the cut heals, Dr. Lynch says. But don't attempt to use any creams or ointments with these bandages, he says, because they won't stay in place if you do.

DAB ON A PETROLEUM-BASED ANTIBIOTIC OINTMENT.
Once the bleeding has stopped, the best way to speed healing is to apply a petroleum-based antibiotic ointment to the injured area, Dr. McDaniel says. He has tested one popular brand, Neosporin, in its new, "faster-healing" formula and found that it did indeed make cuts and scrapes heal up to 50 percent faster, depending on the severity of the injury. And along with the faster healing comes a reduction in scarring, according to Dr. McDaniel. This formula contains various antioxidants including vitamin E, a nutrient with reputed wound-healing and scar-reducing properties.

APPLY ALOE. Keep an aloe plant on your kitchen windowsill in case of burns or cuts, suggests John Heggers, Ph.D., professor of plastic surgery, microbiology, and immunology at the University of Texas Medical Branch and director of clinical microbiology at the Shriners Burns Institute, both in Galveston. "Aloe vera is used extensively to help to heal burns and reduce scarring," he says. "It contains a number of active ingredients that are useful in wound healing. It helps reduce inflammation, swelling, and itching, and it attracts and maintains moisture at the wound or burn site, which also promotes healing."

Fresh is best. Simply cut off a piece of the leaf, squeeze out the gel, and apply it to the wound. (Don't worry, the plant heals itself very nicely, too.) Do this three or four times a day to new cuts or burns, or more often if it soothes your pain, says Dr. Heggers. You can leave the area open or cover it lightly with a bandage or gauze.

Dr. Heggers also likes a product called Dermaide Aloe, which contains a high concentration of aloe. This product is available through mail-order from Dermaide Research Corporation, 7600 West College Drive, Palos Heights, IL 60463.

STAY IN THE SHADE. Healing wounds tend to darken if they are exposed to the sun while they are healing. So keep the wound covered, if you are outside, for two weeks beyond the time that it appears healed, Dr. McDaniel says. Use an adhesive bandage or, once it has healed enough to tolerate it, a sunscreen with a sun protection factor of 15 to 30, which provides protection from both kinds of ultraviolet rays: UVA and UVB. If you are going to the beach, use both, in case the bandage falls off.

LEAVE THAT SCAB ALONE. When you pull off a scab before it is ready to fall off, you pull out a divot of skin in the middle of the wound, which makes it more likely that the wound will heal with a depression, Dr. McDaniel says. If you just can't keep your hands off it, cover it up with an adhesive bandage.

PUT PRESSURE ON BURNS. Burns, too, can develop thick, red, raised scars. Special pressurized bandages are often applied in burn units to help prevent this, Dr. Lynch says. At home, you can wrap the area with an elastic bandage, or if the burn is on your hand, wear a tightly fitted, elasticized glove, such as an Isotoner.

CREAM IT WITH CARE. Hydrocortisone creams may also help, but they shouldn't be used for more than a week without medical supervision, Dr. Lynch says. The reason is that they can thin the scar so much that it weakens and tears.

KNOW WHEN TO GET STITCHES. Most people know enough to go to the emergency room to get stitches for big, deep cuts. But often, folks let smaller cuts that could benefit from stitches just heal by themselves. You should go to the emergency room and get a medical opinion on any cut that gapes, pulls open with movement, or has jagged skin on its borders, according to Dr. McDaniel. This is especially important if the injury is on your face, he says.

INSIST THAT A PLASTIC SURGEON DO THE HONORS. A plastic or dermatologic surgeon, and particularly one who specializes in cosmetic surgery, has the skills and knows the tricks to minimize scars, Dr. McDaniel says. Unlike a general practitioner, who will simply sew you up with one row of stitches, or worse yet (but even quicker) staple you shut, a cosmetic surgeon will often use both a row of dissolvable stitches below the surface of the skin and an additional layer of top stitches. The top layer comes out in just a few days, after the skin edges adhere, and the underlying stitches keep the wound closed until it is completely healed.

KEEP AN EYE OUT FOR KELOIDS. To prevent scarring, you have to pay close attention to your wound and how it is healing. If your cut seems to be healing nicely but then becomes red and raised, see a doctor right away. You are developing a keloid, a raised scar caused by the overgrowth of tissue, Dr. Lynch says. The doctor can inject a small amount of hydrocortisone into the scar tissue to dissolve the keloid.

IF YOU HAVE AN UGLY SCAR, DON'T WAIT TO SEEK HELP. The old rule of thumb—to wait a year after an injury to have a scar fixed—is wrong, Dr. McDaniel says. "In fact, with laser resurfacing or dermabrasion, for many scars we see a dramatic improvement in the results if the scar is revised six to eight weeks after the injury," he says.

SCIATICA
Be Gentle on Your Nerve

The sciatic nerve is a whole lotta nerve. Running from the base of your spine down into your legs, the sciatic is the thickest nerve in your body (about as wide as your thumb), and one of the longest. Any pressure on this mega-nerve can cause sciatica, a sharp, shooting pain or a tingling numbness that radiates out from the buttocks and down the legs.

Pressure on the sciatic nerve can have many causes, including trauma. But most often, it is caused by some sort of back problem. In people under the age of 50, usually a bulging or herniated disk chokes the nerve, says Kevin Reilly, D.C., a certified chiropractic sports physician and owner of Reilly Chiropractic Health and Fitness in Columbus, Ohio. In people over 50, sciatica is frequently a result of spinal stenosis, a stiff-disk condition where arthritis builds up and starts squeezing the nerve.

Sciatica is quite common and quite painful, but anything you do to strengthen your back and improve your flexibility can be counted as prevention. That's why it is a

Treat Sciatica Seriously

A lot of people wait too long before they go to the doctor, says Kevin Reilly, D.C., a certified chiropractic sports physician and owner of Reilly Chiropractic Health and Fitness in Columbus, Ohio. That is a big mistake. Many times, sciatica can be managed successfully if it is caught early enough and if you control or eliminate the underlying cause.

Doctors will use some combination of lifestyle changes, physical therapy, spinal adjustments, anti-inflammatory medications, and other noninvasive treatments. But if it is not treated early on, sometimes sciatica becomes so severe that surgery is the only option for relief. Generally, the worse sciatica gets, the further down the leg the pain or numbness goes, says Dr. Reilly. He urges that people not wait until they feel sciatica in the bottom of their feet to seek help.

good idea to take care of your back, even if there is no hint of a problem yet. Here's how.

FIT IN FITNESS. "You have to exercise to keep your back healthy," says Bruce Dall, M.D., an orthopedic spine surgeon at K-Valley Orthopedics in Kalamazoo, Michigan. The better your muscle tone, the better the support for your back. Toned muscles will take a lot of the pressure off your spine, reducing your chances of getting sciatica.

Just be sure to start out slowly, especially if you are out of shape or are already prone to sciatica. "If you do things the wrong way or go out too hard too fast, you are vulnerable to injuring yourself and your back," says Dr. Reilly. If you are unsure of how to begin a sound exercise plan, you would benefit from talking to a physician or physical therapist first, he adds.

"Walking is the best general, all-around exercise for

the back," says Dr. Dall. That is because it is low-impact and helps strengthen the spinal and abdominal muscles needed for back support.

Wearing supportive shoes is important whenever you walk. In addition, treadmills and well-paved level surfaces are recommended for beginners, says Dr. Reilly.

GET WET. To keep your back healthy and protect your sciatic nerve, go jump in the pool. "Swimming is very good exercise that can help keep muscles toned," says Dr. Reilly. Swim often—the more, the better if your back is in good shape.

If your back is already giving you some trouble, Dr. Dall recommends water physical therapy rather than swimming because some people tend to overarch their spines when they swim. For water physical therapy, you perform traditional exercises such as jogging or leg lifts in chest-high water. Because the water makes you buoyant, the spine isn't stressed by gravity.

STRETCH FOR PROTECTION. "Stretching is key to any sciatica prevention program," says Dr. Reilly. Muscles tighten up when your body is left in a stationary position for too long, especially if you are seated. Doing some simple stretching exercises can help loosen up the muscles that surround the sciatic nerve, he says.

Here's one stretch that you can do for the sciatic region. Lie down on your back, grab one knee, and slowly bring it up and over toward the opposite shoulder, says Dr. Reilly. Hold that position for five seconds, then gently return to the lying position. Repeat the stretch with the other leg. As you get better at this exercise, you can increase the amount of time in the knee-holding position.

LEAN TOWARD YOGA. Many of the stretches done in yoga can also help fend off sciatic problems. "It is a great way to stretch and put your spine through a safe range of motion," says Dr. Dall.

"I've heard lots of people with sciatica say that yoga

has helped them," Dr. Reilly concurs. Many yoga classes are now offered through adult night-school classes and YM/YWCAs as well as at yoga centers.

BUILD YOUR BACK THROUGH YOUR BELLY. "Healthy abdominal muscles make for a healthy back," says Dr. Reilly. The muscles in your stomach provide support for your spine. Patients with large guts and weak abdominal muscles often complain about back pain and sciatica flare-ups, he says. A gentle series of abdominal crunches done several times a week will help build those stomach muscles.

Dr. Reilly recommends partial situps. Lie on your back with both knees bent, feet flat on the floor, and arms crossed and resting on your chest. Curl up, bringing your elbows toward your thighs, until your shoulders are slightly off the floor. Exhale while curling up and inhale while slowly lowering your shoulders to the floor again. Work up to a minimum of three sets of 15 repetitions, suggests Dr. Reilly.

POSSESS GOOD POSTURE. Good posture means standing up straight, with your shoulders back and head directly over your body. To get a taste of perfect posture, try standing erect with your back against a wall. This is the position that can help prevent the pain of sciatica. Slouching puts more strain on your back than standing straight, says Dr. Dall. Standing, sitting, and walking tall takes pressure off your back, and it works more muscles of the body. "It's like exercising your back all day long."

USE YOUR HEAD, NOT YOUR BACK, WHEN YOU LIFT. Here is where lots of people can do their spines a favor. Whenever you lift something that weighs more than a few pounds, keep the object close to your body so that you don't strain the disks in your spine, says Dr. Dall. For the same reason, never twist or turn your torso while you are lifting an object. If you have to change direction, turn with your feet and legs instead. If you have to pick up a heavy item from the floor, make sure that you bend at the knees, not at the waist, he adds.

SIT LESS, SIT SMARTER. "When you tell someone to avoid sitting, it sounds funny, but it is good advice," says Dr. Reilly. That is because sitting for more than two hours at a time puts a lot of stress on your spine. If you have to sit a lot to make your living, make an effort to get up and move around every hour or two, he says.

When you do sit down, do it right. A firm chair is always preferred, says Dr. Reilly.

FAVOR FLAT FEET. When you are sitting, try to avoid letting your feet fall on their sides into a V-shape, cautions Dr. Reilly. This foot position—what he calls duck feet—contributes to tight muscles in your back and buttocks. Instead, keep your feet flat on the floor.

BECOME AN "ARCH"-IST. Maintain the arch in your back while you sit, says Dr. Dall. If you slump, the pressure on your disks goes sky-high. Try putting a back support pillow or a rolled-up towel in the small of your back to help with your sitting posture. "I sometimes take a heavy pair of winter gloves and jam them down into the hollow of my back," says Dr. Dall, who suffers from sciatica himself.

GET DOWN AT THE KNEES. Sit on the edge of your chair and lower your knees down below the edge of the seat. This will force you to balance yourself on the chair, which will maintain the arch in your back, says Dr. Dall.

BE CAREFUL IN THE DRIVER'S SEAT. Sitting for more than two hours at a time in the driver's seat can put your spine in a horrible position, especially if you overextend your right leg to step on the gas and the brake, says Dr. Reilly. Many car seats today are constructed so that the sides are higher than the middle of the seat. When you move over to the right to hit the gas and brake pedals, one part of your backside is put higher than the other, and stress on your back can occur, he says. Make a conscious effort to keep your rump in the center of the seat, even if it means repositioning your seat from your favorite setting.

Relieve Yourself of Pain-in-the-Butt Finances

Money can't buy happiness, but it can aggravate your sciatica. Men who stow their wallets in their back pockets and then sit down on their billfolds all day can worsen their pain, says Kevin Reilly, D.C., a certified chiropractic sports physician and owner of Reilly Chiropractic Health and Fitness in Columbus, Ohio. To avoid this problem, he suggests stashing your cash in a money clip in your front pocket or, better yet, carrying your wallet in your coat pocket, shirt pocket, briefcase, or glove compartment.

GIVE YOUR BACK A GOOD NIGHT'S REST. Sleeping on your stomach can irritate your back and sciatic nerve because it really arches your spine, says Dr. Dall. It is best for your back if you sleep in the fetal position—on your side with your hips and knees flexed. Or you can sleep on your back with a pillow under your calves so that your hips and knees are bent.

LIGHTEN YOUR LOAD. Add this to your list of reasons for losing weight: Carrying around a lot of extra pounds will only load down your spine and make you more prone to degenerative changes of the spine associated with sciatica, says Dr. Reilly.

FEED YOUR SPINE. "There is a nutritional side to the nervous system, no doubt about that," says Dr. Reilly. Certain nutrients are essential for a healthy sciatic nerve. If you want to avoid sciatica, make sure that you are getting enough of them, he advises.

The B vitamins help regenerate sciatic nerve tissues, says Dr. Reilly. In addition, antioxidants, such as vitamins C and E, protect against free-radical damage to these tissues—the aging process that occurs at the cellular level. Taking a good multivitamin can ensure that you are getting at least the Daily Value of most vitamins, but don't count on supplements too much, he cautions. Eating lots of produce and other whole foods is still important. Nutrients are plentiful in and usually readily absorbed from whole foods, as are countless bioflavonoids (substances that have been found to help reduce inflammation of nerve tissue).

DON'T LET HIGH HEELS HURT YOU. Don't let style dictate how you treat your back, says Dr. Reilly. High-heeled shoes are always out of style when it comes to sciatica. "You are basically rocking forward in high-heeled shoes on a permanent basis and putting too much pressure on your lower back and pelvis. Supportive footwear is essential to a stress-free sciatic nerve," he says.

That means no heels higher than two inches. You really want to wear a shoe with a low, wide heel, says Dr. Dall.

Platform or lift shoes are probably okay, provided that the heel of the foot is not more than an inch or two higher than the toes, says Dr. Reilly.

SHINSPLINTS
Tread Lightly in Your Workouts

A stronger heart, firmer thighs, a thinner waist—these are common workout goals. Most people trying to get into shape don't give their shins any thought. But when shinsplints show up, their lower legs quickly become a concern.

Shinsplint is a general term for a dull ache that usually occurs in the inner front part of the lower leg, says Richard Simon, M.D., an orthopedic surgeon and sports medicine specialist at the Orthopaedic Center of South Florida in Plantation. The pain is caused by too much pounding of the lower leg. Repeated impact, usually from running, can cause strains in the muscles and tendons. Sometimes, the connective tissue in the lower leg gets inflamed.

Though beginning runners and joggers are most likely to get this overuse injury, you don't have to be a neophyte to get shinsplints. Anybody who does a sport that requires a fair amount of running (such as soccer or tennis) can get them, too, says Mark Veenstra, M.D., an orthopedic surgeon at K-Valley Orthopedics in Kalamazoo, Michigan.

If you have had shinsplints, you know the pain can put you out of commission for a while. To avoid another go-round, get defensive. Here are the top shinsplint-prevention tips.

BE A TORTOISE, NOT A HARE. Many people get shinsplints when they suddenly decide to start working out and try to do too much too soon. If you are just taking up running or tennis, for example, be sure to start slowly. The best approach is to build up your muscle strength little by little. This will help avoid irritating the tissues around your shins. Take your workouts slow and steady, says Dr. Veenstra.

If you are just taking up running, Dr. Veenstra recommends that you start out by walking the distance that you want to eventually run. Next, mix in a few short jogging spurts. Gradually make the jogging time last longer than the walking time, until you are running the whole distance. The entire process should take about a month or so, depending upon how far you set your first distance goal and the kind of shape you are in, he says.

LET TIME HEAL ALL WOUNDS. Exercise is a process of breaking down and building up muscle tissue, says Dr. Simon. To avoid shinsplints, he suggests taking a day off between hard workouts, especially if you are a beginner.

STRETCH TO SHUN SPLINTS. Avoiding tightness in your legs will help you avoid shinsplints, says Dr. Simon. Loosen up before you work out. Warm up your muscles with a short walk or light calisthenics, then do 5 to 10 minutes of stretching before you start running.

To prevent shinsplints, the calves are the most important muscles to stretch, Dr. Simon says. Try this easy preventive stretch.

Face a wall, standing 18 to 24 inches away from it. With your knees straight and your hands resting on the wall at chest level, bend your arms as you let your body weight go into the wall. Keep your heels as flat on the floor as possible. You should feel a stretch in the back of your lower leg. Hold for a count of 10 to 15, and repeat 10 times.

You can also stretch your calves by standing with just the toes and balls of your feet on a bottom step. While holding on to the railing for balance, let your heels drop below the level of the step. Feel the stretch in your calf muscles. Hold for a count of 10 to 15, then raise yourself up again. Repeat the stretch 15 times.

No stretching exercises should ever involve bouncing or sudden movements. They should only cause a pulling sensation, never pain, says Dr. Simon. If you are unsure of how to perform a stretch, ask a physical therapist, doctor, or certified personal trainer to show you.

IF THE SHOE FITS, WEAR IT. Investing in a good pair of athletic shoes is important to avoid shinsplints, says Dr. Veenstra. You will need a comfortable fit and plenty of shock absorption. You should replace old shoes when you can see about a quarter-inch of wear on the inside edge of the heel, he says.

BE SPORT-SPECIFIC WITH YOUR SHOES. Get shoes specifically designed for the kind of exercise you do most often. Don't play tennis in running shoes or go running in tennis shoes, Dr. Veenstra advises.

SEEK OUT A SMART SALESCLERK. Next time you shop for athletic shoes, try to find a salesclerk who seems knowledgeable about the differences between athletic shoes. If you can't get advice that you trust in a store, ask a personal trainer or maybe the high-school athletic trainer for suggestions.

CONSIDER QUALITY. "When it comes to running shoes, you get what you pay for," says Dr. Veenstra. So consider the fit and support before you spring for a shoe with a rock-bottom price. He says that spending about $75 to $100 should get you a good pair.

AVOID SURFACE STRESS. Running on hard roads made of concrete or asphalt is harder on your shins than running on softer surfaces like grass, cushioned tracks, and gravel, says Dr. Veenstra.

Even treadmills are better-cushioned than roadways, says Dr. Simon. If you do have to run on a road, be sure to switch directions now and then. Over time, the slant of the street can encourage shinsplints if one leg is a little higher and the other one is taking most of your weight.

BE SOFT ON YOURSELF. Whether you are a runner or walker, do some other kinds of sports or workouts as well. Swimming is ideal since there is no banging to your lower leg, says Dr. Simon. Riding a bike is good, too. These workouts give you plenty of exercise but will limit the impact on the tendons and soft tissues in your legs.

LIGHTEN YOUR LOAD. Being overweight puts more pressure on the connective tissues around the shins, says Dr. Simon. If you can shed pounds, you are less likely to get shinsplints.

SIDE STITCHES
Stand, Stretch, and Rub

Take the same attention-grabbing pain of a calf cramp and stick it right below your rib cage. That's a side stitch. Experts can't agree precisely on what causes them. Some say that side stitches are caused by cramps in the diaphragm, the sheet of muscles below your lungs that help you breathe. Others say that the cramp is actually in the abdominal muscles. And a few don't believe side stitches are caused by cramps at all. They suggest that side stitches may be caused by intestinal ischemia, reduced blood flow to the intestines during exercise, says Lewis Maharam, M.D., president of the Greater New York Regional Chapter of the American College of Sports Medicine and medical director of the Metropolitan Athletics Congress in New York City. In fact, there may be more than one variety of what we call side stitches.

Luckily, there is much more general agreement about what it takes to prevent the pain. In fact, most people naturally take steps to stop side stitches at the first sign of a twinge. They slow down, breathe deeply, stretch upright, and press in hard where it hurts with their fingers.

Here are some strategies to blunt those stitches before they start stabbing you.

WARM UP. Take time to warm up before your workout. Most side stitches occur within 10 to 15 minutes of beginning exercise. That is especially true if you run hard, which stresses the abdominal muscles. "Warming up properly allows the small blood vessels in your muscles to dilate, providing them with the blood they need to exert themselves," explains Alan Mikesky, Ph.D., director of the Human Performance and Biomechanics Laboratory at Indiana University–Purdue University in Indianapolis. "This benefits every muscle in your body, including the muscles you use to breathe." Take a full 5 to 10 minutes to slowly step up your pace, and consider it time well-spent.

KNOW YOUR STOMACH. A full stomach can cause a side stitch. "Elite athletes have pre-competition eating down to a science," says Stephen Nicholas, M.D., associate director of the Nicholas Institute of Sports Medicine in New York City and team physician for the New York Jets and Islanders. "They know how their bodies react, they know how far ahead of time they need to eat, and they know what to eat," he says.

If you have had a full meal, wait at least 2 1/2 hours before you exercise. "Lighter foods like fruit or a bagel tend to be handled pretty well by the digestive system, so you can eat those close to the time you start exercising," he says. Wait about 1 hour after eating bread, any other carbohydrate, or fruit.

STAY HYDRATED. Muscle spasms of all kinds are more likely if your body runs low on fluids, Dr. Mikesky says. Drink about 2 cups of water 45 minutes or so before you start to exercise. Then drink 1/2 to 1 full cup of water for every 20 minutes during exercise.

DO SOME BELLY BREATHING. "It's the rapid panters—

those breathing in a shallow, staccato fashion—that get into side-stitch trouble," says Dr. Nicholas.

Instead, take long, deep breaths through both your nose and your mouth at the same time to get enough oxygen. If you do that, you won't have to pant. "The best track runners breathe this way, and they focus even more on deep, relaxed breathing to help stop a side stitch," Dr. Nicholas says.

STRETCH IT OUT. If you start to get a side stitch, you can still take measures to stop it. First stand up straight. If that doesn't help, bend so that you are slightly stretching the side with the stitch, Dr. Nicholas says. Still bending over, move around until you find a position that best relieves your pain. That kind of stretching helps put the muscle at rest.

SINUSITIS
Breathe Free and Prevent Pain

Germs are opportunistic troublemakers. There is probably no better proof of this than sinusitis. Bacteria and viruses wait for the normally air-filled nasal cavities in your head to become blocked, then they dig in and run amok. Sinuses may clog due to allergies, an obstruction (such as a polyp or deviated septum), or the common cold—the germs don't really care. If a single sinus is blocked, these invaders seize the opportunity to create a stuffy, painful infection.

Sinusitis results when mucus-blocked sinuses allow infection and inflammation to form, says Edmund Pribitkin, M.D., an otolaryngologist at Thomas Jefferson University Hospital in Philadelphia. As the lining swells, fluids no longer drain out of your sinuses.

With the buildup of pressure, you feel pain in your face, says Jack B. Anon, M.D., chairman of the nasal and sinus committee of the American Academy of Otolaryngology/Head and Neck Surgery and an otolaryngologist in Erie, Pennsylvania.

Another telltale sign is thick, discolored mucus. You may also have a low-grade fever, a cough, or nasal obstruction, says Dr. Pribitkin.

There are actually several different types of sinusitis, says Dr. Pribitkin. Acute sinusitis is a single episode of infection that usually lasts more than 10 days, which is longer than a cold. In contrast, chronic sinusitis lasts for more than three months, although it may not be severe the whole time. Allergic sinusitis is the kind that affects people who have chronic allergies that open the way to sinus infection.

Doctors can successfully treat sinusitis with medications and, in some cases, outpatient surgery. Prescription antibiotics can combat bacteria if they are causing the infections, but there is a downside to the overuse of these drugs. Antibiotic-resistant infections may develop later. So preventing sinusitis in the first place is best, says Dr. Pribitkin. Here is what you can do in the prevention department.

WASH YOUR HANDS EARLY AND OFTEN. Viruses and bacteria can often hitch a ride to your sinuses on your hands. Go all day without washing your hands, and all you have to do to get infected is touch your mouth or nose. So wash your hands with soap and water to prevent transmission, says Richard Mabry, M.D., professor in the department of otorhinolaryngology at the University of Texas Southwestern Medical Center at Dallas. And make a point of washing your hands before you eat.

BE A FUSSY PHONE USER. Use a public phone, and sinusitis germs can ambush you while you wait for the tone, Dr. Mabry warns. If you carry around a travel pack of moist alcohol wipes, you can discreetly rub down the mouthpiece of a public phone. If you borrow office equipment from someone—pens, calculators, or computer keyboards—give them a wipe-off (preferably with a sanitary wipe) before you start using them, he says.

DON'T SHARE OTHER'S FOOD. Don't swap food, utensils, or plates with other people, especially if they might have a cold, says Dr. Pribitkin. That little taste of whatever you are eating isn't worth a trip to the doctor's office for sinusitis treatment.

FIGHT WITH FLUIDS. If you do have a cold, drink at least eight eight-ounce glasses of noncaffeinated, nonalcoholic fluids a day. Your best choice is water. "Hydration is a hallmark of sinus therapy," says Dr. Pribitkin.

"If mucus can get thick, it can clog up sinus openings, and then it is like a cesspool in there," says Dr. Mabry. As long as the liquids are flowing, there is less chance of the infection settling in.

SURRENDER THE SMOKES. Smoking damages tiny hairlike projections in the sinuses called cilia that sweep mucus out, says Dr. Mabry. Without healthy cilia, your sinuses are much more likely to become clogged and infected.

Smoking may also alter sinus secretions in a way that makes them less effective at clearing out the viruses and other particles that you breathe, says Dr. Pribitkin.

Even secondhand smoke can make you more susceptible to sinusitis, says Dr. Mabry. So stay away from other people who smoke.

CONSIDER SOME ZINC. Cold-Eeze cough drops, made with a special zinc compound, may be helpful in fighting viruses when you have a cold, says Dr. Pribitkin. They may also limit the length of a cold.

ATTACK ALLERGY SYMPTOMS. Preventing allergic reactions—and with them, stuffy sinuses and nasal passages—can help prevent inflamed and infected sinuses, says Dr. Pribitkin. Many types of allergy shots and medications are available. Check with your allergist to see what is best for you.

USE THE RIGHT STUFF TO UNSTUFF. If you have an ordinary cold and want to cut your risk of getting sinusitis, try a mucus-thinning decongestant product, says Dr. Mabry. Steer clear of antihistamines, however, which dry up the sinuses and nose, leaving them open to infection. You can use a saline nasal spray, which will rinse the thick mucus from your sinuses but won't cause swelling of the nasal membranes or damage your cilia as some other products can, he says.

Avoid nasal sprays, however, other than the plain saline products because they can become addictive, says Dr. Pribitkin. If your allergies are causing stuffiness, ask your doctor about topical steroid nasal sprays. These sprays can help reduce the swelling around the opening of the sinuses, he says.

GET SHOT. Flu shots can help reduce your risk for sinusitis. "They give your immune system a good kick in the pants," says Dr. Mabry. That way, your body is conquering germs before they can make you sick. Flu shots also help ward off sinusitis by immunizing the body against flu viruses. Ask your doctor about seasonal flu immunization.

Build Your Defenses

If you let your general condition slip, your sinuses will be more vulnerable to infection. Here is how you can power up your resistance.

LOAD UP ON FRUITS AND VEGETABLES. A healthy diet full of nutrient-packed produce will help keep your system sharp. A good multivitamin can fill in gaps in your healthy eating plan, says Dr. Mabry.

A small preliminary study done in the Netherlands indicates that a food compound called glutathione may help in the fight against sinusitis. Found in fruits and vegetables such as watermelon, grapefruit, oranges, peaches, asparagus, potatoes, and broccoli, glutathione may help keep the lining of the respiratory tract healthy. It is far too early to recommend any specific amount of glutathione, says Charles Gross, M.D., professor of otolaryngology and pediatrics at the University of Virginia Health Sciences Center in Charlottesville, but eating a diet rich in fruits and vegetables is a good way to fortify your immune system so that you can better resist infections.

KEEP FIT. Regular exercise increases the blood supply to the sinuses, which can help keep them healthy and open. "Have you ever noticed that as your heart rate goes up, your nose runs, thereby cleaning the nose and sinuses? It is the same principle," says Dr. Gross.

He emphasizes that exercise is a preventive strategy, not a cure. If you have an existing sinus infection, don't go out and run a few miles or work out for an hour. Rest or engage in only light exercise, then once you are over a bout of sinusitis, start a regular exercise plan to help ward off future episodes.

DON'T LET STRESS GET THE BETTER OF YOU. "Fifty years ago, research showed that stress causes the nose to stop up," says Dr. Mabry. Learning better ways to manage stress could help.

A positive attitude, says Dr. Anon, has also been linked to a stronger immune system.

CRANK UP THAT HUMIDIFIER. "I tell people to start using their humidifiers when they turn the heat on in their houses, and not to turn them off until the heat is turned off," says Dr. Mabry. A humidifier or vaporizer in your home or office will help keep your nose and sinuses from drying out. Humidifiers need to be cleaned thoroughly, per the manufacturers' instructions, to keep molds and other allergens from being sprayed into the air. If you have a cold-mist humidifier, you may need to clean it weekly with a solution of 1 part bleach to 10 parts water, he says.

GET INTO THE CLEAN-AIR ACT. "Sinusitis is much more common today than it was a few decades ago. I think it has to do with all the chemicals we have introduced into our environment," says Kenneth F. Garay, M.D., director of

---

No Nose Deserves This

Marriage, overseas investments, and water. These are three things you should never jump into feet first. But only the third has been linked to sinusitis.

"One thing I see here a few times a year are kids who go jump into a pool or lake feet first and drive contaminated water up into their sinuses," says Richard Mabry, M.D., professor in the department of otorhinolaryngology at the University of Texas Southwestern Medical Center at Dallas. The unlucky swimmers get abscesses in their sinuses and a bad case of painful sinusitis.

People are just not aware of the kind of force that drives water into the sinuses in situations like that, he says. Dr. Mabry suggests that you take the cautious approach and wade in, especially if you are not sure how clean the water is.

---

the Center for Sinus and Nasal Disease in New York City. He notes that he sees more and more kids with this problem than he did 15 years ago, and they have more severe cases. Unfortunately, moving to a less-polluted area isn't an option for everyone. If you think that pollution may be irritating your sinuses enough to create a sinusitis risk, spend more time out of doors in the areas that have the cleanest air. If your local weather forecaster gives reports on the air quality, pay attention and try to limit your time out on exceptionally smoggy days.

COVER UP. Chemicals and environmental factors at the workplace can contribute to sinus troubles, according to Dr. Pribitkin. Gypsum dust is a common problem for people who work in construction, for example. People exposed to such impurities may have to wear protective gear over the nose and mouth.

Cold or Sinusitis? Here's How to Tell

If you have sinusitis, you need to see a doctor right away. But how do you know if what you have is a sinus problem or a cold? Well, only a doctor can tell you for sure, but these signs can help you decide how to proceed, says Edmund Pribitkin, M.D., an otolaryngologist at Thomas Jefferson University Hospital in Philadelphia.

SYMPTOM	COLD?	SINUSITIS?
Thin, clear, runny mucus	yes	no
Green or yellow mucus	no	yes
Facial pressure or pain	no	yes
Clears up in 10 days or less	yes	no
Fever	no	yes
Persistent cough in children	no	yes

BREEZE THROUGH. If you suspect that chemicals inside your home or office are irritating the lining in your nose and sinuses, you may want to open the windows regularly and air out the place. Invest in an air purifier, says Dr. Pribitkin, and discuss your concerns with an otolaryngologist.

TAKE CARE OF THOSE PEARLY WHITES. Dental abscesses can result in sinus infections if left untreated, says Dr. Pribitkin. That's just one more reason not to neglect your teeth.

SKIN CANCER
Seek Shade and Do Inspections

What do Sunbelt retirees, Australian construction workers, and bikini-clad beach bunnies the world over have in common? They are more likely to develop skin cancer than librarians from St. Paul or soldiers who man missile silos.

True, genetics plays a role in skin cancer. The fairer your natural complexion, the more easily you burn and the higher your risk. But most often, at the root of skin cancer is simply catching too many rays.

For most of the one million or so people who get skin cancer each year, the condition won't be particularly threatening. The most common types are highly curable basal- and squamous-cell cancers. But another type of skin cancer, melanoma, is far more serious. This type develops in the pigment cells of the skin and can spread through the body. Each year, more than 40,000 Americans will develop melanoma, and 7,300 will die from it.

Of course, we can't live indoors. And we need the joy that comes with being outside. But even as we enjoy the outdoors, we can take easy preventive precautions for ourselves and for our families.

PREVENT YOUR KIDS FROM GETTING SCORCHED. We accumulate nearly 80 percent of our lifetime sun exposure before we graduate from high school, researchers say. And people who develop melanoma often recall having severe sunburn decades earlier during childhood and adolescence, says Arthur J. Sober, M.D., professor of dermatology at Harvard Medical School and associate chief of dermatology at Massachusetts General Hospital, both in Boston.

While you are avoiding sunburns yourself, make sure that the young ones in your family don't overdose on the beach time and playground time in burning sunlight. Babies should be kept out of the sun completely. Experts advise minimizing the sun exposure of children over the age of six months, especially during the hours of 10:00 A.M. and 3:00 P.M., by covering them well and keeping them in the shade as much as possible. If they are going to be out in the sun, apply lots of waterproof sunblock 20 minutes before exposure and reapply every two hours.

PICK THE RIGHT SUNSCREEN. If you are fair-skinned, use a sunscreen with a sun protection factor (SPF) of 30. If you are dark-skinned, SPF 15 may suffice, says David H. McDaniel, M.D., assistant professor of clinical dermatology and plastic surgery at Eastern Virginia Medical School of the Medical College of Hampton Roads in Norfolk and director of the Laser Center of Virginia in Virginia Beach.

Choose a sunscreen that offers protection from both types of harmful ultraviolet rays: UVB and UVA. All sunscreens offer UVB protection, but some don't offer protection from UVA. Look for one that contains one of these ingredients: zinc oxide, titanium dioxide, or Parsol. The container should say that it offers full-spectrum or broad-spectrum UVA protection, Dr. McDaniel says. And choose waterproof sunscreen, he adds. It stays on longer. Examples of sunscreens that contain the recommended ingredients are Basis (zinc oxide), Bull Frog (titanium dioxide), and Ombrelle (Parsol).

MAKE THE SUNSCREEN PART OF YOUR DAILY ROUTINE.
Use sunscreen every day, applying it in the morning to your entire face and the tops of your hands, Dr. McDaniel says. Any other part of your body that may be exposed to the sun should also be covered, including the tip of your nose, your cheeks, the tops of your ears and hands, and exposed scalp.

PUT PROTECTION BEFORE MAKEUP. Put sunscreen on before you put on makeup, says Dr. McDaniel. Apply it after you clean your skin, then leave it on while you brush your teeth and comb your hair. This will give the sunscreen a few minutes to absorb before the makeup goes on the skin.

DON'T BE STINGY. Most people apply far too little sunscreen, Dr. McDaniel says. Apply it liberally and uniformly, and let it settle in for a while before you go out into the sun and start sweating.

COVER YOUR LIPS, TOO. Lips require extra sun protection because they have less melanin, the specialized pigment that is the skin's natural defense against the sun. The lower lip, especially, is a common site of squamous-cell cancer, and cancer at this site has about a 20 percent chance of spreading to other parts of your body. So apply sunscreen to your lips when you do the rest of your face, advises Dr. McDaniel. Or use a sunscreen lip balm with an SPF of at least 15, such as Banana Boat and Chap Stick. Carry one with you to reapply throughout the day.

DON A SOMBRERO. Every inch of brim trims your facial skin-cancer risk by 10 percent, says Darrell Rigel, M.D., clinical professor of dermatology at the New York University School of Medicine in New York City. Wear a hat with a wide four-inch brim all the way around, and you will reduce the risk of developing skin cancer on your face by 40 percent.

WEAR MORE THAN A WET T-SHIRT. Once a shirt is wet, its ability to block the sun is dramatically reduced, Dr. McDaniel says. And the looser the weave of a fabric, the less sun-blocking power it has. If you are going to be outdoors, you need a dry, loose-fitting, tightly woven shirt to cover your arms and shoulders, not just a wet T-shirt.

TAKE VITAMIN E. There is some scientific evidence that taking the natural form of vitamin E can decrease the damage done by the sun to the skin, says Karen Burke, M.D., Ph.D., a dermatologist in private practice in New York City. So it may help prevent the conditions that could lead to skin cancer. She recommends a vitamin E supplement of 400 IU (international units) a day as a dose that may help with protection. Be sure to get the natural form of the vitamin—it should say so on the label and will contain d- (not dl-) alpha tocopherol, or d-alpha tocopheryl acetate or succinate, says Dr. Burke. But if you are considering taking amounts above 200 IU, discuss this with your doctor first.

APPLY VITAMIN C TO YOUR SKIN. Vitamin C acts as a free-radical-neutralizing antioxidant, but you need to apply it topically, says Sheldon Pinnell, M.D., the J. Lamar Callaway professor of dermatology at Duke University Medical Center in Durham, North Carolina. Ascorbic acid is the only form of vitamin C that the body can use, and to be effective, it must be formulated properly, he says. It is found in several products, including SkinCeuticals Topical Vitamin C High Potency Serum 15. These products are available without prescription from dermatologists, plastic surgeons, and licensed skin-care professionals, according to Dr. Pinnell.

"Vitamin C can't block the sun, but it can help reduce damage from the rays that do get through your sunscreen," Dr. Pinnell explains. It also helps to reduce the weakening of the skin's immune system from overexposure to the sun, a problem that has been found in more than 90 percent of people who get skin cancer.

After you apply the topical vitamin C product, allow it to dry briefly. Then proceed with your skin-care regimen. Be sure to apply a sunscreen that blocks UVA and UVB rays, says Dr. Pinnell.

SLEEP APNEA
Prepare for Better Bedtime Breathing

Sleep is nature's restorer. When everything is working right, we snooze and rest, breathing easily in and out, getting ready for more tomorrow. But sleep apnea destroys our nocturnal tranquillity. If you have it, you actually stop breathing while you are sleeping, and you wake up gasping for air. In the most severe cases of sleep apnea, this happens dozens, even hundreds, of times in the course of a night. Sleep apnea can be tricky because sometimes you are not even aware that you awakened.

Sleep apnea is caused by the dramatic narrowing of air passageways. As your air passages constrict, the air flow slows down. That is when tissues rattle in the breeze, and snoring results. And when your air passages get narrowed *a lot*, oxygen can't get through. Your brain shouts, "Hey, wake up!"

There are several factors that cause the narrowing of the throat. Fat is the leading cause. People who are overweight may have too much tissue in the airway, narrowing it and making it difficult to breathe properly. Alcohol and sleeping pills as well make breathing pauses more frequent—and those pauses are more prolonged in people with sleep apnea.

Sleep apnea itself doesn't pose any immediate threats to your health. But the leading consequence of it—fatigue—puts you at higher risk for plenty of bad things. People who have sleep apnea are about twice as likely to have car accidents as people who sleep through the night. Furthermore, people who are constantly tired are not usually the most effective employees or the most understanding spouses and parents. Indirectly, sleep apnea, left untreated, can get you fired, divorced, or alienated from your kids. Right there, you have reasons enough to prevent it.

But there are even more reasons. Over the long haul, sleep apnea can put you in physical danger, too. If your body isn't getting the oxygen it needs, all of your tissues and organs suffer, and your heart works harder than it should.

Sleep apnea has been associated with high blood pressure, heart disease, and stroke, according to James Rowley, M.D., assistant professor of medicine at Wayne State University School of Medicine and medical director of the Harper Hospital Sleep Disorders Center, both in Detroit. Obviously, these aren't conditions that you can treat lightly, so if you have sleep apnea, be sure to seek treatment. To prevent apnea, most doctors will prescribe the use of a device named CPAP (Continuous Positive Airway Pressure). This machine, featuring a compressor and a specially designed nose mask, pumps air into your nose and throat. The continuous stream of air holds open the passageway.

In some cases, doctors may recommend surgical procedures that ensure an open airway. But, of course, you don't want to go that far to treat apnea if you can possibly avoid it other ways. Here are some tips to help you get a restorative night's sleep.

DO SOME SLIMMING. The heavier you are, the more likely you are to get sleep apnea, says Barbara Phillips, M.D., medical director of the Samaritan Hospital Sleep Apnea Center and director of the University of Kentucky Sleep Clinic, both in Lexington. Not only do airways become more narrow because of fatty tissues but all that stop-and-go night breathing is more taxing on your heart if you have excess fat.

"The single most important risk factor for sleep apnea is obesity," says Dr. Phillips. In fact, neck circumference is the best indicator that sleep specialists have in predicting the condition, she says, since that is one telltale area where fat accumulates. She says that if you can get down to your ideal weight, you may reduce the chances of developing sleep apnea.

CRUSH THE PUFFING HABIT. Research has shown that smoking is linked to sleep apnea, says Dr. Phillips. Smoking can cause swelling of the tissues in the back of the throat and mouth as well as an increase in mucus production. These effects shrink the size of your airway, making an excellent sleep-apnea environment, she says. If you quit smoking (or better yet, never start), you will reduce your risk for sleep apnea.

SAY NAY TO NIGHTCAPS. Alcohol makes your throat tissues so relaxed that they tend to sag and don't keep your airway wide open when you sleep, says Dr. Rowley. To help prevent bouts of mild sleep apnea, he recommends not having any alcoholic beverages for at least four hours before you go to bed.

SLEEP ON YOUR SIDE. People who sleep on their backs have an increased risk for both snoring and sleep apnea, says Dr. Phillips. When you lie face-up, your tongue falls back, which can block your airway. Sleep on your side instead, she says.

WATCH YOUR BLOOD PRESSURE. Just like the great chicken-or-the-egg debate, researchers aren't sure which comes first, high blood pressure or sleep apnea. They only

Don't Ignore a Snore

You may not think that snoring is a big deal, and it may not be. But persistent snorers need to be checked for sleep apnea, says James Rowley, M.D., assistant professor of medicine at Wayne State University School of Medicine and medical director of the Harper Hospital Sleep Disorders Center, both in Detroit.

If you don't have a bedmate to tell you details about your snoring, you will have to take notes on your own, says Barbara Phillips, M.D., medical director of the Samaritan Hospital Sleep Apnea Center and director of the University of Kentucky Sleep Clinic, both in Lexington. You can do this by putting a tape recorder next to your bed. Set the timer on the recorder so that it will turn on during the wee hours of the morning, preferably about two hours before you normally wake up. That is when your sleep is the deepest—and when your snores are most likely to be sounding like a rhino's mating call.

If you suspect that you have sleep apnea, you will need to see a doctor about it. Here are some signs to look for, according to Dr. Rowley.

- Snoring is loud, frequent, and irregular sounding
- Snoring keeps others awake, even people in other rooms
- There are pauses in snoring that sound as if you have stopped breathing
- You wake from sleep with a gasping or choking sensation
- You wake up nonrefreshed or with a headache
- You are exceedingly sleepy during the day—and doze off in highly inappropriate and even dangerous situations, such as at your desk right after lunch or behind the wheel while waiting for a red light

A Dickens of a Problem

Sleep apnea isn't a new discovery. Severe sleep apnea was recorded as far back as Charles Dickens's *Pickwick Papers*. In one of the Dickensian tales, a red-faced, fat boy snores while he sleeps, and he is constantly drowsy while awake. No wonder the most extreme form of sleep apnea is called pickwickian syndrome. It refers to cases where people, usually obese, have trouble breathing in their slumber and while awake. They are also exceedingly sleepy all the time and have signs of heart failure such as swelling at the ankles.

know that when you have one condition, you stand a greater chance of having the other. Dr. Phillips suggests that anyone who is concerned about sleep apnea should check their blood pressure regularly. Since high blood pressure is also a risk factor for stroke and heart disease, lowering high blood pressure levels, regardless of whether you have sleep apnea or not, is a smart move, she says.

SMELL AND TASTE LOSS
Steps for Keeping Those Senses Sharp

The smell of spring flowers. The taste of fresh-baked cookies. What if these basic pleasures were muted or cut off completely? Life would sure be less exciting.

Some loss of our smell skills is common with age, says Richard L. Doty, Ph.D., professor in the department of otorhinolaryngology/head and neck surgery and director of the Smell and Taste Center at the University of Pennsylvania School of Medicine in Philadelphia. In fact, half of all people over the age of 65 have some reduced olfactory function, and 75 percent of people over 80 have a major loss of smell.

But other factors besides age can dull the sense of smell. If you have chronic nasal and sinus infections, the tissues that line your nose get damaged by repeated inflammation, and a sweet-smelling rose may begin to seem blah to your damaged senses. Occasionally, a head trauma can cause smell loss by cutting off or damaging some of the olfactory nerves that send messages to the brain.

True taste loss is much less common. On occasion, a middle-ear infection left untreated can result in decreased taste sensation or even phantom tastes. But what most people experience when they say that they have taste loss is actually diminished flavor distinction, caused, at least in part, by the loss of smell. These people can distinguish salty from sweet, but not sugar from honey, for example.

Of course, these losses don't happen all at once, and you may wonder whether you need to take any steps at all to prevent the demise of taste or smell. As an early warning signal, you can actually test yourself.

Dr. Doty developed the University of Pennsylvania Smell Identification Test (UPSIT), a scratch-and-sniff test to help to determine if patients are suffering from smell and flavor loss and to what degree. You can get more information on ordering a modified 12-item version of this test, called the CC-SIT, by writing to Sensonics, 125 Whitehorse Pike, Haddon Heights, NJ 08035.

Sound too complicated? Then try this simple at-home test suggested by Alan R. Hirsch, M.D., neurological director at the Smell and Taste Treatment and Research Foundation in Chicago. Cover your eyes and have someone wave two different fragrant foods under your nose, such as a slice of hot pizza and a piece of chocolate cake. Does your nose know the difference? If you want to test your flavor perception, cover your eyes again and have someone give you a taste each of chocolate and vanilla ice cream. Can you tell them apart?

Diminished smell and taste sensations aren't a big threat to your physical well-being. They can, however, put you at greater risk from gas leaks, smoke, poisonous fumes, or spoiled foods, which you may not be able to detect. But the real downside of smell and taste loss is in the quality of life. If you can't smell autumn in the air or taste pesto sauce on your linguine, life isn't all it should be. Here are tips to prevent the erosion of your senses.

NIX THE SMOKES. Smoking damages the tissues that are responsible for taste and smell functions. "It is well-documented that smokers have lower sensitivity to both taste and smell," says David V. Smith, Ph.D., professor and vice chairman of the department of anatomy and neurobiology at the University of Maryland School of Medicine in Baltimore. So add sensory deprivation to the list of reasons not to smoke.

Once you stop smoking, you can regain some of the sensual acuity that you have lost. How long that takes, however, is usually related to how long and how much a person smoked prior to quitting.

STEER CLEAR OF GERMS. Getting a lot of colds, bouts of the flu, and sinus or nasal infections—over years—can also be a factor in smell loss, says Dr. Doty. The repeated germ assaults on the olfactory tissues in your nose can compromise them.

Keep your hands clean and avoid close contact with sick people, says Dr. Hirsch. It isn't always possible to stay the recommended 10 feet away, but be aware of distance when exposed to cold-inflicted people. If you know that you're being exposed to germs, wash your hands often, he says.

AVOID ALLERGENS. If you must dust, for example, wear a mask or bandanna over your nose and mouth when roundin' up those fuzzy tumbleweeds under the bed, says Dr. Hirsch. Anything that causes your mucous membranes to swell puts you at an increased risk for colds, flu, or sinus infections.

DON'T BRING HOME THAT DOGGIE IN THE WINDOW. If you know that you have allergies, before falling for a pet, consider the long-term olfactory doom it can impose. If you already have sneeze-inducing furry friends, symptoms can be minimized by rubbing Fido or Fifi down with Allerpet by Farnam, Dr. Hirsch suggests. This product is available at many pet stores and works by reducing the dog's or cat's dander.

Can Estrogen Help You Smell the Coffee?

For postmenopausal women considering hormone-replacement therapy, researchers have sniffed out one side benefit that comes as a surprise. The hormone estrogen seems to help maintain the olfactory membranes in older women.

In a study of more than 750 postmenopausal women who reported smell loss, the women taking estrogen showed significantly more smell function than women who didn't take it, according to Richard L. Doty, Ph.D., professor in the department of otorhinolaryngology/head and neck surgery and director of the Smell and Taste Center at the University of Pennsylvania School of Medicine in Philadelphia.

GET IMMUNE POWER. The U.S. Department of Agriculture Food Guide Pyramid's recommended three to five daily servings of vegetables and two to four daily servings of fruit is nothing to sneeze at. A good healthful diet that is heavy on the fresh fruits and vegetables goes a long way toward boosting your immune system and helping your body resist infections. Fewer infections keep your sniffer in shape, reminds Dr. Hirsch.

A number of plant foods contain substances called flavonoids, which can help prevent germs from taking hold, adds Joseph V. Formics, Ph.D., professor of microbiology at Virginia Commonwealth University, Medical College of Virginia School of Medicine in Richmond. Flavonoid-rich foods include apples, tomatoes, tea, onions, and kale.

BRING IN REINFORCEMENTS. While the right foods can steer your immune system in the right direction, it also helps to have some extra supplements. Vitamin A helps strengthen your body's defenses, while vitamin C helps the immune system go on the attack. This two-pronged approach provides powerful protection against incoming germs.

Researchers aren't sure how much of these vitamins you need to maximize immunity. For vitamin A, the Daily Value of 5,000 IU (international units) is probably enough. For vitamin C, you should probably try to get more than the Daily Value of 60 milligrams, especially when you are sick, says Frances Tysus, a registered dietitian and consultant to the Cleveland Clinic Foundation.

TRY TO HEAL QUICKLY. Treating chronic sinusitis promptly and aggressively is important if you want to protect your sense of smell, says David Kennedy, M.D., professor and chairman of the department of otorhinolaryngology/head and neck surgery at the University of Pennsylvania School of Medicine in Philadelphia. So be sure to take steps to prevent sinusitis.

WATCH OUT WHERE YOU WORK. While the research at this point is only suggestive, long-term exposure to environmental chemical irritants is believed by experts to be hazardous to your olfactory membranes. Dr. Doty and his colleagues observed smell loss in workers in a plastics manufacturing plant who were exposed to industrial chemicals throughout their careers.

If your job puts you in contact with pesticides, manufacturing chemicals, or other questionable materials, try to limit your direct exposure, says Dr. Kennedy. Wearing a respirator or other government-recommended safety gear should be part of your employer's policy.

TAKE TIME TO SMELL THE ROSES. Stopping for a moment every now and then to deliberately smell things around you can help improve your olfactory acuity, says Dr. Hirsch. Just like your muscles and your mind, your olfactory membranes need a workout in order to stay sharp. So take a moment to bend over and sniff the flowers in your yard. Savor the scent of that cup of herbal tea or that pile of freshly washed laundry. It doesn't matter what you get a whiff of, just so long as you use your olfactory senses.

BUCKLE UP. Traumatic head injuries can result in permanent smell loss, so make sure that you wear your seat belt every time you are in the car. Because the nerve membranes that are responsible for smell run through the bones in your nose, they can easily be damaged or severed if you hit your head very hard. "Head trauma is the number one cause of smell loss, after you factor out aging," says Dr. Hirsch.

DON A HELMET. Besides car accidents, other head injuries can also result in a loss of smell and flavor sensation. Wear a helmet while you ride a bike or motorcycle or go inline skating, says Dr. Hirsch.

SNORING
Ward Off Nighttime Noise

Here are the three great unanswerable questions of our time: What was the purpose of Stonehenge? Did Oswald act alone? Why does a snorer only wake his wife up and never himself?

Though science still isn't sure how a person can rattle the rafters and keep right on snoozing, the cause of snoring is clearly understood.

When your air passageways constrict, the air flowing through them picks up speed, just the way a lazy river turns into whitewater when the riverbed narrows. The faster the air, the more turbulence. Greater turbulence vibrates the soft tissues in your throat—especially the back of your palate and your uvula, the thing that hangs down in the back of your mouth. Snoring is the sound of those tissues flapping in the accelerated breeze, says Hector P. Rodriguez, M.D., assistant professor of clinical otolaryngology/head and neck surgery at the Columbia University College of Physicians and Surgeons and director of the division of rhinology at Columbia-Presbyterian Medical Center, both in New York City.

The snoring-prevention secret is keeping those airways as wide open as possible. Here are some steps toward silent nights.

LIGHTEN UP. Your typical snorer is overweight. Carrying around a lot of excess pounds can mean that the person has fatty throat tissues, thus a smaller airway, says Barbara Phillips, M.D., medical director of the Samaritan Hospital Sleep Apnea Center and director of the University of Kentucky Sleep Clinic, both in Lexington. "The vast majority of patients who are willing to lose excess weight find that it helps," she says. Sometimes losing as little as 10 to 15 pounds can make a difference.

DON'T LIGHT UP. Smoking narrows air passages in two ways: by making the tissues swell and by increasing mucus production. Smoking is often connected to snoring, says Dr. Phillips.

DON'T DRINK AND DOZE. Since alcohol relaxes the muscles in your airway, it makes them loose enough to vibrate and causes them to be floppy, partially closing off the opening, says James Rowley, M.D., assistant professor of medicine at Wayne State University School of Medicine and medical director of the Harper Hospital Sleep Disorders Center, both in Detroit. Avoid alcoholic beverages for at least four hours before you go to bed.

STEER CLEAR OF SEDATIVES. Sleeping pills and diazepam (Valium) relax your muscles and slacken tissues in the back of the throat, says Dr. Phillips. Don't use sedatives if you can help it, and you will be less inclined to snore through the night.

GET OFF YOUR BACK. People who sleep on their backs are more likely to snore than those who don't, says Dr. Rowley. When you are on your back, your tongue falls toward your throat, and your airway can be partially blocked.

Try changing positions so that you sleep on your side

or stomach instead, says Dr. Phillips. To ensure that you stay that way, you can literally train yourself with the help of a tennis ball and a T-shirt with a vest pocket. Just put the tennis ball in the pocket and put the shirt on backward before you go to bed. If you roll over onto your back, the discomfort of the tennis ball will wake you up, and you will automatically seek a more comfortable position on your stomach or side.

DON'T GO SHORT ON SLEEP. Sleep deprivation makes snoring worse, says Dr. Rowley. Going to bed overly tired—either from lack of quality sleep or from too much physical activity—can cause snoring. If your airway muscles are tired, they will loosen up and vibrate.

EAT EARLY OR LIGHT. Heavy meals right before you go to sleep can contribute to snoring, says Dr. Rodriguez. Try not to eat anything in the hour before you hit the sack. If you have to eat a late dinner, at least make it a light one— like soup and a sandwich.

RAISE YOUR HEAD. Dr. Phillips says that if you are experiencing nose congestion, sleeping with your head elevated slightly higher than your feet may help prevent the obnoxious night noises. "Two or three pillows might do the trick. In some cases, sleeping in a fully opened recliner works as a temporary snore deterrent," she says.

JOIN THE NFL. Ever notice those adhesive-bandage-like strips that football players wear across the tops of their noses? The theory is that they open nasal passages and let the athletes get more air, which helps them pulverize their opponents more effectively. They may help prevent snoring, too, says Dr. Phillips. Marketed under brand names such as Nozovent and Breathe Right, these nasal strips have been proven effective for some people who have snoring problems.

UNPLUG THAT PROBOSCIS. Allergies and colds can clog up your nasal passages, forcing you to breathe through your mouth when you sleep. People with stuffed noses often snore. Steroidal nasal inhalers (like Rhinocort or Nasacort) and other fast-acting prescription allergy treatments can help, says Dr. Rowley. If you are allergy-prone, ask your doctor about sinus-clearing medications that might help. Taken an hour or so before bed, fast-acting medications can usually help you sleep quietly.

CHECK WITH YOUR DOCTOR FOR RISK OF APNEA. If you have tried everything and you are still snoring loudly and persistently enough to send your partner packing, you might have sleep apnea. With this condition, the amount of oxygen you take in decreases because your airway gets too narrow, says Dr. Phillips. Here are some signs that it is time to call your doctor.

- Your snoring is loud and frequent, sounds irregular, and keeps other people awake.
- Your partner hears pauses in your snoring that sound as if you are not breathing.
- When you awaken, you often have a headache and don't feel refreshed.
- You are sleepy during the day and catch yourself dozing.

SORE THROAT
Keep a Happy Swallow

Don't take sore throats lightly. The father of our country did, and his indifference may have cost him his life. George Washington had a sore throat before he died, which was caused by complications from an infected oral abscess. Had he paid closer attention to his throat, it might have altered the course of history.

Some sore throats are caused by physical irritants. But usually scratchy throats are the result of upper respiratory infections and postnasal drip. Any nasal airway blockage—such as that caused by allergies—can lead to throat pain because the detour of breath from nose to mouth creates an irritated, dry climate inside your throat. "Your nose is designed to humidify, filter, and warm the air as you breathe in," says Deborah Loney, M.D., an otolaryngologist in private practice in Sterling, Virginia. "But your mouth can't do any of this as effectively."

Once you have a sore throat, drinking warm liquids and using over-the-counter throat sprays and lozenges can

Work toward a Reflux Reduction

Sometimes a sore throat can be caused by gastroesophageal reflux disease (GERD), a condition where stomach contents, including the acid, splashes back up into the throat, says Sanford Archer, M.D., associate professor of otolaryngology/head and neck surgery at the University of Kentucky College of Medicine in Lexington. Caffeine, smoking, alcohol, and greasy or spicy foods can all aggravate the condition.

One way to prevent the backlash is to avoid eating anything one to two hours before you go to bed. When you do have a flare-up, liquid antacids work better than chewable ones, says Dr. Archer. Over-the-counter antacids contain about half the strength of their prescription cousins, he adds.

If reflux in bed is a problem, Dr. Archer recommends propping up the head of your bed about six inches by placing two cinder blocks under the legs at the headboard. This will keep stomach acid where it belongs. While you might expect a bunch of pillows to do the trick, Dr. Archer says that you need your whole bed raised. Pillows only raise up your head, without changing the angle from stomach to throat.

GERD can be a sign of a greater problem, such as esophageal precancerous condition (Barrett's esophagus) or a peptic ulcer, says Walter J. Hogan, M.D., professor of medicine and radiology in the division of gastroenterology and radiology at the Medical College of Wisconsin in Milwaukee. Continued acid-reflux problems can also erode your tooth enamel, he says. If you have several sore throats a year that may be accompanied by heartburn, hoarseness, or regurgitation (a bad taste in the mouth), contact your physician.

help lessen the pain, says Sanford Archer, M.D., associate professor of otolaryngology/head and neck surgery at the University of Kentucky College of Medicine in Lexington. You may also want to try gargling gently with a tall glass of water, a pinch of salt, plus a pinch of baking soda. Sucking on ice cubes or frozen fruit-juice pops can also help numb the sore tissues.

But, of course, the best treatment is prevention. Better to thwart sore throats before they get started. Here are some tips for keeping the nasal passageways nice and clear so that your nose can do the work it was meant to do—moistening and warming the air.

GAIN CONTROL OF YOUR ALLERGIES. You and your doctor should determine what medications work best to control the postnasal drip caused by your allergies, says Dr. Archer. If they are seasonal allergies brought on by pollen, maybe you just need to stay indoors with the air-conditioning on when the offensive pollen is really bad.

BE BOLD WITH MOLDS. If you are sensitive to molds, installing allergy air filters on your furnace can help, provided they are cleaned regularly, says Dr. Archer. To help halt creeping versions of mold, repair all doorways and windowsills that leak water. And run a dehumidifier in moist places, such as the basement and any crawl spaces, he suggests. To prevent mold growth within the dehumidifier, remember to empty it frequently.

DO AWAY WITH DUST. People who are allergic to dust mites are in for a tough battle at home. Steam-cleaning your carpets and furniture every three months or so will reduce the dust collection. Get allergy covers for your mattress and pillows, says Dr. Archer, and use the hot-water setting when you launder your sheets and pillowcases. Wearing slippers around the house instead of going barefoot also helps since dust mites live off the skin scales that your feet shed.

TUMBLE DRY YOUR TEDDY BEARS. Stuffed animals can accumulate a lot of dust, too. Provided they don't have a lot of plastic parts, you can put yours in the dryer with the temperature set low for 20 minutes, says Dr. Archer. No need to wash—it is the heat that kills the dust mites.

WASH YOUR PETS. If you are allergic to dog or cat dander, you probably don't have to get rid of the family pet to prevent sore throats. "Washing your pet with shampoo and warm water twice a month will substantially reduce the amount of dander," says Dr. Archer.

TREAT YOUR TOOTHBRUSH. If you share a bathroom with somebody who has a viral or bacterial infection, don't let them use your toothbrush, says Dr. Archer. It is an easy way to share the germs that can cause a sore throat. If all the family toothbrushes shack up in a communal holder, protect yourself by soaking your brush in some Listerine to kill the germs, he says. And be sure to throw out old, ratty toothbrushes as soon as they turn into has-beens (every three to six months, or as soon as the bristles begin to bend outward). If you keep them around, they can become breeding grounds for germs.

GET STEAMED UP. If you feel a scratchy throat coming on, try running hot water in the bathroom sink while you lean over it with a towel draped on top of your head, says Dr. Loney. Then inhale deeply through your mouth. Do this for five minutes and repeat the procedure a few times a day to help humidify your throat.

CRANK UP THE HUMIDIFIER. When your home heating system is on, it is possible for you to wake up in the morning with a sore throat, especially if you tend to breathe through your mouth when you sleep. Use a cool-mist humidifier in the living areas and bedrooms to help make the air inside your home less dry, says Dr. Loney. Just be sure that you clean it frequently since it can begin to harbor mold and create an irritating environment if you don't follow the cleaning directions on the humidifier.

WASH DOWN TROUBLE. Mucus can be fairly thick and irritating in the back of the throat, says Dr. Archer. Drinking a lot of fluids, preferably water, will help thin the mucus out and make it less abrasive. Eight to 10 eight-ounce glasses a day will do the trick, he says. But keep away from caffeine-containing drinks since they are diuretics that can actually cause you to lose more fluid and worsen your mucous problem.

CLEAN UP YOUR ACT. "Germs get passed around on people's hands easily," says Dr. Loney. Wash your hands frequently, especially before meals, to reduce the risk of getting an infected throat.

TAKE A MULTI, AND MAYBE MORE C. "A good, balanced vitamin and mineral supplement is a healthy thing to take daily," says Dr. Archer. Some studies have indicated that you may reduce the chance of infection if you take 500 milligrams of vitamin C at regular intervals four times a day. "It can't hurt you at that dosage since vitamin C that isn't used by the body gets excreted through your urine," he says. "So if someone were constantly battling colds and wanted to try it, I'd say go ahead." Be aware that excess vitamin C may cause diarrhea in some people.

COME IN OUT OF THE COLD. Cold winter air may not feel like the desert, but it is just as dry as an Arizona mesa. And when air is that dry, it parches your throat. In a humid, warm climate, you reduce your chance of getting a sore throat, notes Dr. Archer. If you live where winters are cold and dry, "at least try to limit the amount of cold air you expose your throat to," he says. Wrapping a scarf around your mouth when the temperature plummets may help.

STOMACHACHE
Take Care of Your Belly

The company party roars on into the night. With an open bar, appetizers, filet mignon for dinner, and chocolate cheesecake for dessert, you know that you are overdoing it, but frankly, you don't care.

If prevention were your primary concern, you could stop potential tummy trouble right there—"No more, thank you!" But often, a turbulent tummy seems like a small price to pay for such good eats. So you go on, knowing better all along.

But not all stomachaches can be prevented with mere culinary self-control. "Many things fall into the category of stomachache," says Geoffrey C. Lamb, M.D., associate professor of internal medicine at the Medical College of Wisconsin in Milwaukee. In fact, what we usually describe as stomach pain may have little or nothing to do with the stomach.

According to Dr. Lamb, stomach pain could be coming from a number of places in the abdominal region, including the stomach, liver, gallbladder, pancreas, and intestines. Symptoms range from a dull ache to full-blown cramps to a burning, acidy pain. Common culprits include indigestion, heartburn, lactose intolerance, gallstones, stress, ulcers, irritable bowel syndrome, and overeating. So when you want to prevent recurrent stomachache, get a checkup from your doctor. But if you are just trying to avoid the most common causes of stomach turmoil, here are some prevention tips.

ALLAY THE ACID. H_2-blockers (histamine-blockers), such as Tagamet HB 200, Zantac 75, or Pepcid AC, suppress acid at its source and prevent it from irritating the lining of the stomach. Use them to prevent an acid stomach if you know that you are going to be eating foods that have caused you heartburn in the past, particularly rich, spicy, or fatty foods, suggests Dr. Lamb. Follow label directions for recommended dosages.

DITCH THE DAIRY. If drinking milk or eating ice cream seems to fuel your intestinal distress, you could be lactose intolerant. That means your body isn't producing enough of the lactase enzyme to break down lactose, the sugar found in milk and other dairy products.

Most adult Blacks, Asians, Native Americans, and some Whites have difficulty digesting milk because they have little or no lactase. To discover whether lactose intolerance is causing your discomfort, eliminate all dairy products from your diet. Wait three days, then add an eight-ounce glass of nonfat milk to your diet. If you can safely drink that glass of milk every day without any adverse reaction, it is all right to slowly reintroduce other dairy products such as nonfat yogurt and cheese, adding a new food every few days. If discomfort returns, you may have found your problem, says Dr. Lamb.

Relief is available in the form of dietary supplements that make dairy foods more digestible such as Lactaid and Dairy Ease. Lactaid also makes milk that has been pretreated with the lactase enzyme. It is available in most major grocery stores in the dairy section.

SAY GOODBYE TO CHOCOLATE. Eating chocolate can cause heartburn, especially when it follows a big meal, says Dr. Lamb. That is because chocolate relaxes the valve connecting the esophagus to the stomach. When the valve loosens, acid splashes up into the esophagus, causing heartburn.

GO EASY ON THE PAIN RELIEVERS. Aspirin, ibuprofen, and other nonsteroidal anti-inflammatory drugs (NSAIDs) can irritate the stomach lining and break down its protective mucous layer, causing discomfort, says Dr. Lamb. In the long term, overuse can lead to ulcers or kidney problems.

"An aspirin a day to prevent strokes or heart attacks is safe and remains a good idea. A few people, however, will have irritation with just a few doses," he says.

TAKE A YOGA CLASS. Is your stomach in turmoil over something that happened at the office? Yoga offers one solution for preventing stomachaches and other symptoms of stress "because it puts us in close touch with our bodies and our minds and warns us when stress is looming," says Richard Miller, Ph.D., a clinical psychologist in San Rafael, California, and co-founder of the International Association of Yoga Therapists, based in Mill Valley, California. Because of this early warning, we can intervene with breathing, meditation, massage, and other relaxation strategies. Many yoga classes are offered through adult night-school classes, at fitness centers, and through organizations such as the YM/YWCA.

STOMACH CANCER
Eat Smart to Stay Cancer-Free

Today, stomach cancer is one-fourth as common as it was in 1930. In the United States, it ranks seventh behind lung, breast, colon, and other cancers (although it remains a leading cause of cancer death worldwide).

Why the dramatic turnaround? One reason is the widespread use of refrigeration, which has improved our diets by making fresh fruits and vegetables available to more people year-round, says Pelayo Correa, M.D., professor of pathology at Louisiana State University in New Orleans. Americans are also eating less salted and smoked foods, which have been found to be risk factors for stomach cancer.

Improved sanitation also may have played a role in stomach cancer's decline. The *Helicobacter pylori* bacteria can spread from person to person when conditions are crowded and unsanitary. Since *H. pylori* is one of the major risk factors for developing certain kinds of stomach cancer, the disease has become less prevalent as sanitary conditions have improved in countries like the United States.

Can Meat Cause Stomach Cancer?

Nothing signals summer like the annual firing up of the barbecue. But could this backyard ritual be hazardous to your health? In a study conducted by the National Cancer Institute's Division of Cancer Epidemiology and Genetics, researchers found a link between individuals with stomach cancer and the consumption of meats that were cooked at high temperatures. They discovered that those who ate their beef medium-well or well-done had more than three times the risk of stomach cancer than those who opted for rare or medium-rare. They also found that people who ate beef four or more times a week had more than twice the risk of stomach cancer than those eating it less often.

One culprit may be heterocyclic amines (HCAs), which are carcinogenic chemicals formed from the cooking of muscle meats such as beef, pork, fowl, and fish. HCAs form when amino acids and creatine react at high cooking

Although stomach cancer has declined overall, one particular type of stomach cancer, cardia stomach cancer, has been increasing at an alarming rate. Cardia stomach cancer occurs in the part of the stomach next to the esophagus.

"Over the last 10 to 15 years, epidemiology researchers at the National Cancer Institute have noted a significant increase in stomach cancers that appear in the upper portion of the stomach," says Richard Alexander, M.D., head of the surgical metabolism section, surgery branch, at the National Cancer Institute.

Researchers are stumped as to why cardia stomach cancer is on the rise. But they do know that it appears most often in overweight white men from the middle and upper-middle classes.

Here are some preventive tips to cut your risk of cardia stomach cancer as well as the other kinds of stomach cancer.

temperatures. Frying, broiling, and barbecuing produce the largest amounts of HCAs because the meats are cooked at very high temperatures. Oven roasting and baking, which are done at lower temperatures, create lower levels of HCAs. Stewing, boiling, and poaching meats create only negligible amounts.

Eating undercooked meats can be hazardous to your health as well, as evidenced by recent breakouts of *E. coli* and other infectious bacteria. So what's a person to do? The National Cancer Institute suggests partially cooking meats in the microwave before you fry, broil, or barbecue. Meats that were microwaved for two minutes prior to cooking had a 90 percent decrease in HCA content. You will lose even more HCA if you pour off the liquid that forms during microwaving.

Finally, don't make gravy from meat drippings. The researchers found that gravy made this way contains a hefty amount of HCAs.

PREEMPT WITH A TEST. If you have a family history of stomach cancer, consider getting tested for *H. pylori*, says Julie Parsonnet, Ph.D., associate professor of medicine and of health research and policy at Stanford University. Long-term infection of the stomach with this bacterium may lead to a possible precancerous change in the lining of the stomach.

Don't be overly alarmed if you find that you have the bacteria. About 50 percent of the U.S. population does. Your risk of stomach cancer may be higher if you have a family history of stomach cancer in combination with *H. pylori*. The infection is treatable with antibiotics.

FILL YOUR PLATE WITH FRESH FRUITS AND VEGE-TABLES. A balanced and varied diet that is rich in fresh fruit and vegetables may provide protection against stomach cancer, says Dr. Correa. These foods contain powerful antioxidants such as vitamins C and E and beta-carotene. The antioxidants help protect cells from free radicals, which are unstable, high-energy molecules that can damage healthy cells and set the stage for many diseases, including cancer. Follow the National Cancer Institute guidelines by eating at least five servings of fruits and vegetables every day, he says.

SKIP THE SALT. Don't season with salt when you are cooking or eating, says Dr. Correa. Excessive salt consumption has been linked to higher incidences of stomach cancer. Pickled foods, which are high in salt, are considered a risk factor.

STOP SMOKING. Cigarette smoking appears to play a role in the early development of stomach cancer. Tobacco and tobacco smoke contain N-nitroso compounds and other carcinogens that may affect the mucous membrane of the stomach. Tobacco can also slow down the emptying of the stomach, causing food to remain there for longer periods. This may be a risk factor for cancer.

DRINK IN MODERATION. Like tobacco, alcohol can delay the time it takes for the stomach to empty, allowing food to remain too long in the stomach. Alcohol may contribute to the development of inflammation. That inflammation may damage the inner layer of the stomach, which is a risk factor for stomach cancer.

EAT YOUR ALLIUMS. Onions, garlic, and other members of the allium family of vegetables could help prevent stomach cancer. In the Netherlands Cohort Study, which began in 1986 with 120,852 men and women, researchers found a strong relationship between onion consumption and declining cancer rates in nearly all parts of the stomach. Those who ate the most onions, it turned out, had the lowest rates of stomach cancer. Although the Netherlands study did not find similar cancer-protective benefits in garlic and leeks, other studies have. Allium vegetables are traditionally known for their antibacterial and fungicidal benefits. They also may have anti-carcinogen compounds.

An Apple a Day Recipe

Cancer-Protective Quesadillas

The onions in these quesadillas are alliums—vegetables that can help prevent stomach cancer.

- 1 teaspoon olive oil
- 2 medium onions, thinly sliced
- 1 large tomato, chopped
- 1/3 cup chopped fresh cilantro or parsley
- 1 jalapeño chile pepper, seeded and finely chopped (wear plastic gloves when handling)
- 8 flour tortillas (12" diameter)
- 3/4 cup shredded reduced-fat Monterey Jack cheese

Warm the oil in a medium nonstick skillet over medium heat. Add the onions and cook for 8 minutes, or until the onions are golden brown. Add the tomato, cilantro or parsley, and pepper. Cook and stir for 5 minutes.

Preheat the broiler.

Place 4 tortillas on a large baking sheet. Divide the onion mixture among them. Top with the Monterey Jack and the remaining tortillas.

Broil the quesadillas for 1 to 2 minutes, or until the cheese melts. Cut into wedges.

Makes 16 wedges. Per wedge: 133 calories, 3 g. fat

TAKE TIME FOR TEA TIME. Green tea may be a powerful weapon in the fight against stomach cancer. A study in Shanghai, China, where green tea is consumed by more than 80 percent of tea drinkers, showed that green-tea drinkers had a lower risk of stomach cancer than those who didn't drink green tea. Green tea contains polyphenols, antioxidative substances that can inhibit the formation and growth of a variety of tumors, including stomach cancer.

But if you want the full beneficial effects from green tea, don't add milk to it. Proteins in milk may bind with the beneficial compounds in tea and inhibit the tea's antioxidant properties.

DON'T EAT PRESERVED FOODS. Bacon, hot dogs, cooked sausages, cured pork, lunchmeats, deviled ham, smoked fish, and beef jerky all contain nitrates, preservatives that break down in the body into nitrites and cancer-causing nitrosamines. Excessive consumption of nitrates has been identified as a risk factor for stomach cancer, says Dr. Parsonnet.

TAKE SOME NUTRITIONAL INSURANCE. Multivitamins can't replace the healthy benefits of fresh fruits and vegetables, but they can provide extra assurance that you are getting adequate nutrients from your diet. And those added nutrients have been shown to help prevent stomach cancer. Dr. Parsonnet recommends a standard multivitamin/ mineral supplement with 100 percent of the Daily Value for most nutrients.

STRESS
It's Hard to Be Easy

As a magazine editor, Liz Ludlow knows stress intimately. Working against ever-looming deadlines, she spends her days in and out of meetings, editing and writing copy, and managing her expanding staff of writers and editors. "Because I manage a department, I have to give the impression that I'm under control and not panicking," says Ludlow. "But I tend to internalize that anxiety, so I have had to create ways in my life to channel that energy."

Three years ago, Ludlow turned to yoga to help her prevent stress and the tension headaches that often accompanied it. She now applies the relaxation, breathing, and focusing techniques that she has learned in her yoga classes to her hectic work schedule. "I think of my mind now as a muscle, and that muscle is in shape," she says.

It may seem inevitable that operating the command center of a monthly magazine would invite stress. But many people don't realize that stress is something that you can prevent—no matter how intense your occupation or how fast-paced your daily life. And every ounce of prevention can help prevent other conditions.

Stress has been linked to dozens of physical ailments, from heart disease to dizziness, and it undermines our mental health as well. Stress can lead to depression, anxiety, irritability, and other emotional problems, says Georg Eifert, Ph.D., professor of clinical psychology at West Virginia University in Morgantown.

To prevent stress and ward off its negative impact on your health, take some tips from the stress experts.

Pass the pasta, please. The next time you are forced to eat a late-night dinner after a particularly long and frustrating day, make yourself a pasta or rice dinner, suggests Jack Groppel, Ph.D., an exercise physiologist and vice president of L. G. E. Sport Science Center in Orlando, Florida.

Foods that are high in carbohydrates bring about a rise in the level of the brain chemical serotonin, which has a calming effect on the body, Dr. Groppel explains.

Don't have a beef. Conversely, if you are feeling particularly frazzled, you may want to avoid high-protein meals. Protein releases an amino acid called tyrosine that stimulates the development of two potentially troublesome hormones, norepinephrine and dopamine. Although Dr. Groppel usually promotes the energy benefits of a protein meal, these hormones can lead to elevated blood pressure, hyperactivity, and even anxiety, all of which are unfriendly to an already-stressed system. So if you usually eat a couple of eggs for breakfast, chicken salad for lunch, and a steak dinner, he recommends some mealtime revisions.

Become a strategic snacker. Low blood sugar can intensify emotional stress, irritability, and anxiety, says Dr. Groppel. To keep your blood sugar from sinking, snack on something healthy such as fruit every 2 to 2 1/2 hours between moderate-size meals, he suggests.

Take out a multivitamin/mineral insurance policy. Physiological and emotional stress can rob the body of

An Apple a Day Recipe

Soul-Soothing Pasta

Pasta and beans combine for maximum complex carbohydrates, which have a calming, relaxing effect. The fresh greens make this a light alternative to heavy pasta entrées.

8 ounces ziti, penne, or rigatoni pasta
4 teaspoons olive oil
4 cloves garlic, thinly sliced
½ teaspoon red-pepper flakes
2 medium heads escarole or 1 bag (10 ounces) spinach, leaves torn in half

2 cans (15 ounces) cannellini beans, rinsed and drained
Freshly ground black pepper
1 tablespoon lemon juice
2 tablespoons grated Parmesan cheese

Cook the pasta in a large pot of boiling water according to the package directions. Drain.

Meanwhile, warm the oil in a large nonstick skillet over medium heat. Add the garlic and red-pepper flakes. Cook for 3 minutes, or until the garlic is golden. Add the escarole or spinach and cook, stirring often, until the greens begin to wilt. Add the beans and cooked pasta. Season with the black pepper. Heat, stirring gently, for 5 minutes, or until the beans are hot. Sprinkle with the lemon juice and Parmesan.

Makes 4 servings. Per serving: 506 calories, 7 g. fat

important nutrients, including antioxidant vitamins, says Dr. Groppel. In times of stress, free radicals—unstable molecules of harmful chemicals—increase and pillage the body's healthy molecules for replacement electrons, leaving more free radicals and damaged cells and tissues in their wake. Antioxidants, most notably vitamins C and E and beta-carotene, protect the body's healthy molecules by sacrificing their own electrons to neutralize free-radical invaders. To arm yourself against a stress-induced free-radical invasion, take a daily multivitamin/mineral supplement, he says.

DO A "STRESS" REHEARSAL—WITH EXERCISE. Exercise plays a key role in minimizing the damage that stress does to our health, says James E. Loehr, Ed.D., a sports psychologist and president of L. G. E. Sport Science Center and author of *Stress for Success: The Proven Program for Transforming Stress into Positive Energy at Work*. Exercise acts as a stress rehearsal for other kinds of stress. "If the body gets used to dealing with the flood of hormones that get released during exercise, then it learns to respond better to all kinds of stress in the future," he says.

Exercise also triggers the release of endorphins, brain chemicals associated with pain relief and euphoria. "Endorphin levels rise significantly both in the brain and in the body as a result of exercise," says Dr. Loehr. When we make exercise a constant in our lives, our elevated endorphin levels can make us calmer.

For stress prevention, Dr. Loehr suggests interval exercise. Interval exercise simply means varying the intensity of exercise throughout your workout. For example, if you walk, start slow, then increase your speed, slow down again, speed up, and so forth. This surge-and-recover approach imitates the normal stress pattern in life, so it makes us better at coping. This change-of-pace strategy can be used with an exercise bicycle, treadmill, aerobic workout, or whatever type of exercise you choose.

BREATHE EASY. Yoga increases self-awareness and makes us acutely sensitive to physiological and psychological stressors in our lives, says Richard Miller, Ph.D., a clinical psychologist in San Rafael, California, and co-founder of the International Association of Yoga Therapists, based in Mill Valley, California. If we can perceive the source of our stress early on, then we can intervene with deep breathing, which is an important component of yoga. "Breathing intervention is worth gold," he says.

Try this simple breathing exercise suggested by Dr. Miller. Sit comfortably on the floor or in a chair, unless you prefer to stand or lie down. Take note of your inhalations and exhalations. Now shift your breathing pattern so that the exhalations are twice as long as the inhalations. The breathing should feel comfortable, long, smooth, and stable. When you exhale, feel the breath move out of your abdomen, sides, and lower back.

Do this exercise for 10 to 15 minutes daily. On different days, alternate between sitting, lying down, and standing. To build this technique into your daily life, check in with your breathing pattern throughout the day for 15 seconds and reassert this technique whenever necessary, says Dr. Miller.

SEEK HERBAL RELIEF. Siberian ginseng and Panax ginseng support the adrenal glands and reduce feelings of stress and anxiety, says Hyla Cass, M.D., assistant clinical professor of psychiatry at the University of California, Los Angeles, School of Medicine and author of *Saint-John's-Wort: Nature's Blues Buster*. The adrenals are two small glands above the kidneys that are responsible for producing the fight-or-flight hormone, adrenaline. The adrenals also influence blood sugar, blood volume, and sexual development.

Siberian and Panax ginseng are adaptogenic tonics. Adaptogens such as ginseng have a normalizing effect on physiological functions (such as bringing high blood pressure down and low blood pressure up), which enhances

Go Where Your Mind Takes You

Daydreaming has always gotten a bum rap. You can probably hear the echoes of your first-grade teacher telling you to pay attention, but daydreaming can be useful. Through a technique known as guided imagery, we can direct our daydreams and deliberately create images that promote wellness and give us a sense of calm.

"Guided imagery takes the mind to a purposeful fantasy or memory," explains Belleruth Naparstek, a licensed psychotherapist in Cleveland Heights, Ohio, and author of *Your Sixth Sense* and the *Health Journeys* guided imagery audiotape series. The idea behind guided imagery is simple. Think back to a time when you felt warm, safe, and loved, and invoke the sense memories of that time. If you can conjure the sights, sounds, tastes, smells, and feelings, your mind and body will respond accordingly. "If you visualize a time when you felt safe and prized, the body begins to reproduce the same stress-reducing biochemical response you had at that time," says Naparstek.

To guide your own imagery toward relaxing thoughts, Naparstek recommends the following steps.

• Wait until everyone is asleep or out of the house, then find a quiet space that you can call your own. If

---

resistance to stress. Ginseng can be incorporated into a daily nutritional regimen with other nutritional and herbal supplements, and it may actually enhance the other supplements' effects, according to Dr. Cass.

For stress prevention, take 100 milligrams of Siberian or Panax ginseng in any standardized form, three times daily, says Dr. Cass. *Standardized* means that the herbal product has been processed to guarantee an appropriate possible, turn off the ringer on the phone and add some soothing background music.

- Sit comfortably and think of a time when you felt very safe, loved, and protected. Perhaps you have memories of sitting on your grandmother's lap and hearing your favorite story. Or recall walking along the beach at sunrise. Whatever it is, take that memory and relive it in all of its sensory detail. If it is the beach scenario, for example: Was there water lapping at your ankles? Was cold sand squishing through your toes? Did the air smell salty? What sounds did you hear?
- Allow yourself to fantasize. Guided imagery doesn't have to be based on actual events in your life.
- Don't think that you have blown it if your mind drifts away from the scene you are recreating. Just gently guide your attention back to the original sensory details. Your level of concentration will improve over time.
- Practice guided imagery twice a day for 10 to 15 minutes each time, preferably when you are waking up and falling asleep, says Naparstek.
- Put your hands in the same position on your body (for example, your stomach) every time you try guiding your imagery. That way, when you feel yourself getting stressed, you can put your hands on that spot, take a couple of breaths, and immediately cue your body to destress, says Naparstek.

level of one or more of the major active ingredients. Look for Siberian ginseng that is standardized at 1 percent of the active ingredient eleutheroside and Panax ginseng containing a minimum of 15 milligrams of the active ingredient ginsenoside. It is best to start with a daily dose of 100 milligrams once a day and build up to three doses, if needed, paying attention to your reaction. Too much ginseng may be overstimulating in highly sensitive individuals, causing anxiety, insomnia, increased blood pressure, or menstrual irregularities, cautions Dr. Cass. If these occur, lower the dosage or discontinue usage.

LET NATURE NURTURE YOU. Nature can be a tremendous aid in preventing stress, according to Valerie Gennari Cooksley, R.N., a teacher and lecturer in Issaquah, Washington, and author of *Aromatherapy: A Lifetime Guide to Healing with Essential Oils.* And you can find nature in some unexpected places: the plant store, a local park, or even outside your own office. Some simple suggestions: Fill your home and work space with lush, living plants; put a fish tank in your office; stroke your pets for at least 15 minutes every day; and walk outdoors on your lunch hour instead of hanging around the office or lunchroom. At the minimum, place nature-inspired artwork in your surroundings.

MAKE SCENTS OF YOUR STRESS. Imagine walking in a lush, colorful garden, breathing in the soothing aroma of roses or lavender. With aromatherapy, you can bottle up those evocative scents and breathe them in whenever you are feeling stressed-out or blue. Aromatherapy is the use of essential oils for physical and emotional health. Essential oils are distilled from flowers, leaves, fruit, bark, and roots of plants. To prevent stress, they can be inhaled directly or dispersed in a scented mist using a special device called a diffuser. Essential oils can also be diluted in vegetable or nut oils, such as sweet almond, sunflower, and olive, and applied to the skin through a bath, a massage, lotions, and compresses. But pregnant women should avoid essential oils, Cooksley cautions.

MIX A STRESS-PREVENTING BATH. It is easy to add essential oils to your bath, says Cooksley. The warmth of the bathwater, combined with the aromatic essential oils, will help to ease muscle tension and soothe the mind.

Choose a relaxing essential oil such as bergamot, chamomile, geranium, juniper, lavender, lemongrass, rose, or ylang-ylang, Cooksley suggests. Next, add 6 to 10 drops, at the most, of the essential oil to what is called a carrier—that is, the material that helps carry the aroma. Since the oils enter the bloodstream, children and the elderly should only use half of the adult amount, Cooksley cautions. To avoid phototoxicity (skin pigmentation), do not use bergamot if you are going to be exposed to the sun after bathing with this oil.

For bathwater, she recommends using one of the following carriers: one-half cup of whole milk, one-quarter cup of sea salt or Epsom salts, or two tablespoons of honey. When the tub is full of warm bathwater, add the oils with the carrier, hang out the "Do Not Disturb" sign, close the bathroom door, and enjoy.

OIL UP TO STOP WORK STRESS. Aromatherapy also has a home in the workplace, says Cooksley. Keep a bottle of essential oil in your desk drawer, and from time to time, take a whiff of the calming scent of your choice. Before you go into a business meeting, place a few drops of the oil on a tissue or notepad and bring it along, she advises.

SAY NO TO FUTURE STRESSORS. Learn to say no to new responsibilities when your plate is already full. "One of the main reasons why people feel stress is that they take on too many tasks at once and underestimate how much time they will need to complete them," says Dr. Eifert. "If they were more realistic in estimating how much time they need to spend on certain activities, they would probably feel less stress."

STROKE
Keep the Blood Flowing Freely

Strokes happen in the brain, but they strike at the heart. The stroke victim may lose the ability to speak clearly. Memory fades. Often, there is some paralysis. Stroke is the leading cause of disabilities and the third-leading cause of death in the United States, according to the U.S. Public Health Service Office of Health Statistics.

While there is no way to prevent a stroke for sure, every step you take to keep your arteries healthy is a stroke-prevention measure. A stroke happens when the blood supply to the brain is interrupted, either because of a blockage or, much less commonly, a leak in blood vessels. An occlusive stroke, the kind caused by blockage, is most likely to happen in people with clogged arteries, especially the arteries in their necks. But it can also occur when a blood clot that formed somewhere else in the body breaks loose, travels to the brain, and gets stuck in some smaller artery. Here are the heart-smart protection strategies that also minimize your chances of stroke.

MAINTAIN NORMAL BLOOD PRESSURE. High blood pressure (above 140/90) makes you much more likely to have a stroke, says Murray Goldstein, D.O., director of the United Cerebral Palsy Research and Education Foundation and a member of the board of directors of the National Stroke Association. It can cause small tears in blood vessels, which can then clot or completely blow out. Your doctor can suggest medication to control your blood pressure, but there are lots of other things that you can do to keep blood pressure normal. You should try to get to and maintain your ideal weight. It is important that you watch your diet. Minimize your salt intake and get adequate amounts of potassium, magnesium, and calcium, Dr. Goldstein advises. Potassium is found in most raw vegetables and dried fruits, magnesium in nuts and whole grains, and calcium in dairy products and green, leafy vegetables.

DRINK BLACK TEA. A study from the Netherlands found that men who drank more than 4.7 cups of black tea a day were 69 percent less likely to have a stroke than men who drank less than 2.6 cups a day. Black and green teas contain bioflavonoids, compounds that increase capillary strength, says Barry Taylor, a naturopathic doctor with the New England Family Health Center in Weston, Massachusetts.

AVOID FAT. The same high-fat diet that clogs up your coronary arteries can impede blood flow through the arteries in your neck, which raises your odds of having a stroke. Pay particular attention to eating less saturated fat, by choosing lean meats and low-fat salad dressings and low-fat dairy products.

GET SOME OF THE "GOOD" OILS. You may want to substitute saturated fat in the diet with monounsaturated or polyunsaturated fat, says Joel Simon, M.D., assistant professor of medicine at the University of California, San Francisco, School of Medicine.

He found that men with high concentrations of alpha-linolenic acid (a polyunsaturated fatty acid in the same

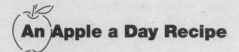

An Apple a Day Recipe

Bioflavonoid Spiced Iced Tea

Bioflavonoids are compounds in foods that have multiple health benefits, including warding off stroke. This apple-spiced iced tea (or any type of black tea) contains these beneficial bioflavonoids. Researchers recommend at least 4 cups of tea a day for maximum benefits.

⅓ cup apple juice
½ cup brewed
  orange-flavored
  black tea, chilled

1 apple slice
1 sprig fresh mint

Pour the apple juice and tea over ice in a tall glass. Garnish with the apple slice and mint sprig, if desired.

Makes 1 serving. Per serving: 40 calories, 0.1 g. fat

family of fatty acids as fish oil) in their blood had a lower risk of stroke. "Alpha-linolenic acid may decrease the risk of a stroke by affecting blood viscosity and clotting," Dr. Simon explains. Important sources of alpha-linolenic acid are flaxseed, canola, soybean, and walnut oils.

FEED ON THE FRUIT OF THE LAND. Harvard researchers found that eating more fruits and vegetables cuts the risk of a stroke. This protective effect is independent of fat intake, blood cholesterol levels, and blood pressure, says Matthew Gillman, M.D., associate professor of ambulatory care and prevention at Harvard Medical School and Harvard Pilgrim Health Care, both in Boston, and the main author of the study.

The Warning Sign of Stroke

"Like chest pains before a heart attack, stroke also often gives warning signals," says Murray Goldstein, D.O., director of the United Cerebral Palsy Research and Education Foundation and a member of the board of directors of the National Stroke Association. These warning signals are short periods of reduced blood flow to the brain, called transient ischemic attacks, or TIAs.

The symptoms may include short-term confusion, temporary loss of vision or blurred vision in one eye, tingling or weakness in an arm or leg, or a bit of drooling from one side of the mouth. An attack is most likely to occur first thing in the morning, and people often don't realize the symptoms are serious since they often disappear in a minute or two.

It is vital not to overlook even the briefest of TIAs, Dr. Goldstein says. "A TIA may mean a stroke is imminent. It is a medical emergency, and you should call your physician immediately." If you can't see your doctor right away, get to the emergency room for immediate medical treatment.

People who are having a stroke caused by a blockage—as opposed to one caused by a leak—can be given fast-acting, clot-dissolving drugs that may stop or even reverse a stroke. If a loved one has any of the symptoms of a TIA, you may be able to get the drug in time to prevent a stroke. So call your physician as soon as you recognize the signs.

"Antioxidants such as vitamin C and carotenoids may help," says Dr. Gillman. Both of these antioxidants are found in yellow and orange fruits and vegetables, such as carrots and peaches, and in dark green, leafy vegetables, such as spinach. "And the folate in fruits and vegetables helps reduce levels of homocysteine, a protein fragment that new evidence suggests may be as much a risk factor for stroke as it is for heart disease."

Look for pressure valves. There is a lot of evidence that stress contributes to high blood pressure. If you have a particularly stressful life *and* high blood pressure, find ways to relax, says Dr. Goldstein. Try meditation or imagery. An engrossing hobby can help: Woodworking or gardening may take your mind off the stressors in your life.

A beagle can lower your blood pressure, too. A number of studies have shown that interacting with pets can help put people at ease. Pet ownership changes your perspective and directs your attention to affectionate interactions, says Dr. Goldstein.

Ask your doctor about aspirin. Daily doses of aspirin have been proven effective in reducing the risk of stroke—but not for everyone. Aspirin may be appropriate for you if you have had a heart attack or an occlusive stroke or if you have a false rhythm of the heart called paroxysmal arrhythmia, Dr. Goldstein says.

Talk with your doctor about the right amount to take. "Amounts used in studies vary, but evidence suggests that an amount from 162 to 320 milligrams a day is sufficient," Dr. Goldstein says. That range is the equivalent of one-half to one adult aspirin daily.

Keep on moving. It is a well-accepted fact that regular exercise reduces your risk of having a heart attack. Well, same goes for stroke. In one study, even easy exercise—20 minutes a day of walking, gardening, dancing, or golf—cut stroke risk by more than half. And strenuous exercise reduced risk by two-thirds.

"Exercise inhibits the production of blood clots and raises blood levels of high-density lipoprotein (HDL), the 'good' cholesterol," explains Ralph L. Sacco, M.D., director of the Northern Manhattan Stroke Study at the Columbia-Presbyterian Medical Center in New York City.

HEED THE WARNING LABELS ON CIGARETTES. Smokers are more likely to have a stroke than someone who doesn't smoke, Dr. Goldstein says. "Smoking damages blood vessel walls, speeds up the clogging of arteries, raises blood pressure, and makes the heart work harder."

IF YOU SMOKE, BE CAUTIOUS ABOUT THE TYPE OF ORAL CONTRACEPTIVES YOU USE. Birth control pills can increase the blood's tendency to clot. When you combine smoke damage with the side effects of certain types of oral contraceptives, it is a one-two blow to your arteries. These two habits combined contribute to strokes in younger women, Dr. Goldstein says. Make sure that you discuss your smoking habit with your doctor when he prescribes contraceptives for you.

EXPLORE ESTROGEN. There is evidence that hormone-replacement therapy (HRT), sometimes used to help women through menopause, may reduce stroke risk slightly. But HRT is controversial. Women should consult their doctors about whether it may be a preventive option.

DON'T OVERDO THE HARD STUFF. Moderate drinking is associated with a reduced risk for stroke, possibly because small amounts of alcohol raise the level of a naturally occurring "clot-buster" in the blood, Dr. Goldstein says. In studies related to stroke, moderate drinking is defined as no more than one daily serving of a 12-ounce beer, a 4-ounce glass of wine, or a cocktail containing 1 ounce of alcohol. "Binge drinking, though, has a strong association with stroke, possibly because of spikes in blood pressure," he says.

WATCH YOUR NECK. People sometimes have strokes after their necks have been hyperextended or twisted. That movement can tear the lining of one of the four arteries going to their brains, causing a clot to form inside the artery. "This kind of stroke has been reported in women whose neck has been extended over a sink at the hairdresser, in drivers who sharply turn their necks, and rarely, as a result of chiropractic neck adjustment," Dr. Goldstein says.

At the hairdresser, make sure that you have a pillow under your neck, or you may prefer to lean forward over the sink, instead of backward. When driving, turn your head slowly. If you experience any light-headedness during your chiropractic adjustment, ask the doctor to stop immediately.

TMD
Taking a Bite Out of Jaw Pain

You may be surprised to know that the strongest muscle in your body, pound for pound, is your jaw muscle. That's why overworking it by clenching your jaw and grinding your teeth can lead to a painful problem known as TMD (temporomandibular disorder).

TMD affects the jaw joint and the muscles that control chewing. With this disorder, some people can't open their mouths freely. Others can't close their mouths fully. Sometimes, TMD throws your upper and lower teeth out of alignment. It can create powerful headaches and even cause your jaw to make a popping or grinding sound every now and then. But you can help prevent jaw pain if you avoid straining your jaw muscle and joint. Here are ways to avoid that gnawing pain.

USE IT SPARINGLY. If you are prone to jaw pain, don't crunch on ice or chew gum, pencils, or your fingernails. These habits can cause more pain than you realize, says

Thomas R. Feder, D.D.S., a dentist in private practice in Santa Monica, California.

BE A PICKY EATER. Taking huge bites of a sandwich can put your joints at risk for TMD. "When you are eating, don't open your jaw wider than is necessary," says Dr. Feder.

Cut your food up into small pieces, adds Ira Schneider, D.C., a chiropractor in private practice in Santa Monica and Thousand Oaks, California. Steer clear of chewy, crunchy foods that may traumatize your jaw joint, he says.

BITE RIGHT AT NIGHT. You may be a jaw-clencher without being aware of it. Lots of people clench their jaws and grind their teeth when they are asleep. A dental appliance called a bite guard or night guard can help. "A bite guard widens the space between the teeth slightly so that the muscle can't clench as tightly," says Dr. Feder. If your dentist agrees that this device may help you, he can prescribe one that will fit your mouth properly.

RUB YOUR MUSCLE. Massaging your jaw joint often helps to relieve the tightness that can lead to TMD pain. "Massage across the muscle on the outside of your jaw," says Dr. Schneider. Feel for the hinged area on either side of your jaw close to your ears. "Then, insert your index finger inside your mouth and use it to gently massage the interior part of the muscle where it feels tender," he adds.

DO SOME RUBBERNECKING. Sometimes, massaging the muscles on either side of the neck also helps prevent the tension that can lead to TMD pain, says Dr. Schneider. Using your fingertips, just massage the muscles gently, especially near the jawline, to ease tension in the face and jaw.

GIVE YOUR JAW A POTATO BREAK. Relaxing your jaw whenever possible relieves clenching and muscle tension and helps prevent pain. Try relaxing with moist heat. "Boil a potato, wrap it in a towel, and hold it against your cheek for 10 to 15 minutes to relax the muscle," suggests Dr. Schneider. Just be careful to let it cool a bit first so that you don't burn yourself.

TOOTH SENSITIVITY
Cherish Your Choppers

Tooth care is a real pain. It is one of those relentless, long-term health obligations that just keeps demanding maintenance attention. It takes discipline to keep at it because you can't actually see the results of dental diligence, but you can feel them. If you are doing a good job of caring for your teeth, something *won't* happen. You won't be wincing in pain from tooth sensitivity.

Teeth are easy to take for granted. We chew away without giving them a second thought. Until we have a problem, that is. Then tender teeth become a royal nuisance. They can undermine your quality of life by keeping you from enjoying favorite foods. And you may even smile less often even though you're not conscious of it because you are thinking about hiding your teeth.

Tooth sensitivity is often a sign of gum disease, which can make you prone to many infections. While the prevention strategy is pretty simple—good dental hygiene—the road to hygiene is paved with distractions. Here is the dental dogma for keeping your incisors insensitive and your molars ready to mash.

BEWARE TRAUMATIC FOODS. Most tooth sensitivity is caused by tooth decay and gum disease. But sometimes you can wound a tooth or tear the gum around it by making it chew a particularly hard or crunchy food. If you have touchy teeth, steer clear of hard pretzels, peanut brittle, or any food that requires jaw power, says Charles H. Perle, D.M.D., a dentist in Jersey City, New Jersey; a spokesperson for the Academy of General Dentistry; and a member of the Council on Communications of the American Dental Association (ADA).

CHOOSE THE RIGHT TOOL. "Use a soft-bristle nylon toothbrush," says Dr. Perle. A hard toothbrush may actually be too tough on the gums, he explains. Look for one of the many toothbrushes on the market that carry the ADA's seal of acceptance, he adds.

BRUSH UP ON YOUR BRUSHWORK. Brushing teeth up and down is not the right way to brush. "This technique can increase periodontal disease because food particles are being brushed into the gums," says Joffie Pittman, D.D.S., general director and medical administrator of the Henry J. Austin Health Center in Trenton, New Jersey.

Dentists suggest that you start with some up-and-down brushing to be sure that you clean out the crevices at the gum line but that you finish with some side-to-side strokes. "Move the toothbrush in and out along the gum line, tilting it at a 45-degree angle against your gum. You have to be sure to brush the particles of food away from the gum," says Dr. Pittman. Don't forget to brush the lingual side of the teeth, which is the inside area of your teeth that your tongue touches.

BE PICKY ABOUT YOUR PASTE. If you have had problems with tooth sensitivity in the past, try using a toothpaste specifically formulated for sensitive teeth. "This can help give you temporary relief," says Dr. Perle. Check the drugstore for brands that are specifically labeled for sensitive teeth (like Sensodyne) and that carry the ADA's seal of acceptance. Or ask your dentist what brand he recommends, he suggests.

RINSE, PLEASE. A topical fluoride rinse helps keep teeth in tip-top shape. "It can make teeth less sensitive," says Dr. Perle. Fluoride rinses combine with material inside the tooth to seal up pores, he adds.

Dr. Pittman stresses that fluoride rinses are an adjunct, not a replacement, for brushing and flossing. You should look for brands that contain fluoride or check the labels of rinses carried at drugstores for the ADA's seal of acceptance.

GLOSS WITH FLOSS. Flossing prevents decay between teeth and keeps the gums healthy. "If the gums are healthy," says Dr. Perle, "you don't get gum recession and, consequently, tooth sensitivity."

VITALIZE WITH VITAMIN C. Vitamin C is one of the essential vitamins that work for the growth and regeneration of normal tissues. "Vitamin C helps fight gum disease," says Dr. Pittman. He recommends that people get the recommended Daily Value of 60 milligrams to gain the greatest benefit from it. Good sources of vitamin C include citrus fruits and vegetables such as broccoli and red peppers.

BEWARE CHEWABLE C. Some studies suggest that chewable vitamin C tablets can damage tooth enamel. The evidence isn't decisive. But take a nonchewable supplement to be on the safe side, Dr. Perle recommends.

CEASE THE SMOKE. Cigarettes have a bad reputation for discoloring teeth, turning them yellowish, but their ingredients may do other damage as well. "Smoking increases the amount of tartar that builds up on your teeth, which causes more plaque to build up," says Dr. Pittman. "When this occurs, you are at greater risk of bone loss and tooth sensitivity."

EAT TEMPERATELY. If your teeth are giving you pain,

don't eat hot with cold. "If you do, you are just asking for tooth sensitivity," says Dr. Perle. Avoid combinations like cold ice cream followed by hot coffee. You may be able to avoid an excruciating tooth experience just by being wary of such combinations.

TOOTH STAINS
Keep Your Teeth Looking Their Best

Advertisers would have us believe that our teeth should be white as the driven snow. But since snow and teeth have nothing in common, there is no reason why any set of teeth—even good ones—should resemble a glistening alpine snowfield.

The fact is that dentin, the layer of our teeth beneath the clear enamel is *naturally* grayish or yellow. Tooth enamel often thins out as we age, letting the underlying colors of the dentin come through. And our teeth pick up colors from things we eat, drink, or smoke and from bacteria in our mouths. Still, nice, bright teeth are definitely a cosmetic plus.

Keeping your teeth clean can go a long way toward preventing permanent discoloration. Here is what dentists and dental hygienists recommend to get rid of unwanted stains before they decide to stay forever.

POLISH WITH A BIT OF BAKING SODA AND PEROXIDE. "Mix a bit of baking soda and hydrogen peroxide into a slurry the consistency of toothpaste," suggests Alan A.

Winter, D.D.S., of Park Avenue Periodontal Associates in New York City.

To make the slurry, use about a teaspoon of baking soda and a little less than one-half teaspoon of hydrogen peroxide. "Dab a cotton swab into it, and then use the swab to rub the stain off the tooth. The baking soda acts as an abrasive, while the hydrogen peroxide is somewhat of a bleaching agent," he explains.

This technique, however, should only be used for special occasions, not as a weekly routine, cautions Dr. Winter. Using baking soda too often will actually thin the enamel.

CHASE STAINS WITH GUM OR WATER. After you eat or drink something that stains—coffee, tea, blueberry pie—pop a piece of sugarless gum into your mouth and let your saliva rinse away stain-causing juices, suggests Carol Beidleman, a registered dental hygienist practicing in Allentown, Pennsylvania. Or you can just rinse out your mouth with water after you have eaten a food that leaves stains.

TRY BLEACHING, BUT ONLY WITH YOUR DENTIST'S SUPERVISION. Beware of the at-home bleaching kits that you pick up at the drugstore. They can cause gum irritation because the bleaching tray may not properly fit your mouth, says Harald A. Heymann, D.D.S., professor and chairman of the department of operative dentistry at the University of North Carolina at Chapel Hill. When you bleach your teeth under a dentist's supervision, the bleaching tray is custom-tailored.

STRAIGHTEN UP AND BRUSH RIGHT. People tend to be careless when they brush their teeth. This makes for sloppy, inefficient brushing, Beidleman says. "You can't just push the toothbrush around. You need to make sure to brush up along your gumlines at a 45-degree angle, and you need to brush each section longer than you probably do," she says. Brush about two to four minutes per toothbrushing, spending 30 to 40 seconds in each area of your mouth.

USE A STAIN-REMOVING TOOTHPASTE. One product in

particular, Topol, marketed to smokers, helps to remove stains, Beidleman says. Most stain-removing toothpastes are safe to use every day for one of your brushings. Use a regular toothpaste with fluoride for your other daily brushings.

TRY FULL DISCLOSURE. Your dental hygienist can get you chewable disclosing tablets. When you chew them, they will reveal by color where plaque is sticking to your teeth, Beidleman says. "Those are spots where your teeth will stain first unless the plaque is removed. This is a great aid to home care. It lets you see exactly where you are missing when you brush."

START BRUSHING WHERE STAINS ARE THE WORST. The most noticeable discoloration is usually in the front lower teeth. "If you start at your trouble spot, you are less likely to miss this area when you brush," Beidleman says.

GO ELECTRIC. If you have arthritis or some other problem that prevents you from using a regular toothbrush as well as you would like, use an electric one, Beidleman suggests. One new electric toothbrush she recommends is Sonicare, by Optiva, which is available in department stores and some drugstores. "It has a sonic vibrating action that actually helps break up stains and shake them off," she explains. "Used on a daily basis, this will help control your stains."

USE A MOUTHWASH THAT DISSOLVES STAIN-CATCHING PLAQUE. Anything that helps stop the growth of the bacteria that cause dental plaque will reduce your tendency to pick up stains, Beidleman says. She recommends an antibacterial rinse like Listerine or fluoride rinses like Listermint, ACT, or Fluorigard. Any of these rinses will help inhibit the attachment of plaque, restore needed minerals to areas in the early stages of decay, and relieve tooth sensitivity caused by gum recession.

GET PROFESSIONALLY CLEANED MORE OFTEN. Instead of every six months, Beidleman recommends that you get a cleaning every three or four months.

DON'T WEAR AWAY YOUR SMILE. Just as you wouldn't use an abrasive scouring powder on a countertop, you don't want to overdo it with polishing compounds or an overly abrasive toothpaste aimed at whitening your teeth. That is because these products can wear off tooth enamel, Dr. Heymann says. Unfortunately, there is no good rule of thumb on how much is too much, he adds. "Certainly, though, you have gone overboard if your teeth become sensitive to hot or cold."

ULCERS
Let Sleeping *H. Pylori* Lie

Not long ago, the best advice for preventing ulcers was the Never-Eat-Anything-Fun Wellness Program. Tacos, pizza, even orange juice, were verboten for anybody worried about getting an ulcer. Even worry itself was deemed worrisome because it implies stress, and stress was thought to cause ulcers.

Well, reschedule the chili fest. Science now knows that although pepperoni and pressure are not good for your health, they are not entirely to blame for ulcers. Stress may well be an aggravating factor, and if you have an ulcer, you should seek ways to minimize your stress. Stress, however, is not the true ulcer culprit. The real cause of ulcers is a bacteria—*Helicobacter pylori*, to be precise. It is found in the stomach of nearly all people with duodenal ulcers and in four out of five people with gastric ulcers. A duodenal ulcer is an irritation in your duodenum, the upper part of the small intestine. A gastric ulcer is on the wall of the stomach itself.

It is pretty tough to avoid infection with *H. pylori*. In the United States, up to 50 percent of the population harbors the organism. Fortunately, only about 20 percent of this group develops an ulcer. There is evidence that most people get infected as children, and the bacteria just doesn't kick into destructive gear until years later. Here are some steps that you can take to minimize the chances that *H. pylori* will wake up and turn against you.

BE SMOKE-FREE. "Smoking increases the potential for ulcers in people who are predisposed to them," says Lawrence S. Friedman, M.D., associate professor of medicine at Harvard Medical School and associate physician in the gastrointestinal unit at Massachusetts General Hospital, both in Boston.

Not only does smoking increase your risk of developing ulcers, but smokers are more likely to sustain serious ulcer complications like perforation. Furthermore, the antibiotic treatment that fights *H. pylori* is less effective for smokers as compared to nonsmokers, and once healed, a smoker's ulcer is more likely to recur.

LIMIT YOUR ALCOHOL. Alcohol alone generally won't cause ulcers, but avoid alcohol in excess because it can damage the stomach lining, says Dr. Friedman.

"If you think you have an ulcer, drinking alcohol is most unwise," according to Malcolm Robinson, M.D., clinical professor of medicine at the University of Oklahoma and medical director of the Oklahoma Foundation for Digestive Research, both in Oklahoma City.

FORTIFY WITH FIBER. There is some evidence that a high-fiber diet may be helpful in preventing ulcers, according to Dr. Friedman. A study by Harvard researchers found that people who averaged 30 grams of fiber a day cut their risk of duodenal ulcers in half. Though it isn't clear if fiber can inhibit the recurrence of ulcers, it is worth trying since a high-fiber diet has plenty of other health benefits, he says.

Some good sources of fiber? Dried pears, apples, and

An Apple a Day Recipe

Onion-Hearty Relish

The sulfur compounds in onions help neutralize the harmful bacteria that can cause ulcers. Relishes and salsas are a delicious way to serve onions and get their health benefits. Try this apple-onion relish on grilled pork or chicken, or as an accompaniment to bean dishes. Sweet onions such as Vidalia, Walla Walla, or Texas Sweet taste best here. Freeze leftover relish for up to six months.

2 teaspoons olive oil
3 large onions, chopped
2 apples and/or pears, seeded and chopped
¼ cup cider vinegar
¼ cup honey
¼ cup raisins
¼ cup frozen orange juice concentrate, thawed
½ teaspoon ground cinnamon
¼ teaspoon ground cloves

Warm the oil in a medium saucepan over medium heat. Add the onions and cook for 10 minutes, or until golden brown. Add the apples and/or pears, vinegar, honey, raisins, juice concentrate, cinnamon, and cloves. Bring to a boil.

Reduce the heat to medium-low and cook, stirring frequently, for 25 minutes, or until the relish is thick.

Makes 3 cups. Per 2 tablespoons: 36 calories, 0.5 g. fat peaches and many different kinds of beans, including lima beans, kidney beans, navy beans, and black beans.

BECOME AN ONION-LOVER. Not only is this pungent food not harmful to ulcer sufferers, it is actually beneficial as an ulcer preventive. Scientists believe the sulfur compounds in onions attack the bacterium *H. pylori*. Experts suggest that eating half an onion a day may be beneficial, so try to include it whenever possible in your salads, sandwiches, and cooking.

SAY NO TO THE NSAIDs. Beware of taking non-steroidal anti-inflammatory drugs (NSAIDs), like aspirin or ibuprofen. These drugs increase your risk of ulcers even if you don't have *H. pylori*. In fact, they are the only significant cause of ulcers besides the bacteria. If you do carry the bacteria, taking these medications can put you at even greater risk, according to Dr. Robinson.

For aches and pains, try acetaminophen instead, suggests David A. Peura, M.D., professor of medicine and associate chief of the division of gastroenterology and hepatology at the University of Virginia in Charlottesville.

URINARY TRACT INFECTIONS
Preventing Plumbing Problems

Riding sidesaddle inside your pelvis area, you have an array of tunnels and tubes that work on one basic drainage project, carrying urine away from your bladder and out the exit.

Most of the time, all goes smoothly in that region. A number of times each day, you get the urge, go, and that's that. But every once in a while, you may find yourself paying more attention than you would like to that simple process. Could be that your bladder feels full even when it isn't. Or you have to visit the bathroom more often, but when you urinate, you get a burning sensation. Sometimes, you might see traces of blood in your urine.

Any of these symptoms would be enough to send you straight to the doctor—and it is quite understandable since they are all signs of urinary tract infections (UTIs). These infections can't be taken lightly since the whole urinary system performs so many essential clean-up functions. And what starts as a mild infection can ultimately put your kidneys at risk if it isn't treated.

Call in the Cranberry

For years, doctors have suspected that cranberry juice could help stop urinary tract infections and bladder infections by acidifying the urine. They believed the acidic makeup of cranberries created an environment where the bladder was inhospitable for bacteria. Recently, however, researchers learned that a substance in cranberries stops bladder infections by preventing *E. coli* bacteria from attaching to the bladder wall.

Women can prevent recurrent infections by drinking two six-ounce glasses of cranberry juice twice a day, according to Paul Barney, M.D., adjunct professor at Weber State University and a family practitioner in Layton, Utah, who has studied the effect of cranberries on bladder infections. Drinking the cranberry juice found in supermarkets will work just fine, he says. Or you can take a cranberry supplement that can usually be found in health food stores.

In his experiments, Dr. Barney tested the supplement brand CranActin and found that it reduced the overall incidence of recurrent bladder infections by 70 percent among the women who took it. Although all brands don't necessarily have the same potency of active ingredient, Dr. Barney recommends that his patients take one 400-milligram cranberry pill in the morning and one in the evening. If you follow that advice and are free of bladder infections for several months, he suggests reducing the dosage to one a day. And if you are still free of infections for another few months after that, you can reduce the dosage to one every other day.

Both men and women can experience bouts of incomplete urination that cause UTIs, says Larrian Gillespie, M.D., a retired urologist in Los Angeles and author of *You Don't Have to Live with Cystitis*. Women statistically get these infections much more frequently than men. But after men hit the age of 50, they begin to catch up, particularly since enlarged prostates can obstruct the flow of urine.

Fortunately, there are many ways to help prevent UTIs in the first place and avoid a painful nuisance that could lead to an even more serious health problem. Consider these two big prevention principles: First, keep those bacteria out of the urethra, the tube that drains the bladder. Second, make sure that the whole urinary tract flows strongly and freely to wash out any bacteria that make it that far.

DON'T GET A SHRINK. The decongestants that people take for colds and allergies have the power to shrink swollen nasal membranes by constricting tiny blood vessels inside the nose. The problem is that they can also constrict the neck of your bladder. This side effect cuts down the flow of urine and sets you up for a bladder infection.

"When there is a high pollen count, doctors will see a wave of cystitis. That's because people are taking decongestants," says Dr. Gillespie. If you have an allergy, she suggests talking to your doctor about one of the new allergy medicines that do not contain decongestants.

FILL THE CANALS. To keep your urinary tract humming, drink eight eight-ounce glasses of water a day, says Paul Barney, M.D., adjunct professor at Weber State University and a family practitioner in Layton, Utah.

DON'T FLOOD THE SYSTEM. It is possible to overload on water and weaken your bladder. "I had patients who were drinking 12 to 20 glasses of fluids a day because they were petrified of having another bladder infection, and they stretched their bladders out to the point where they could not void as efficiently," says Dr. Gillespie.

To see whether you are getting enough water in your system, watch the color of your urine, she advises. If it is clear or very pale, you are probably getting enough water; if it is dark yellow, you are not, she says.

LIMIT YOUR ALCOHOL INTAKE. People who are prone

to bladder infections should limit their intake of alcohol to no more than one drink per day, says Dr. Gillespie. (That's one 12-ounce glass of beer, 5 ounces of wine, or 1½ ounces of hard liquor.) That's because alcohol "temporarily interferes with the brain chemical that causes the bladder muscles to contract efficiently."

GO WHEN YOU GOTTA GO. When you don't urinate frequently enough, bacteria stays in your bladder and has a chance to multiply, says Dr. Gillespie. A couple of bathroom breaks a day is not enough, she adds. If you feel the need to urinate, don't put it off.

Specifically for She Systems

Most UTIs in women are caused by *E. coli* bacteria that find their way from the rectum, where they live harmlessly, up to the urethra, where they start to create itchiness and other problems. Twenty percent of all women are likely to have at least one outbreak during their lifetimes. And for the women who get one, there is an 80 percent chance of getting one again within two years.

Even though women are very prone to UTIs, all the equipment is in place to help prevent these infections. According to Dr. Gillespie, a woman's urinary tract has a highly efficient cleansing mechanism, perfectly designed to remove bacteria from the bladder and its surroundings. If you help it to work at peak efficiency, it can protect you from the inconvenience and pain of bladder infections.

In addition to the advice suggested above, here are some tips, expressly designed for women, for thwarting the *E. coli* that often cause UTIs and sometimes lead to bladder infections.

VISIT THE LOO AFTER L'AMOUR. If you urinate after sex, you wash away any bacteria that may have been moved from the rectal or vaginal area into the urethra, says Alice

An Apple a Day Recipe

Cranberry Hot Toddy

Looking for a different kind of warm beverage? This nonalcoholic hot toddy is spiced just right. Plus, the cranberry juice can help prevent urinary tract infections. Some cranberry juices are full of sugar or high-fructose corn syrup, so be sure to read labels and purchase 100% pure juice.

3 cups cranberry-apple
juice (100% juice)

3 cups apple cider

1 cinnamon stick, broken
into pieces

1 teaspoon whole cloves

⅛ teaspoon ground
nutmeg

Peel of 1 orange, cut
in 1 continuous strip

In a large saucepan over medium-high heat, combine the cranberry-apple juice, cider, cinnamon stick, cloves, nutmeg, and orange peel. Bring to a boil. Reduce the heat to low, cover, and simmer for 10 to 15 minutes. Remove from the heat.

Strain the mixture, discarding the solids.

Makes 6 cups. Per cup: 107 calories, 0 g. fat

Stollenwerk Petrulis, M.D., professor of medicine at Case Western Reserve University in Cleveland. If you have some foresight about sex on the horizon, get a quick drink of water before the romancing begins. That way, you are sure to have the urge to urinate afterward.

COACH YOUR GUY. Dr. Gillespie says that the standard

Does a Strong Back Mean a Healthy Bladder?

To maximize your urinary performance and minimize your risk of urinary tract infections, take good care of your back, advises Larrian Gillespie, M.D., a retired urologist in Los Angeles and author of *You Don't Have to Live with Cystitis*. The nerves that control the operation of your bladder originate in the section of the spine that constitutes your lower back, the lumbar curve. When the lower back becomes weak, she says, the nerve currents to the bladder are also reduced. "Like a weak battery, the current-deprived bladder does not function well. It does not empty efficiently and may leave residual urine, which can lead to infections," she says. Here are some everyday back strainers to avoid.

Stairclimbing machines. "Stairclimbing machines are not designed properly for the female pelvis," says Dr. Gillespie, "and they cause side-to-side weakening in the spine. I get a lot of women off the stairclimbers, and their bladder infections stop." (These machines don't affect men the same way.)

Vacuuming. Don't push and drag the vacuum with your arm, advises Dr. Gillespie. Instead, walk forward and backward with the machine so that you are not bending over and straightening.

High heels. High heels are fine for some women, says Dr. Gillespie. In fact, some women actually stand straighter when they are wearing high-heeled shoes. But for others, the added height results in an additional curve to the lower back, called lordosis. If you are experiencing back pain, experiment with not wearing high heels, and see if that makes a difference.

missionary position for sex can increase the chances of bladder infections if the man is too high up on a woman's pelvis. In that position, he puts pressure on the opening of the urethra, and the up-and-down thrusting motion also drags the urethra up and down. "It quickly becomes sore and swollen," she says.

To avoid this problem, she recommends more of a rocking motion. The most bladder-friendly missionary position is "hipbone to hipbone," with the man rocking forward into the woman and then back, according to Dr. Gillespie.

DOUBLE-CHECK YOUR DIAPHRAGM. About a decade ago, says Dr. Gillespie, many women were being fitted with large diaphragms to more effectively block sperm. Unfortunately, these big diaphragms also obstructed the urethra, impeding the flow of urine, which can lead to a UTI.

Don't get a diaphragm larger than 65 millimeters in circumference, Dr. Gillespie advises. And make sure that your diaphragm has a soft rim, which compresses more easily when you urinate and puts you at less risk for a bladder infection than diaphragms that are rigid. If you are using a diaphragm that is too large or too rigid, talk to your gynecologist about changing, she suggests.

TAKE OUT THE TAMPON. Do you get a bladder infection around your period? The problem may be your tampon. "The super-size tampons can compress or obstruct the neck of the bladder, altering the urinary flow rate so that you can't void efficiently," says Dr. Gillespie. The solution, she says, is to remove the tampon before every urination.

VARICOSE VEINS
Keeping the Flow Going

Veins are the channels that carry blood from all parts of your body back to your heart. When they are in good shape, the valves inside them urge the blood on its way. If your vein walls are weakened, however, the veins can dilate, pulling the valves apart. So the little flaps on the valves no longer form an effective seal, and gravity causes the blood to leak backward. And the blood tends to pool in the place where gravity wants it—down in your legs. The result? Those bulging varicose veins and those pink or blue spidery veins.

Although the tendency for vein walls to weaken and dilate is hereditary, biology is not destiny. There are steps that you can take to thwart varicose veins. The key is to focus on good circulation and to take up some habits that can help keep your blood flowing smoothly.

People who stand for prolonged periods of time are more likely to get varicose veins than other people, says Dee Anna Glaser, M.D., assistant professor of dermatology in the department of dermatology at the St. Louis University

School of Medicine. "Standing in one place for a long period of time without moving your muscles allows for the pooling of blood." Not surprisingly, people who are constantly on their feet—like hairdressers, factory workers, and grocery checkout clerks—are especially susceptible. If you have a job that keeps you on your feet but not moving around a lot, think up some ways to move your legs periodically.

DO A FOOT FLEX. "For about 10 minutes every hour throughout the day, flex your ankles up and down (5 minutes per foot)," says Dr. Glaser. "This causes your calf muscles to contract, thereby forcing the blood upward." Muscle contraction is the very best way to help the blood get back up to the heart, she adds.

BE A STROLLER. Another good way to use the calf muscles is to take little walks periodically. "The best thing that you can do at work is to walk around whenever you can," says Mitchel P. Goldman, M.D., associate clinical professor of dermatology at the University of California, San Diego.

RAISE 'EM HIGH. Elevating your feet at the end of the day also helps take pressure off your veins and reduces swelling. So when you get home at the end of the day, make a point of taking your shoes off and swinging your legs up on the couch or footstool, recommends Dr. Glaser.

EAT UP THE MILES. Regular walking is probably the best defense against varicose veins. When the leg and foot muscles contract, the blood heads toward the heart. Dr. Goldman recommends a 20-minute brisk walk every day— or at least three times a week.

SPIN AND SPLASH. Biking and swimming are good low-impact muscle contractors. Ride a bike the next time you are going on an errand. Or add a gentle twice-a-week swim to your workout routine, suggests Alan Kanter, M.D., medical director of the Vein Center of Orange County in Irvine, California.

ESCHEW EXERTION. Intense exercise that pushes blood downward in the legs may actually help cause varicose veins. "Excessive straining during overly vigorous weight training is also detrimental to your veins," says Dr. Glaser. Additionally, anything that increases abdominal pressure, like abdominal exercises with your legs below your heart, is very bad for varicose veins because it makes it more difficult for blood to get back to your heart.

Sometimes modifying an exercise can help reduce the local pressure. "If you want to do abdominal crunches," says Dr. Goldman, "have your legs elevated in the air."

HELP WITH HOSIERY. "Graduated compression stockings can help increase the efficiency with which the calf muscle pumps blood back to the heart," says Dr. Goldman. Unlike regular stockings, this special type of hosiery is tighter at the ankle and gradually becomes less tight as it goes up your leg, so it encourages the blood to flow upward. Although you can buy them over the counter at drugstores, the most effective types are available by prescription. If you get the kind offered in drugstores, make sure the box is labeled "graduated compression stockings," he advises.

The stockings also give additional support to the valves that tend to fail. "The ones that are marginal will be supported to the point where they will last longer, which means that you will probably see fewer new veins appearing over time," explains Dr. Kanter.

He recommends that women with varicose veins or a family history of them wear graduated compression stockings during pregnancy since the hormones and abdominal pressure associated with pregnancy aggravate and bring out varicose veins. "Women will have fewer problems *after* pregnancy as well if they wear the stockings while they are pregnant," says Dr. Kanter.

WATCH YOUR WEIGHT. "Excess weight puts more pressure on the veins and retards the flow of blood from your legs to your heart," says Dr. Kanter. Keeping your weight down is an important part of keeping varicose veins under control.

SCRAP THE STILETTOS. Wear low-heeled or flat shoes

and avoid high heels. "When you walk in high heels, you use your buttock muscles more and your calf muscles less," says Dr. Goldman. And that is not a prescription for smooth legs. When it comes to preventing varicose veins, active calf muscles are important, he points out.

HOLD THE HORMONES. "The hormones of pregnancy are the greatest kick-start to vein disease," says Brian McDonagh, M.D., founder and medical director of Vein Clinics of America in Chicago. "Then, after pregnancy, when hormone levels decrease, we see improvement." This is one of the indicators that hormones play a role in bringing out varicose and spider veins. So if you are considering hormone-replacement therapy, be aware that high levels of hormones may increase your chances of getting varicose veins.

"Birth control pills are another source of high hormone doses. If a woman wants to do everything possible to prevent the development of varicose veins, it would be wise not to use birth control pills," says Dr. Goldman.

WARTS
Warding Them Off

In days of yore, when unsightly skin bumps known as warts appeared, their origin was thought to be mystical. And so were the "cures." Rubbing a cut potato on them and then throwing it over the fence was one old wives' remedy. Stealing a used washcloth, rubbing it on the warts, and then burying it was another.

Now we know that the cause of warts has nothing to do with evil spells. It is something much less exotic—a common virus called human papillomavirus. The key premise for wart prevention is making your skin less vulnerable to this pesky virus. Here are some ways to ward off warts.

GO HAND IN GLOVE. The papillomavirus most easily invades broken or cut skin. Wearing protective gloves while doing physical work reduces the chances that it will get cozy. If you garden, work in the kitchen, or have a job where you get nicks and cuts on your skin, you may be more susceptible to the virus. "Wear gloves to protect your hands and avoid cuts," advises Robert F. Garry, Ph.D., a virologist and professor of microbiology and immunology at Tulane Medical School in New Orleans. And gloves can help protect your skin from the drying, abrasive effect of cleansers and other chemicals.

WASH AWAY WARTS. Just like the common cold, the wart virus can be picked up from any surface touched by other hands. Doorknobs, bowling balls, and public telephones are loaded with germs and viruses. Be aware of what you touch in public places and make sure that you wash your hands with soap and water often. If you have been exposed to the virus, "washing your hands will help keep you from spreading it to other parts of your body," says Nicholas G. Popovich, Ph.D., professor of pharmacy practice at Purdue University in West Lafayette, Indiana.

NIX THE NIBBLING. If you are a nail-biter, you may be making your fingers vulnerable to warts. Biting your nails often leaves microabrasions that are openings for the papillomavirus. "The virus will use any kind of open avenue where it can get in," says Dr. Popovich.

Furthermore, "if you already have warts around your fingernails, biting at them can spread the virus to your lips," says Stephen M. Schleicher, M.D., clinical instructor of dermatology at Graduate Hospital and co-director of the Dermatology Center, both in Philadelphia.

SHIELD WITH SLIPPERS. Pools and locker rooms are breeding grounds for the type of wart that grows on the bottom of the feet, known as plantar warts. "Wearing protective footwear such as sandals or flip-flops in these areas instead of going barefoot can protect you from plantar warts," says Dr. Popovich.

SAVE YOUR SKIN. In cold weather, your skin can become dry, chapped, and irritated, creating tiny fractures in your skin. "The microabrasions that occur allow the papillomavirus to be absorbed into the skin," says Dr. Garry.

Besides wearing gloves in cold weather, use moisturizer to keep your skin nice and supple, Dr. Garry suggests.

The fewer cracks in your epidermal armor, the less vulnerable you may be to warts.

HUMIDIFY YOUR HIDE. Dry air is a skin-parcher. If you use a humidifier in your house, especially in your bedroom, you will enhance your skin's protective power, says Dr. Popovich.

WATER RETENTION
Keeping the Fluid in Motion

Feeling puffy? Swollen? Waterlogged? Water retention may be the cause of your discomfort.

But what is the cause of water retention? Experts agree that when water is retained in the body, it is usually retained with salt. Many women experience water retention about a week before the start of their periods. When your body realizes that the egg has not been fertilized, the level of the hormone progesterone drops. This causes your body to store excess salt and fluid.

In its more serious forms, water retention can be due to kidney disease, liver disease, or even heart failure. But many otherwise healthy women find that it is an inevitable sideshow to the monthly cycle, a result of the change in hormone levels that occurs prior to their periods.

But there are natural ways to help prevent it. Below, the experts offer some tips that "hold water," so you won't have to.

EAT THE APPLE. Stick with other naturally grown foods as well. "Nature has blessed us with a generally low-salt environment," says Charles Tifft, M.D., associate professor of medicine at Boston University School of Medicine. Choosing natural foods should enable you to keep your sodium intake at a healthy level. Eat fresh fruits, vegetables, grains, and such, but avoid processed foods.

"Processed foods are the major source of sodium in our lives," says Dr. Tifft. Chips, canned goods like soup, and any products with added salt should be limited. "When sodium is restricted, the total amount of water is less of an issue because the sodium helps hold the water in the body."

PUMP AWAY PUFFINESS. One of the common consequences of water retention is the swelling, or edema, of the leg area, particularly the ankles. "Standing around and being generally sedentary can cause you to feel puffy around the ankles by the end of the day," says Dr. Tifft. With exercise, you can keep the excess fluid moving throughout the body, thereby reducing the edema. "Exercise is one of nature's ways to mobilize swelling from the lower extremities."

Walking, running, biking, stairclimbing, and aerobic dancing are all good ways to accomplish this. "These exercises allow your calf muscles to contract, squeeze the veins, and pump the excess swelling out of the legs," says Dr. Tifft. "The excess fluid can then flow back into the bloodstream so that the organs can get rid of it." Be sure to check with your physician before undertaking any new exercise regimen. Some conditions could be aggravated by unsupervised exercise.

VITALIZE WITH VITAMINS. Some people may find that vitamin B_6 will help get rid of retained fluid. "Vitamin B_6 is considered a natural diuretic and can be helpful, especially prior to a woman's period," says May M. Wakamatsu, M.D., an instructor at Harvard Medical School and a urogynecologist at Massachusetts General Hospital, both in Boston. She recommends that people take it in doses of 100 to 500 milligrams per day. You can also get your B_6 through foods. The best food sources of vitamin B_6 are plantains, poultry, avocados, and bananas. Other good sources are

Elevate to Circulate

Gravity is one of the reasons that people get edema in the legs and ankles, suggests Charles Tifft, M.D., associate professor of medicine at Boston University School of Medicine. To help prevent that down flow, try lifting your feet. And when you do, make sure that your legs are raised up above your heart. "This makes it easier for your body to rid the lower extremities of the edema because the fluid can flow into the general circulatory system and then pass out of the body in urine," he says.

"Oftentimes women, especially over 60 years of age, collect fluid in their legs or ankles," adds May M. Wakamatsu, M.D., an instructor at Harvard Medical School and a urogynecologist at Massachusetts General Hospital, both in Boston. She recommends lying down anywhere you are comfortable. You can lie on a couch with a book on your lap or recline on a rug in front of the television. Just make sure that you are nearly flat on your back with your legs elevated. "A reclining chair won't do, unless it is a chair that allows the body to be nearly flat with the legs elevated," she says.

Try to spend at least one to two hours in this position. "The longer you lie this way," says Dr. Wakamatsu, "the more the fluid is going to pass out of your ankles so that your body can get rid of it."

spinach and lean meats. Sweet potatoes and figs also provide small amounts of B_6.

Caution: People may experience an unstable gait and numb feet if they take more than 50 milligrams of vitamin B_6 over an extended period of time.

PULL UP YOUR SOCKS. Wearing support hose can help you "bail out" the problem of water retention in your legs. You can find support hose in most hospital equipment stores. Pull them on first thing in the morning, before your ankles have a chance to swell, advises Dr. Tifft.

If you find that over-the-counter support hose aren't doing enough, talk to your doctor. You might need compression stockings, which apply more pressure and can help relieve water retention that rises as high as the calf or knee. These sturdier stockings aren't available over the counter, however, so you will need a prescription.

EAT THE LEAN OF THE LAND. Eating sufficient amounts of protein can help you avoid water retention. "Although not a common problem in America, if you have a low protein intake, you may get a low protein concentration in the blood plasma. That low concentration will cause bloating or edema in the tissue," says Brian Wallace, Ph.D., director of research, applied physiology, and nutrition at L. G. E. Sports Science International in Orlando, Florida.

Dr. Wallace recommends eating lean meats, like turkey and chicken. He also recommends egg-white omelets as a way of getting good protein intake without high saturated-fat content.

"If you are a vegetarian," says Dr. Wallace, "it is a bit harder because you have to get your protein intake by combining different balances of amino acids." Vegetarians must balance incomplete proteins to form a complete protein to be properly used by the body, he notes. Foods that make complete proteins when eaten together include cereal and milk, pasta and cheese, rice and beans, and tofu and sesame seeds.

FUNNEL MORE IN. Although you may think that drinking water while you are retaining it sounds counterproductive, it isn't. Hydration is one of the most important concerns that a body has. This makes perfect sense when you consider that the body is made up of 70 percent water. "People often do not get enough water," says Dr. Wallace, "and this can cause more problems than anything." He suggests that people drink 8 to 10 glasses of water per day and more if they are involved in exercise.

WRINKLES
Slowing the Sands of Time

The romantic version of wrinkles goes like this. They are souvenirs of laughter, worry, and all our days in the sun. Wrinkled wizards like painter Georgia O'Keeffe and poet W. H. Auden wore that hard-won wisdom in the lines on their faces.

But the truth about wrinkles goes like this. Wisdom, shmisdom. Everybody would rather look young than wise.

Short of cosmetic surgery, you can't stop the dermatological clock. But you sure can slow it down. Here is some advice from experts on keeping your skin youthful, preventing your pelt from looking prematurely wise.

BE SELECTIVE ABOUT SUNSHINE. When it comes to wrinkles, the sun is probably public enemy number one. Prolonged exposure can prematurely age your skin. "Skin has some ability to regenerate itself if you really avoid the sun and use sunblock," says David H. McDaniel, M.D., assistant professor of clinical dermatology and plastic surgery at Eastern Virginia Medical School of the Medical College of Hampton Roads in Norfolk and director of the Laser

Center of Virginia in Virginia Beach. You can't stay inside all day, but you can take care to limit how much time you spend in the sun and take other skin-protecting precautions listed below.

MAKE SUNSCREEN ROUTINE. This can help slow down the wrinkling process, says Dr. McDaniel. Apply sunscreen as habitually as you brush your teeth in the morning. Put it on after you wash. Give it a couple of minutes to be absorbed on your face before you apply makeup, he advises.

PICK THE RIGHT SUNSCREEN. If you are fair-skinned, use a sunscreen with a sun protection factor (SPF) of 30; if you are dark-skinned, SPF 15 may suffice, Dr. McDaniel says. And make sure that it offers protection from both kinds of ultraviolet rays, UVB and UVA.

Look for a sunscreen that contains zinc oxide, titanium dioxide, or Parsol. The right sunscreen should offer full-spectrum or broad-spectrum UVA protection, he says. If your skin doesn't break out, use a waterproof type. It will stay put longer.

IF YOUR EYES BURN, READ LABELS. If regular sunscreen makes your eyes burn, look for a product that contains microfine transparent zinc oxide, known as Z-Cote. "Zinc oxide has over a three-hundred-year history of mildness," says Sheldon Pinnell, M.D., the J. Lamar Callaway professor of dermatology at Duke University Medical Center in Durham, North Carolina. It has been used to treat diaper rash for years, and it is safe and nonirritating, even on skin sensitive to other sunscreen ingredients (especially chemical sunscreens). It is also best to use a fragrance-free sunblock around your eyes. Read the labels to find out if you are choosing a product with this ingredient.

GET GOOD COVERAGE. Lots of people forget important spots when applying sunscreen. Be sure to cover the tip of your nose, the tops of your ears and hands, and any part of your scalp that will be exposed to sun, Dr. Pinnell says.

USE A SUNBLOCK LIP BALM. Look for one with an

SPF of 15, and carry it with you so that you can apply it as needed, Dr. McDaniel says. Make sure that it covers the skin on both lips, and pay particular attention to the outer half of your lower lip, a common site of skin cancer.

CUT SQUINTS WITH SHADES. Squinting causes wrinkles around the eyes. If you wear dark sunglasses, however, you will reduce sunlight glare and reduce squinting, Dr. McDaniel says. "I have seen people's fine squint lines disappear within six to eight months once they started wearing dark sunglasses."

BLOCK THE UVs. Since ultraviolet (UV) light is a major culprit causing wrinkles, be sure to get glasses that block UV light, advises Dr. McDaniel. For prescription or regular sunglasses, ask for the anti-UV coating.

STAY AWAY FROM TANNING SALONS. Despite what salon owners may tell you, there is no such thing as a healthy tan, Dr. McDaniel says. "We have examined young women who have used tanning booths for only a short period of time and found that they appear to accumulate years' worth of sun damage to their skin," he says.

BECOME THE CAT IN THE HAT. The less exposure you have to sun, the better off you are in terms of resisting wrinkles. Wear hats with brims, suggests Dr. McDaniel. Baseball caps are good and straw hats provide protection, too. "A three- to four-inch brim all around is best," he says.

MIRROR YOUR EXPRESSIONS. Over time, your face develops wrinkles where it is being crinkled up the most. If you are prone to scowls or you furrow your brow, wrinkles may become permanent. To prevent that, put a mirror by your phone and watch yourself as you talk, Dr. McDaniel suggests. This lets you identify—and stop making—the expressions that cause your muscles to form wrinkles.

APPLY VITAMIN C. Vitamin C does two things in skin to help prevent wrinkles. It helps to neutralize damage from the sun's rays, and it also helps the skin produce collagen, the protein that gives skin its strength.

Just eating vitamin C isn't enough to counteract the harmful effects of sunlight, cigarettes, and pollution on skin. Some dermatologists now recommend daily application of a topical vitamin C (L-ascorbic acid) skin-care product to help protect against UV damage. Equally effective against both the short UVB (burning) and UVA (aging) rays, topical vitamin C reduces the sun's damage, says Dr. Pinnell.

"Vitamin C is the body's major antioxidant, and it protects skin from damage by neutralizing free radicals that break down and even mutate cells. This process, oxidation, causes iron to rust, tires to dry out, and skin to wrinkle," Dr. Pinnell explains.

But only one kind of vitamin C (L-ascorbic acid) is chemically stable enough to be used topically. Researchers at Duke University developed the technology that delivers more vitamin C into skin than is possible by diet. Now patented, this high-powered vitamin C is available without a prescription from doctors, dermatologists, plastic surgeons, or licensed skin-care professionals. So check with your doctor. To be effective, topically applied vitamin C should be allowed to dry briefly before applying sunscreen or other skin-care products, says Dr. Pinnell.

KEEP YOUR WEIGHT STEADY. Gaining and losing even small amounts of weight can create fine wrinkles because of the constant stretching and tightening of skin, Dr. McDaniel says. "You can see even a four- or five-pound weight loss in the face because it is one of the first places people seem to lose weight." The result: jowls and a sagging neckline. While these problems can be corrected with surgery, you are better off not developing them in the first place.

LOSE WEIGHT SLOWLY. Exercise to keep weight off. Don't try to get down to some unrealistic, unhealthy weight, Dr. McDaniel advises.

STOP SMOKING. Dermatologists can always pick smokers out in a crowd, even in a nonsmoking area. Smoking constricts capillaries in the face, depriving the skin of blood and decreasing the oxygen supply to the tissues, making it wrinkle-prone, says Neil A. Fenske, M.D., director of dermatology and cutaneous surgery at the University of South Florida in Tampa. Pursing your lips around a butt eventually creates creases on the upper lip. So those who smoke are far more likely to develop a telltale set of wrinkles than those who don't, he says.

FORGET FACE EXERCISERS. There is no good proof that those gadgets you see in magazines can help wrinkles, Dr. McDaniel says. "In fact, most evidence indicates that the more you use the muscles in your face, the more wrinkles you develop."

EXERCISE REGULARLY. That healthy glow you get in your cheeks when you exercise means that blood is flushing your skin. The result is denser, thicker, more elastic skin that resists wrinkling, says James White, Ph.D., exercise physiologist and professor emeritus in the department of physical education at the University of California, San Diego, and author of numerous books, including *Jump for Joy*, a book of exercise programs for people concerned about their skin.

"Actual facial exercises are probably wrinkle-*producing*," says Dr. White. A good overall exercise program, on the other hand, helps your skin and may even reduce bags under the eyes by reducing the fat cells around that area.

But while you are exercising, remember not to become dehydrated. When your cells lose water, they lose strength—even after the water is replaced, Dr. White says.

YEAST INFECTIONS
Creating a Hostile Environment

Yeast has this wholesome, nourishing image. It helps bread to rise and beer to ferment. But if this single-celled organism, which is always present in our bodies, starts to proliferate, it is far from nurturing. It can get downright aggressive and parasitic.

The most common yeast infection is the vaginal yeast infection, with its cottage-cheesy discharge and, usually, lots of itching. But yeast can cause trouble in other places, too. It can grow in your mouth and throat, a condition called thrush, which shows up as creamy-white patches. Yeast can also become a stubborn tenant in your fingernails or toenails. And sometimes, intestinal yeast infections can lead to serious problems—from fatigue and chronic headaches to irritable bowel syndrome.

If you have been bothered with yeast infections in the past, the prevention trick is to make your body as unfriendly an environment as possible for yeast, says Jennifer Brett, a naturopathic doctor in private practice in Stratford, Connecticut. Try these antiyeast preventive tips.

DOUBLE-CHECK YOUR ANTIBIOTICS. Long-term or repeated use of antibiotics is a common cause of yeast problems, says William Crook, M.D., president of the International Health Foundation in Jackson, Tennessee, and author of *The Yeast Connection Handbook*.

"Antibiotics are overprescribed, especially for respiratory infections and for ear infections in children," says Dr. Crook. Try to avoid them when possible. Ask your doctor if an antibiotic is the only answer to your medical problem.

WATCH OUT FOR SUGAR AND UNREFINED STARCH. If you are prone to yeast infections, Dr. Crook advises to cut way down on simple sugars—white sugar, brown sugar, honey, and molasses. If you actually have a yeast infection, you should cut out those sugars entirely until the infection is under control. The same holds true for unrefined starches—like pasta and white bread—because they break down into simple sugars in the intestines. "Yeast thrives on sugar and starches," he says.

EASE UP ON ALCOHOL. Yeast loves alcohol almost as much as it loves sugar, Dr. Crook says. "Alcohol is easy for yeast to break down and digest."

AVOID FOODS THAT CONTAIN YEAST. This includes yeast-raised breads, sourdough bread, and fermented foods such as beer and vinegar.

BE WARY OF MOLDS. This includes aged cheeses, mushrooms, dried fruits, fruit juices (unless they are freshly made), peanuts, and peanut butter. "People with yeast overgrowth tend to be hypersensitive to these sorts of foods and can develop a multitude of symptoms when they eat them," Dr. Crook says. It is safe to eat foods that contain proteins such as eggs, lean meat, chicken, and dairy products without sugar.

GO WITH GARLIC—EVERY DAY. Garlic has impressive

antifungal properties, says Barry Taylor, a naturopathic doctor with the New England Family Health Center in Weston, Massachusetts. It is best eaten fresh and raw. Try two cloves a day. Add it to salad dressings or toss it in at the end of cooking a marinara sauce or stir-fry.

LEARN TO LIKE YOGURT. Live-culture yogurt contains "friendly" bacteria that help crowd out yeast. It helps create a slightly acidic environment that discourages yeast growth, according to Dr. Taylor. But because the culture needs to be live, frozen yogurt doesn't help, he notes. Plain unsweetened yogurt can be an important part of a nutritional therapeutic diet. Double-check to make sure that you don't have any milk allergies or are sensitive to milk products.

SHORE UP YOUR IMMUNE SYSTEM WITH VEGGIES. People with chronic yeast overgrowth often develop immune system problems that can show up as frequent infections or allergies, Dr. Taylor says. "For this, I recommend a nutrient-packed diet that includes raw vegetables and juices, such as carrot juice, lots of green leafy vegetables, and other nutritious vegetables, such as winter squash and whole grains."

GO FOR VAGINAL VENTILATION. Vaginal yeast infections are by far the most common variety. One reason is that yeast thrives in warm, moist places. Experts suggest that, when possible, you might want to go without underwear. Sleeping in the buff—or at least without panties under your nightshirt—will help.

TAKE A COTTON TO COTTON UNDIES. A natural fiber like cotton allows for better vaginal ventilation than polyester. Even if you prefer nylon undies, get some that have a cotton crotch. Keep this in mind when you shop for panty hose, too. Look for the kinds that have a cotton crotch. Remember that you want air circulating as freely as possible. More air means that your vagina will be cooler and dryer, which translates into a less hospitable environment for yeast, says Dr. Crook.

LOOSEN YOUR JEANS. Tight pants may show off your

figure, but they are not a good idea if you are prone to vaginal yeast infections. Favor loose-fitting clothes. Dresses and skirts are the best fashion choice for fighting these kinds of infections.

SNUFF THE PUFF. Many dusting powders contain starch. And a fungus like yeast grows well in starch. So you don't want to use any of these powders in the vaginal area.

DOCTORS AND EXPERTS CONSULTED

All the practical health advice in this book is based upon interviews with doctors, researchers, practitioners of alternative medicine, and other well-qualified experts. The following is a complete list of those who contributed their advice and reviewed the medical and health information in *The Doctors Book of Home Remedies for Preventing Disease*.

LOUTFI SAMI ABOUSSOUAN, M.D., a pulmonary disease specialist and assistant professor of medicine at Wayne State University in Detroit

CAROLYN ADAMS-PRICE, PH.D., associate professor of psychology and chairman of the interdisciplinary gerontology program at Mississippi State University in Starkville

DAVID ALBERTS, M.D., professor of medicine in the cancer prevention and control program at the Arizona Cancer Center, a division of the College of Medicine at the University of Arizona in Tucson

Walid H. Aldoori, M.D., Sc.D., a former research fellow in the department of nutrition and epidemiology at the Harvard School of Public Health

Helaine M. Alessio, Ph.D., associate professor of physical education and sport studies at Miami University of Ohio in Oxford

Richard Alexander, M.D., head of the surgical metabolism section, surgery branch, at the National Cancer Institute

Ibtisam Al-Hashimi, Ph.D., director of the Salivary Dysfunction Clinic in the department of periodontics of the Baylor College of Dentistry at Texas A&M University in Dallas

Karen Allen, a senior physical therapist in the office of environmental health and safety at the University of Virginia in Charlottesville

Miriam Alter, Ph.D., chief of epidemiology in the hepatitis branch of the Centers for Disease Control and Prevention

Sonia Ancoli-Israel, Ph.D., professor of psychiatry at the University of California, San Diego, School of Medicine; director of the Sleep Disorders Clinic at the Veterans Affairs Medical Center in San Diego; and author of *All I Want Is a Good Night's Sleep*

James Anderson, M.D., professor of medicine and clinical nutrition at the University of Kentucky and chief of endocrinology at the Veterans Administration Medical Center in Lexington

Richard Anderson, Ph.D., lead scientist at the U.S. Department of Agriculture Human Nutrition Research Center in Beltsville, Maryland

Jack B. Anon, M.D., chairman of the nasal and sinus committee of the American Academy of Otolaryngology/Head and Neck Surgery and an otolaryngologist in Erie, Pennsylvania

Art Antonelli, Ph.D., an extension entomologist at Washington State University at Puyallup

Lawrence J. Appel, M.D., associate professor of medicine, epidemiology, and international health at Johns Hopkins University Medical Institutions in Baltimore

SANFORD ARCHER, M.D., associate professor of otolaryngology/head and neck surgery at the University of Kentucky College of Medicine in Lexington

BAHRAM ARJMANDI, R.D., PH.D., associate professor in the department of nutritional sciences at Oklahoma State University in Stillwater

E. WAYNE ASKEW, PH.D., professor and director of the division of foods and nutrition at the University of Utah in Salt Lake City

M. T. ATALLAH, PH.D., associate professor of nutrition in the department of nutrition at the University of Massachusetts in Amherst

GLENN O. BAIR, M.D., director of the Bair PMS Center in Topeka, Kansas

JAN E. BAKER, an advanced practice registered nurse in the department of obstetrics and gynecology at the University of Utah Hospital in Salt Lake City

BOB BALLARD, M.D., director of the National Jewish/University of Colorado Sleep Disorders Center at the National Jewish Medical and Research Center in Denver

JOSEPH P. BARK, M.D., chairman of the department of dermatology at Saint Joseph Hospital in Lexington, Kentucky, and author of *Your Skin: An Owner's Guide*

ANDREW BARKIN, D.C., a certified chiropractic sports physician in private practice in Valley Stream, New York

THOMAS BARLOON, M.D., associate professor of radiology at the University of Iowa College of Medicine in Iowa City

PAUL BARNEY, M.D., adjunct professor at Weber State University and a family practitioner in Layton, Utah

BARBARA BARTLIK, M.D., a psychiatrist and sex therapist at the New York Hospital/Cornell Medical Center in New York City

LINDY J. BATIS, an aesthetician and owner of Lindy's Healing Facials in Los Angeles and Ojai, California

DONALD BAXTER, M.D., an orthopedic surgeon and clinical professor of orthopedic surgery at the University of Texas Medical School at Houston

CAROL BEIDLEMAN, a registered dental hygienist practicing in Allentown, Pennsylvania

BRADLEY BEISWANGER, D.D.S., professor of oral biology at Indiana University in Indianapolis

VINCENT S. BELTRANI, M.D., associate clinical professor of dermatology at the Columbia University College of Physicians and Surgeons in New York City and a dermatologist in Poughkeepsie

WILMA F. BERGFELD, M.D., head of clinical research in the department of dermatology at the Cleveland Clinic

RON BERMAN, a forensic examiner and a canine behavioral consultant and trainer

ZUZANA BIC, DR.P.H., assistant adjunct professor in the division of hematology and oncology at the University of California, Irvine, and preventive care specialist at the Chao Family Comprehensive Counsel Center in Orange

DIANA BIHOVA, M.D., a dermatologist in private practice in New York City

WILLIAM H. BINNIE, D.D.S., professor and chairman of diagnostic sciences at Baylor College of Dentistry in Dallas

ROBERT W. BIRCH, PH.D., a sex therapist in Columbus, Ohio, and author of *Male Sexual Endurance*

DENNIS BLACK, PH.D., associate professor of epidemiology and biostatistics at the University of California, San Francisco

BRIAN BLAKLEY, M.D., an otolaryngologist in private practice in Winnipeg

MICHAEL BONNET, PH.D., professor of neurology at Wright State University School of Medicine in Dayton, Ohio

EDMUND BOURNE, PH.D., author of *The Anxiety and Phobia Workbook*

ALAN S. BOYD, M.D., assistant professor of dermatology and pathology at Vanderbilt University in Nashville

PATRICIA BRALY, M.D., professor and chief of gynecological cancer at the Stanley S. Scott Cancer Center of the Louisiana State University Medical Center in New Orleans and co-chairman of the National Institutes of Health Consensus Development Statement on cervical cancer

FREDRIC BRANDT, M.D., clinical associate professor of dermatology at the University of Miami School of Medicine and a dermatologist in Miami

RICHARD BRAVER, D.P.M., a sports podiatrist and director of the Active Foot and Ankle Care Center in Englewood and Fair Lawn, New Jersey

MARC A. BRENNER, D.P.M., a podiatrist at the Institute for Diabetic Foot Research in Glendale, New York

JENNIFER BRETT, a naturopathic doctor in private practice in Stratford, Connecticut

SYLVIA BRICE, M.D., a dermatologist at the University of Colorado Health Sciences Center in Denver

JOHN BRICK, PH.D., executive director of Intoxikon International in Yardley, Pennsylvania, a company that conducts alcohol and drug research, education, and training

ROSS BRIGHT, M.D., medical director of the Psoriasis Medical Center in Palo Alto, California

DONALD J. BROWN, naturopathic doctor and author of *Herbal Prescriptions for Better Health* and editor of the *Quarterly Review of Natural Medicine*

ROSS BROWNSON, PH.D., professor of epidemiology at the St. Louis University School of Public Health

ARTHUR BROWNSTEIN, M.D., clinical instructor of medicine at the University of Hawaii School of Medicine and director of the Princeville Medical Clinic in Princeville

LINDA BRUBAKER, M.D., associate professor and director of urogynecology at the Rush–Presbyterian–St. Luke's Medical Center in Chicago

PETER BRUNO, M.D., associate professor at New York University School of Medicine in New York City and team doctor for the New York Knicks

CRAIG BUCHMAN, M.D., an otologist in private practice in Miami

GEORGE BUNCE, PH.D., professor emeritus of biochemistry and nutrition at Virginia Polytechnic Institute in Blacksburg

GREGORY BURKE, M.D., an epidemiologist and vice chairman of the department of public health sciences the Bowman Gray School of Medicine of Wake Forest University in Winston-Salem, North Carolina

KAREN BURKE, M.D., PH.D., a dermatologist in private practice in New York City

WESLEY A. BURKS, M.D., an allergist-immunologist and professor of pediatrics at the University of Arkansas for Medical Sciences in Little Rock

JOANNA M. CAIN, M.D., professor and chairman of the department of obstetrics and gynecology at Pennsylvania State University at the Milton S. Hershey Medical Center in Hershey

MICKHAEL CANNON, of Seattle, a recipient of the Paul Mitchell World Medal of Honor in Hairdressing and artistic director at the Worldwide Beauty Store on the Internet

ALBERT CARLIN, PH.D., professor of psychiatry at the University of Washington School of Medicine in Seattle

ANNE CARLON, M.D., an assistant attending obstetrician and gynecologist at New York/Cornell Medical Center in New York City

MARY A. CARSKADON, PH.D., professor of psychiatry and human behavior at Brown University in Providence, Rhode Island

REBECCA CASERIO, M.D., clinical associate professor of dermatology at the University of Pittsburgh

HYLA CASS, M.D., assistant clinical professor of psychiatry at the University of California, Los Angeles, School of Medicine and author of *Saint-John's-Wort: Nature's Blues Buster*

WILLIAM P. CASTELLI, M.D., former director of the famed Framingham Heart Study and medical director of the Framingham Cardiovascular Institute in Massachusetts

JAMES J. CERDA, M.D., professor of medicine at the University of Florida College of Medicine in Gainesville

ERNEST N. CHARLESWORTH, M.D., clinical associate professor of medicine in the department of allergy and the department of dermatology at the University of Texas Medical School at Houston and a staff allergist and dermatologist at Brenham Clinic Association in Brenham

LAWRENCE J. CHESKIN, M.D., a gastroenterologist, associate professor of medicine at Johns Hopkins University, director of the Johns Hopkins Weight Management Center in Baltimore, and author of *Losing Weight for Good*

HARRIS R. CLEARFIELD, M.D., professor of medicine and section chief of the division of gastroenterology at the Allegheny University of the Health Sciences, Hahnemann Division, in Philadelphia

ALEX CLERK, M.D., director of the Stanford University Sleep Disorders Clinic

DAVID E. COHEN, M.D., clinical instructor of environmental sciences at the Columbia University School of Public Health and director of occupational and environmental dermatology at New York University Medical Center, both in New York City

SHELDON COHEN, PH.D., professor of psychology at Carnegie Mellon University in Pittsburgh

VALERIE GENNARI COOKSLEY, R.N., a teacher and lecturer in Issaquah, Washington, and author of *Aromatherapy: A Lifetime Guide to Healing Oils*

J. MICHAEL CORNWELL, D.V.M., a veterinarian at the Glencoe Animal Hospital and the department of veterinary preventive medicine at Ohio State University, both in Columbus, and the developer of a dog-bite-prevention program for children

PELAYO CORREA, M.D., professor of pathology at Louisiana State University in New Orleans

BRUNO CORTIS, M.D., a cardiologist in Chicago and author of the book *Heart and Soul: A Psychological and Spiritual Guide to Preventing and Healing Heart Disease*

ROGER CRENSHAW, M.D., a sex therapist and psychiatrist in private practice in La Jolla, California

WILLIAM CROOK, M.D., president of the International Health Foundation in Jackson, Tennessee, and author of *The Yeast Connection Handbook*

DAVID L. CROSBY, M.D., associate professor of dermatology at the Medical College of Wisconsin in Milwaukee

GARY CURHAN, M.D., Sc.D., director of the Partners Center for Kidney Stone Disease at Massachusetts General Hospital in Boston

BRUCE DALL, M.D., an orthopedic spine surgeon at K-Valley Orthopedics in Kalamazoo, Michigan

RALPH C. DANIEL III, M.D., clinical professor of dermatology at the University of Mississippi in Jackson and a dermatologist in Jackson

JEFF DAVIDSON, a certified management consultant and executive director of the Breathing Space Institute in Chapel Hill, North Carolina, and author of *Breathing Space: Living and Working at a Comfortable Pace in a Sped-Up Society*

MARGO DENKE, M.D., associate professor of medicine in the Center of Human Nutrition at the University of Texas Southwestern Medical Center in Dallas

DOMINICK DePAOLA, D.D.S., PH.D., president of Forsyth Dental Center in Boston

SEYMOUR DIAMOND, M.D., director of the Diamond Headache Clinic and national chairman of the National Headache Foundation, both in Chicago

JOHN P. DiFIORI, M.D., assistant professor of family medicine and a sports medicine specialist in the department of family medicine at the University of California, Los Angeles, and a team physician in the department of intercollegiate athletics

JACK A. DIPALMA, M.D., professor of medicine and director of the division of gastroenterology at the University of South Alabama College of Medicine in Mobile

RICHARD L. DOTY, PH.D., professor in the department of otorhinolaryngology/head and neck surgery and director of the Smell and Taste Center at the University of Pennsylvania School of Medicine in Philadelphia

DOUGLAS A. DROSSMAN, M.D., professor of medicine and psychiatry in the division of digestive disease at the University of North Carolina (UNC) at Chapel Hill and co-director of the UNC Functional Disorders Center

RHETT DRUGGE, M.D., a dermatologist in Stamford, Connecticut, who is president and founder of the Internet Dermatology Society, and chief editor of the *Electronic Textbook of Dermatology*

JAMES A. DUKE, PH.D., master herbalist and retired ethnobotanist and toxicology specialist at the U.S. Department of Agriculture and author of *The Green Pharmacy*

MARY DAN EADES, M.D., vice president of the Colorado Center for Metabolic Medicine in Boulder

CHARLES F. EHRET, PH.D., senior scientist emeritus at Argonne National Laboratory in Clarendon Hills, Illinois, and author of *Overcoming Jet Lag*

GEORG EIFERT, PH.D., professor of clinical psychology at West Virginia University in Morgantown

DOUGLAS EINSTADTER, M.D., assistant professor of medicine at Case Western Reserve University in Cleveland

MARGIE ELLIS, of Highland Village, Texas, a hairstylist for 13 years and the creator of Hair Tips by Margie on the Internet

PAUL ELLNER, PH.D., professor emeritus of microbiology at Columbia University in New York City

JEAN ENDICOTT, PH.D., director of the Premenstrual Evaluation Unit at Columbia-Presbyterian Medical Center in New York City

Robert Ettinger, D.D.Sc., professor at the Dows Institute for Dental Research at the College of Dentistry at the University of Iowa in Iowa City

Walter Ettinger, M.D., professor of internal medicine and public health science, osteoarthritis researcher, and director of the J. Paul Sticht Center on Aging at the Wake Forest University School of Medicine in Winston-Salem, North Carolina

William J. Evans, Ph.D., director of the nutrition, metabolism, and exercise program in the Donald W. Reynolds department of geriatrics at the University of Arkansas for Medical Sciences in Little Rock

William R. Fair, M.D., professor of urologic oncology at Memorial Sloan-Kettering Cancer Center and director of the Prostate Diagnostic Center, both in New York City

Thomas R. Feder, D.D.S., a dentist in private practice in Santa Monica, California

Federico, owner and director of the Federico Hair Salon in Manhattan

Larry J. Feldman, Ph.D., director of the Pain and Stress Rehabilitation Center in New Castle, Delaware

Neal A. Fenske, M.D., director of dermatology and cutaneous surgery at the University of South Florida in Tampa

Karl B. Fields, M.D., professor of family medicine at the University of North Carolina and director of the Family Practice Residency and Sports Medicine Fellowship at Moses H. Cone Memorial Hospital in Greensboro

Kathy Fields, M.D., a clinical instructor of dermatology at the University California Medical Center at San Francisco

Terry Fife, M.D., professor of clinical neurology at the University of Arizona and director of the Balance Center at the Barrow Neurological Institute in Phoenix

Alan B. Fleischer, M.D., associate professor of dermatology at Bowman Gray School of Medicine of Wake Forest University in Winston-Salem, North Carolina

John Folts, Ph.D., professor of medicine and the head of

the coronary thrombosis research laboratory at the University of Wisconsin Medical School in Madison

JOSEPH V. FORMICS, PH.D., professor of microbiology at Virginia Commonwealth University, Medical College of Virginia School of Medicine in Richmond

JAMES M. FOX, M.D., an orthopedic surgeon and knee specialist with the Southern California Orthopedic Institute in Van Nuys and author of *Save Your Knees*

ELLEN S. FREEDMAN, director of the childhood injury prevention program at the Boston Public Health Commission

LAWRENCE S. FRIEDMAN, M.D., associate professor of medicine at Harvard Medical School and associate physician in the gastrointestinal unit at Massachusetts General Hospital, both in Boston

SHELLY FRIEDMAN, D.O., medical director of the Scottsdale Institute for Cosmetic Dermatology in Arizona, president of the American Board of Hair Restoration Surgery, and a medical advisor to the American Hair Loss Council

JAMES D. FROST, M.D., a jet lag specialist and professor of neurology at Baylor College of Medicine in Houston

KENNETH F. GARAY, M.D., director of the Center for Sinus and Nasal Disease in New York City

JAMES G. GARRICK, M.D., director for the Center for Sports Medicine at Saint Francis Memorial Hospital in San Francisco

ROBERT F. GARRY, PH.D., a virologist and professor of microbiology and immunology at Tulane Medical School in New Orleans

MARGERY GASS, M.D., a gynecologist and director of the University Hospital Menopause and Osteoporosis Center at the University of Cincinnati

GLENN GASTWIRTH, D.P.M., executive director of the American Podiatric Medical Association

LILIANA GAYNOR, M.D., clinical assistant professor in the department of obstetrics and gynecology at Northwestern University Medical School in Chicago

ROGER GEBHARD, M.D., a gastroenterologist and professor of medicine at the University of Minnesota School of Medicine in Minneapolis

RAY W. GIFFORD JR., M.D., professor of internal medicine at Ohio State University College of Medicine in Columbus and consulting physician in the department of nephrology and hypertension at the Cleveland Clinic Foundation in Cleveland

HOPE GILLERMAN, a board-certified teacher of the Alexander Technique in New York City

LARRIAN GILLESPIE, M.D., a retired urologist in Los Angeles and author of *You Don't Have to Live with Cystitis*

MATTHEW GILLMAN, M.D., associate professor of ambulatory care and prevention at Harvard Medical School and Harvard Pilgrim Health Care, both in Boston

EDWARD GIOVANNUCCI, M.D., assistant professor of medicine and nutrition at Harvard Medical School and Harvard School of Public Health

DEE ANNA GLASER, M.D., assistant professor of dermatology in the department of dermatology at the St. Louis University School of Medicine

MARCIA GLENN, M.D., a dermatologist in private practice in Marina Del Ray, California

KENNETH GOLDBERG, M.D., founder and director of the Male Health Institute in Irving, Texas

MITCHEL P. GOLDMAN, M.D., associate clinical professor of dermatology at the University of California, San Diego

IRWIN GOLDSTEIN, M.D., professor of urology at the Boston University School of Medicine and co-director of the New England Reproductive Center–Medical Center in Boston

MURRAY GOLDSTEIN, D.O., director of the United Cerebral Palsy Research and Educational Foundation and a member of the board of directors of the National Stroke Association

G. KENNETH GOODRICK, PH.D., a psychologist, assistant professor of medicine at Baylor College of Medicine in Houston, and author of *Living Without Dieting*

DORIAN GRAVENESE, M.D., a dermatologist in private practice in New York City

IAN A. GREAVES, M.D., associate professor of environmental and occupational health at the University of Minnesota School of Public Health in Minneapolis

STEVEN A. GREEN, M.D., chairman of the department of family practice and a family-practice physician at Sharp Rees-Stealy Medical Group in San Diego

ELLIOT GREENE, past president of the American Massage Therapy Association and a massage therapist for 25 years in Silver Spring, Maryland

PETER GREENWALD, M.D., director of cancer prevention at the National Cancer Institute

PATRICIA GREGORY, R.D., a dietitian at Shands Hospital at the University of Florida in Gainesville

ROLAND R. GRIFFITHS, PH.D., professor in the departments of psychiatry and neuroscience at the Johns Hopkins University School of Medicine in Baltimore

ELLEN GRITZ, PH.D., a clinical psychologist chairman of the department of behavioral science at the University of Texas M. D. Anderson Cancer Center in Houston

JACK GROPPEL, PH.D., an exercise physiologist and vice president of L. G. E. Sport Science Center in Orlando, Florida

CHARLES GROSS, M.D., professor of otolaryngology and pediatrics at the University of Virginia Health Sciences Center in Charlottesville

TED GROSSBART, PH.D., an instructor in the department of psychiatry at Harvard Medical School, senior associate and clinical supervisor for the department of psychiatry at Beth Israel Hospital, a clinical psychologist in Boston, and author of *Skin Deep: A Mind/Body Program for Healthy Skin*

GARY GROVE, PH.D., vice president of research and development for the Skin Study Center, an independent testing laboratory in Broomall, Pennsylvania

STEPHEN GULLO, PH.D., president of the Institute of Health and Weight Sciences in New York City and author of *Thin Tastes Better*

JACK GWALTNEY, M.D., professor of medicine and head of the division of epidemiology and virology in the department of internal medicine at the University of Virginia in Charlottesville and one of the world's leading experts on colds

JAMES HAGBERG, PH.D., professor of kinesiology at the University of Maryland in College Park

DOUGLAS HALE, D.P.M., a podiatrist at the Foot and Ankle Center of Washington in Seattle

DALE HAMILTON, PH.D., a microbiologist and director of clinical microbiology at the Alvin C. York Veterans Administration Medical Center in Murfreesboro, Tennessee

GARY HARPER, PH.D., assistant professor of psychology at DePaul University in Chicago and an expert in AIDS prevention

RANDALL HARRIS, M.D., PH.D., director of the School of Public Health at Ohio State University in Columbus

STEVEN T. HARRIS, M.D., clinical professor of medicine and radiology and chief of the osteoporosis clinic at the University of California, San Francisco

JO ANN HATTNER, R.D., a clinical dietitian at Stanford University Medical Center

PETER HAURI, PH.D., director of the insomnia program and co-director of the Mayo Clinic Sleep Disorders Clinic in Rochester, Minnesota

HEIDI K. HAUSAUER, D.D.S., assistant clinical professor in the department of operative dentistry at the University of the Pacific School of Dentistry in San Francisco

GREGORY HEATH, a doctor of health sciences and an epidemiologist and exercise physiologist at the Centers for Disease Control and Prevention

JOHN HEGGERS, PH.D., professor of plastic surgery, microbiology, and immunology at the University of Texas Medical Branch and director of clinical microbiology at the Shriners Burns Institute, both in Galveston

THOMAS HELM, M.D., assistant clinical professor of dermatology and pathology at the State University of New York at Buffalo and director of the Buffalo Medical Group Dermatopathology Laboratory in Williamsville

MICHAEL HERTOG, PH.D., an epidemiologist at the National Institute of Public Health and Environmental Protection in The Netherlands

DARLENE HEWITT, a manicurist and nail technician in Toronto

HARALD A. HEYMANN, D.D.S., professor and chairman of the department of operative dentistry at the University of North Carolina at Chapel Hill

WILLIAM HIATT, M.D., professor of medicine in the section of vascular medicine at the University of Colorado Health Sciences Center and executive director of the Colorado Prevention Center, both in Denver

JOSEPH R. HIBBELN, M.D., chief of the outpatient clinic at the National Institute on Alcohol Abuse and Alcoholism, and a leading expert on the role of omega-3 fatty acids in depression

ALAN R. HIRSCH, M.D., neurological director at the Smell and Taste Treatment and Research Foundation in Chicago

KHIN MAE HLA, M.D., professor in the departments of medicine and preventive medicine at the University of Wisconsin School of Medicine in Madison

WALTER J. HOGAN, M.D., professor of medicine and radiology in the division of gastroenterology and radiology at the Medical College of Wisconsin in Milwaukee

PAUL N. HOPKINS, M.D., associate professor of internal medicine at the University of Utah Cardiovascular Genetics Research Center in Salt Lake City

NICOLETTE S. HORBACH, M.D., a urogynecologist in private practice in Annandale, Virginia

LAWRENCE Z. HUPPIN, D.P.M., a podiatrist at the Foot and Ankle Center of Washington in Seattle

KATHLEEN HUTCHINSON, PH.D., associate professor of audiology at Miami University of Ohio in Oxford

ARTHUR JACKNOWITZ, PHARM.D., chairman of the clinical pharmacy department at West Virginia University School of Pharmacy in Morgantown

PAUL JACQUES, D.SC., an epidemiologist and associate professor of nutrition at Tufts University in Boston

KATHERINE JETER, ED.D., retired executive director of the National Association for Incontinence, a nonprofit consumer organization in Union, South Carolina

CRAIG JOHNSON, PH.D., professor of clinical psychology at the University of Tulsa and director of the eating disorders program at the Laureate Psychiatric Clinic and Hospital in Tulsa, Oklahoma

DAVID E. JOHNSON, M.D., medical director and president of Wilderness Medical Associates in Bryant Pond, Maine

CAROL JONES, R.N., a board-certified enterostomal therapy nurse and a member of the ostomy-wound team at the Methodist Hospital of Indiana in Indianapolis

DAVID JONES, M.D., medical director of the Spine and Sport Medical Center in Orange, Texas

JEFFREY JONES, M.D., director of the department of emergency medicine at Butterworth Hospital in Grand Rapids, Michigan

LENORE KAKITA, M.D., assistant clinical professor in the department of medicine, division of dermatology, at the University of California, Los Angeles

CRAIG KAMINER, founder of Childproofers, a Saint Louis–based company that has installed child safety devices in thousands of homes, and a former paramedic with emergency medical services in New York City

ALAN KANTER, M.D., medical director of the Vein Center of Orange County in Irvine, California

NORMAN KAPLAN, M.D., professor of internal medicine in the hypertension division at the University of Texas Southwestern Medical School in Dallas

WAHIDA KARMALLY, R.D., director of nutrition at the Irving Center for Clinical Research at Columbia-Presbyterian Medical Center in New York City

HAROLD KATZ, D.D.S., director of the California Breath Clinic, which is based in Los Angeles

SEYMOUR KATZ, M.D., clinical professor of medicine at New York University School of Medicine; attending gastroenterologist at North Shore University Hospital, Long Island Jewish Medical Center, and Saint Francis Hospital; and past president of the American College of Gastroenterology

PAUL KECHIJIAN, M.D., clinical associate professor of dermatology at New York University Medical Center in New York City and a dermatologist in Great Neck, New York

DAVID KENNEDY, D.D.S., a dentist and the president of the Preventive Dental Health Association in San Diego

DAVID KENNEDY, M.D., professor and chairman of the department of otorhinolaryngology/head and neck surgery at the University of Pennsylvania School of Medicine in Philadelphia

KATHI KEVILLE, director of the American Herb Association

DHARMA SINGH KHALSA, M.D., president and medical director of the Alzheimer's Prevention Foundation in Tucson, Arizona, and author of *Brain Longevity*

THOMAS KIDDER, M.D., associate professor of otolaryngology and human communications at the Medical College of Wisconsin in Milwaukee

ANDREA KIELICH, M.D., clinical professor of internal medicine specializing in women's health at the Portland Clinic in Oregon

CHARLES P. KIMMELMAN, M.D., professor of otolaryngology at Cornell Medical School and attending physician at Manhattan Eye, Ear, and Throat Hospital in New York City

SHERYL KINGSBERG, PH.D., a clinical psychologist and assistant professor of psychology in the departments of reproductive biology and psychiatry at Case Western Reserve University in Cleveland

DOUGLAS KIRBY, PH.D., a senior research scientist at ETR Associates, a nonprofit health education organization in Santa Cruz, California

MICHAEL KLEEREKOPER, M.D., an endocrinologist and professor in the departments of internal medicine, obstetrics and gynecology, and pathology at Wayne State University in Detroit

LORRAINE KLIGMAN, PH.D., research associate professor of dermatology at the University of Pennsylvania School of Medicine in Philadelphia

DANIEL B. KOPANS, M.D., associate professor of radiology at Harvard Medical School and director of the breast imaging division at Massachusetts General Hospital, both in Boston

RICHARD KOPLIN, M.D., professor of ophthalmology at the New York Medical College in Valhalla and director of the Eye Trauma Center, New York Eye and Ear Infirmary in Manhattan

ANDREA KRISKA, PH.D., associate professor in the department of epidemiology in the School of Public Health at the University of Pittsburgh and an expert in diabetes and exercise

MANFRED KROGER, PH.D., professor of food science at Pennsylvania State University in University Park

ESTA KRONBERG, M.D., a dermatologist in private practice in Houston

GERALD KRUEGER, M.D., professor of dermatology at the University of Utah School of Medicine in Salt Lake City

GEOFFREY C. LAMB, M.D., associate professor of internal medicine at the Medical College of Wisconsin in Milwaukee

MARIANNE K. LANGE, M.D., assistant professor of surgery at Michigan State University in East Lansing and a physician in Grand Rapids

EDWARD R. LASKOWSKI, M.D., co-director of the Sports Medicine Center at the Mayo Clinic in Rochester, Minnesota

MARY GILBERT LAWRENCE, M.D., associate professor of ophthalmology at the University of Minnesota in Minneapolis

BRUCE LEBOWITZ, D.P.M., director of the podiatric clinic of the Johns Hopkins Bayview Medical Center in Baltimore

JOHN G. LEE, M.D., a gastroenterologist and assistant professor of medicine at the University of California, Davis

PAULA LEVINE, PH.D., director of the Anorexia and Bulimia Resource Center in Coral Gables, Florida

GARY LICHTENSTEIN, M.D., associate professor of medicine and director of the inflammatory bowel diseases program at the University of Pennsylvania School of Medicine in Philadelphia

PATRICIA LIEHR, R.N., PH.D., associate professor of nursing at the University of Texas, Houston School of Nursing, and a stress-management consultant at the Hermann Hospital Wellness Center, also in Houston

BRUCE S. LIESE, PH.D., professor of family medicine and psychiatry at Kansas University Medical Center in Kansas City and editor of *The Addictions Newsletter*

KENNETH LIGHT, M.D., medical director of the San Francisco Spine Center

JEROME Z. LITT, M.D., assistant clinical professor of dermatology at Case Western Reserve University School of Medicine in Cleveland and author of *Your Skin: From Acne to Zits*

JAMES E. LOEHR, ED.D., a sports psychologist and president of L. G. E. Sport Science Center in Orlando, Florida, and author of *Stress for Success: The Proven Program for Transforming Stress into Positive Energy at Work*

DEBORAH LONEY, M.D., an otolaryngologist in private practice in Sterling, Virginia

VICKIE LOVIN, M.D., a gynecologist in private practice in Hickory, North Carolina

RUTH LUBAN, a counselor and consultant in private practice in Laguna Beach, California, who specializes in preventing and treating burnout and is the author of the book and audiotape *Keeping the Fire: From Burnout to Balance*

DENNIS J. LYNCH, M.D., chairman of the department of surgery at the Scott and White Clinic, chairman of surgery for the Texas A&M School of Medicine, both in Temple, and president of the American Society of Plastic and Reconstructive Surgeons

MARTIN LYNN, D.P.M., a podiatrist at the Foot and Ankle Center of Washington in Seattle

MARGARET LYTTON, M.D., a family practitioner in private practice in Narberth, Pennsylvania

RICHARD MABRY, M.D., professor in the department of otorhinolaryngology at the University of Texas Southwestern Medical Center at Dallas

THOMAS H. MAGNUSON, M.D., assistant professor of surgery at the Johns Hopkins University School of Medicine in Baltimore and an expert in gallstone disease

LEWIS MAHARAM, M.D., president of the Greater New York Regional Chapter of the American College of Sports Medicine and medical director of the Metropolitan Athletics Congress in New York City

IRWIN MANDEL, D.D.S., professor emeritus, former director of preventive dentistry, and director of clinical research for dentistry at Columbia University School of Dental and Oral Surgery in New York City

JOANN MANSON, M.D., associate professor of medicine at Harvard Medical School and Harvard School of Public Health and an endocrinologist in the division of preventive medicine at Brigham and Women's Hospital, all in Boston

ROBERT E. MARKISON, M.D., associate clinical professor of surgery at the University of California, San Francisco, School of Medicine, and a hand surgeon in San Francisco

JAMES MARKS JR., M.D., professor of medicine in the division of dermatology at the Pennsylvania State University College of Medicine in Hershey

JANE MARKS, R.N., clinical coordinator for the continence program at the Johns Hopkins Geriatric Center in Baltimore

JOSEPH MARZOUK, M.D., an infectious disease specialist at the Infectious Disease Medical Group in Oakland, California

SUSAN TAYLOR MAYNE, PH.D., associate professor of epidemiology and public health and director of cancer prevention and control research for the Yale Cancer Center at the Yale University School of Medicine

BRUCE MCCLENAGHAN, a physical trainer who holds his doctorate in physical education and is director of the physical therapy program and Motor Rehabilitation Laboratory at the University of South Carolina in Columbia

DAVID H. MCDANIEL, M.D., assistant professor of clinical dermatology and of plastic surgery at Eastern Virginia Medical School of the Medical College of Hampton Roads in Norfolk and director of the Laser Center of Virginia in Virginia Beach

BRIAN MCDONAGH, M.D., founder and medical director of Vein Clinics of America in Chicago

JERRY W. MCLARTY, PH.D., chairman of the department of epidemiology and biomathematics at the University of Texas Health Center in Tyler

JOHN MCSHANE, M.D., director of primary care sports medicine at Thomas Jefferson University in Philadelphia

LORRAINE FAXON MEISNER, PH.D., professor of preventive medicine at the University of Wisconsin in Madison and one of the creators of Cellex-C

DEAN D. METCALFE, M.D., chief of the Laboratory of Allergic Diseases at the National Institute of Allergy and Infectious Diseases (a division of the National Institutes of Health)

ALAN MIKESKY, PH.D., director of the Human Performance and Biomechanics Laboratory at Indiana University–Purdue University in Indianapolis

MICHAEL MILLER, M.D., associate professor and director for preventive cardiology at the University of Maryland School of Medicine in Baltimore

RICHARD MILLER, PH.D., a clinical psychologist in San Rafael, California, and co-founder of the International Association of Yoga Therapists, based in Mill Valley, California

ARTHUR MITTELSTAEDT, ED.D., executive director of the Recreation Safety Institute in Ronkonkoma, New York

REED MOSKOWITZ, M.D., clinical assistant professor of psychiatry, founder and medical director of the stress disorders service at New York University Medical Center in New York City, and author of *Your Healing Mind*

STEVEN R. MOSTOW, M.D., professor of medicine at the University of Colorado, chairman of the American Thoracic Society's committee on the prevention of pneumonia and influenza, and chairman of medicine at the Rose Medical Center in Denver

CHRISTEN M. MOWAD, M.D., assistant professor in the department of dermatology at the University of Pennsylvania in Philadelphia

SHEILA A. MUNDORFF-SHRESTHA, associate professor of dentistry with the Eastman department of dentistry in the School of Medicine and Dentistry at the University of Rochester in New York

ANNE MUNOZ-FURLONG, founder and president of the Food Allergy Network in Fairfax, Virginia

MICHAEL T. MURRAY, a naturopathic doctor in Seattle and author of *Natural Alternatives to Prozac*

BELLERUTH NAPARSTEK, a licensed psychotherapist in Cleveland Heights, Ohio, and author of *Your Sixth Sense* and the *Health Journeys* guided imagery audiotape series

DAN NELSON, M.D., associate professor of ophthalmology at the University of Minnesota in Minneapolis and chairman of the department of ophthalmology at the Health Partners–Regions Hospital in St. Paul

MARION NESTLE, PH.D., professor of nutrition and food studies at New York University in New York City

DAVID NEUBAUER, M.D., associate director of the Johns Hopkins Sleep Disorders Center in Baltimore

ALFRED NEUGUT, M.D., PH.D., associate professor of medicine and public health at the Columbia University College of Physicians and Surgeons and director of the university's program in cancer prevention and control at its Herbert Irving Comprehensive Cancer Center, both in New York City

VICTOR NEWCOMER, M.D., clinical professor of dermatology at the University of California, Los Angeles, School of Medicine

GARY NEWKIRK, M.D., clinical professor of family medicine at the University of Washington School of Medicine in Seattle and director of the Family Medicine Residency Program in Spokane

STEPHEN NICHOLAS, M.D., associate director of the Nicholas Institute of Sports Medicine in New York City and team physician for the New York Jets and Islanders

GEORGE NIKIAS, M.D., a gastroenterologist at Hackensack University Medical Center in New Jersey

MICHAEL NORDEN, M.D., a psychiatrist and clinical associate professor at the University of Washington in Seattle and author of *Beyond Prozac*

GARY NOSKIN, M.D., associate professor of medicine in the division of infectious diseases at Northwestern University Medical School in Chicago

RICHARD ODOM, M.D., interim chairman of the dermatology department at the University of California, San Francisco

EUGENE OLIVERI, D.O., professor of medicine at Michigan State University College of Osteopathic Medicine in East Lansing and a gastroenterologist in Milford

PATRICK M. O'NEIL, PH.D., a clinical psychologist and director of the Weight Management Center at the Medical University of South Carolina in Charleston

STEPHEN W. PAINTON, PH.D., associate professor of communication science and disorders at the University of Oklahoma Health Sciences Center in Oklahoma City

HAROLD PALEVSKY, M.D., medical co-director of the program in advanced lung disease and medical director of respiratory care services at the University of Pennsylvania Medical Center in Philadelphia

PETER PANAGOTACOS, M.D., a dermatologist and an expert in hair restoration and hair-loss prevention in private practice in San Francisco

JULIE PARSONNET, PH.D., associate professor of medicine and of health research and policy at Stanford University

DONNA OROFINO PATNO, R.N., a doctor of naturopathy and certified nurse midwife with a clinical doctorate in nursing at the Women's Hormone Center at the Center for Health Studies in Beachwood, Ohio

SCOTT PATTEN, M.D., PH.D., assistant professor in the departments of community health sciences and psychiatry at the University of Calgary in Canada, and a psychiatrist with the Calgary Regional Health Authority

HEATHER PAUL, PH.D., executive director of the National SAFE KIDS Campaign in Washington, D.C.

ROBERT M. PEPPERCORN, M.D., a dermatologist and cosmetic surgeon in private practice in Yuba City, California

CHARLES H. PERLE, D.M.D., a dentist in Jersey City, New Jersey; a spokesperson for the Academy of General Dentistry; and a member on the Council on Communications of the American Dental Association

VICKI PETERS, president of the Peters Perspective, a consulting firm for the nail industry, located in Las Vegas, and author of *Salon Ovations Nail Q and A Book*

MARC PETERS-GOLDEN, M.D., professor of internal medicine in the division of pulmonary and critical care medicine at the University of Michigan Medical Center in Ann Arbor

ALICE STOLLENWERK PETRULIS, M.D., professor of medicine at Case Western Reserve University in Cleveland

DAVID A. PEURA, M.D., professor of medicine and associate chief of the division of gastroenterology and hepatology at the University of Virginia in Charlottesville

BARBARA PHILLIPS, M.D., medical director of the Samaritan Hospital Sleep Apnea Center and director of the University of Kentucky Sleep Clinic, both in Lexington

SHELDON PINNELL, M.D., the J. Lamar Callaway professor of dermatology at Duke University Medical Center in Durham, North Carolina

JOHN PINTO, PH.D., associate professor of biochemistry at Cornell University Medical College and director of the nutrition research laboratory at Memorial Sloan-Kettering Cancer Center, both in New York City

JOFFIE PITTMAN, D.D.S., general director and medical administrator of the Henry J. Austin Health Center in Trenton, New Jersey

ROBERT PLANCEY, M.D., assistant clinical professor of medicine at the University of Southern California in Los Angeles and an internist and allergist in Arcadia

THOMAS PLATTS-MILLS, M.D., PH.D., head of the division of allergy and clinical immunology at the University of Virginia Medical Center in Charlottesville

NICHOLAS G. POPOVICH, PH.D., professor of pharmacy practice at Purdue University in West Lafayette, Indiana

JOEL PRESS, M.D., medical director at the Rehabilitation Institute of Chicago

EDMUND PRIBITKIN, M.D., an otolaryngologist at Thomas Jefferson University Hospital in Philadelphia

JILL MAURA RABIN, M.D., chief of urogynecology and of the division of ambulatory care at Long Island Jewish Medical Center in New Hyde Park, New York

Paul Ratner, M.D., an allergist in private practice in San Antonio, Texas

Arnold Ravick, D.P.M., a podiatrist at Capital Podiatry Associates in Washington, D.C.

Bandaru Reddy, Ph.D., associate director for research and chief of the division of nutritional carcinogenesis at the American Health Foundation in Valhalla, New York

Geoffrey P. Redmond, M.D., director of the Women's Hormone Center at the Center for Health Studies in Beachwood, Ohio

Quentin Regestein, M.D., director of the Sleep Clinic at Brigham and Women's Hospital in Boston

Kevin Reilly, D.C., a certified chiropractic sports physician and owner of Reilly Chiropractic Health and Fitness in Columbus, Ohio

Millard Reschke, Ph.D., a senior scientist for neuroscience at NASA's Johnson Space Center in Houston

Harold Reuter, M.D., clinical assistant professor in the department of otorhinolaryngology at Baylor College of Medicine in Houston

Julie Reynolds, director of public affairs for the National Fire Protection Association in Quincy, Massachusetts

Darrell Rigel, M.D., clinical professor of dermatology at the New York University School of Medicine in New York City

Lawrence Robbins, M.D. assistant professor of neurology at Rush Medical College of Rush University in Chicago, director of the Robbins Headache Clinic in Northbrook, and author of *Headache Help*

William Roberts, M.D., co-director of MinnHealth Sports-Care in White Bear Lake, Minnesota

David Robertson, M.D., professor of medicine, pharmacology, and neurology at Vanderbilt University in Nashville

Donald Robertson, M.D., medical director of the Southwest Bariatric Nutrition Center in Scottsdale, Arizona

Malcolm Robinson, M.D., clinical professor of medicine at the University of Oklahoma and medical director of the Oklahoma Foundation for Digestive Research, both in Oklahoma City

CHERYL ROCK, R.D., PH.D., associate professor in the department of family and preventive medicine at the University of California, San Diego

JOHN S. RODMAN, M.D., associate clinical professor of medicine at Cornell University School of Medicine in New York City and co-author of *No More Kidney Stones*

HECTOR P. RODRIGUEZ, M.D., assistant professor of clinical otolaryngology/head and neck surgery at the Columbia University College of Physicians and Surgeons and director of the division of rhinology at Columbia-Presbyterian Medical Center, both in New York City

JOHN ROMANO, M.D., professor of dermatology at the New York Hospital/Cornell Medical Center and Saint Vincent's Hospital in New York City

DAVID ROSE, M.D., associate director and chief of the division of nutrition and endocrinology at the American Health Foundation in Valhalla, New York

LESTER ROSEN, M.D., a colorectal surgeon in private practice in Allentown, Pennsylvania

RONENN ROUBENOFF, M.D., associate professor of nutrition and medicine at Tufts University and lab chief at the U.S. Department of Agriculture Human Nutrition Research Center, both in Boston

PETER ROWE, M.D., associate professor of pediatrics at the Johns Hopkins University School of Medicine in Baltimore

JAMES ROWLEY, M.D., assistant professor of medicine at Wayne State University School of Medicine and medical director of the Harper Hospital Sleep Disorders Center, both in Detroit

WILLIAM B. RUDERMAN, M.D., a practicing physician at Gastroenterology Associates of Central Florida in Orlando

MACK T. RUFFIN IV, M.D., associate professor of family medicine at the University of Michigan Medical Center in Ann Arbor

WILLIAM H. RUTHERFORD, D.P.M., a clinical instructor in the podiatry section at Howard University School of Medicine in Washington, D.C.

RALPH L. SACCO, M.D., director of the Northern Manhattan Stroke Study at the Columbia-Presbyterian Medical Center in New York City

WILLIAM B. SALT II, M.D., clinical associate professor of medicine at Ohio State University in Columbus, education director in gastroenterology at Mount Carmel Health Hospital, and author of *Irritable Bowel Syndrome and the Mind-Body, Brain-Gut Connection*

TOBIAS SAMO, M.D., an infectious disease specialist at Methodist Hospital in Houston

HUGH SAMPSON, M.D., professor of pediatrics; chief of the pediatric, allergy, and immunology department; and director of the Jaffe Institute for Food Allergy at the Mount Sinai Medical Center in New York City

DENNIS SAVAIANO, PH.D., professor of nutrition and dean of the school of consumer and family sciences at Purdue University in West Lafayette, Indiana

DON SCHAFFNER, PH.D., an extension specialist in food science at Rutgers University Cooperative Extension in New Brunswick, New Jersey

RICHARD K. SCHER, M.D., a nail specialist and professor of dermatology at Columbia-Presbyterian Medical Center in New York City

MICHAEL SCHIKS, executive vice president of Recovery Services for the Hazelden Foundation, a nonprofit organization in Center City, Minnesota

TOD SCHIMELPFENIG, Rocky Mountain School director of the National Outdoor Leadership School in Lander, Wyoming

STEPHEN M. SCHLEICHER, M.D., clinical instructor of dermatology at Graduate Hospital and co-director of the Dermatology Center, both in Philadelphia

IRA SCHNEIDER, D.C., a chiropractor in private practice in Santa Monica and Thousand Oaks, California

LOUISE SCHNEIDER, M.D., medical director of Brigham and Women's Primary Care Associates in Norwood, Massachusetts

ROBERT SCHOEN, M.D., clinical professor of medicine at the Yale University School of Medicine and co-director of the Lyme Disease Clinic in New Haven, Connecticut

LIA SCHORR, a skin-care expert in New York City

MARVIN M. SCHUSTER, M.D., professor of medicine and psychiatry at the Johns Hopkins University School of Medicine and director of the Marvin M. Schuster Center for Digestive and Motility Disorders at the Johns Hopkins Bayview Medical Center, both in Baltimore

FORREST SCOGIN, PH.D., professor of psychology at the University of Alabama in Tuscaloosa

ANTHONY SCOTTI, president of the Scotti School of Defensive Driving in Medford, Massachusetts

JOHANNA M. SEDDON, M.D., associate professor of ophthalmology at Harvard Medical School and director of the epidemiology unit at the Massachusetts Eye and Ear Infirmary, both in Boston

KENNETH SETCHELL, PH.D., professor of pediatrics at the University of Cincinnati School of Medicine

FRED SHEFTELL, M.D., director and co-founder of the New England Center for Headache in Stamford, Connecticut; national president of the American Council for Headache Education (ACHE); and co-author of *Headache Relief for Women*

BARBARA B. SHERWIN, PH.D., professor of psychology and of obstetrics and gynecology at McGill University in Montreal

ANU SHETH, M.D., lead physician at the Egleston Children's Health Care Center in Dunwoody, Georgia

MITCHELL SHIFFMAN, M.D., chief of the hepatology section of the Medical College of Virginia at Virginia Commonwealth University in Richmond

Jonathan Ship, D.M.D., associate professor and vice chairman in the department of oral medicine, pathology, and surgery at the University of Michigan School of Dentistry and director of hospital dentistry at the University of Michigan Medical Center, both in Ann Arbor

David R. Shlim, M.D., medical director of the CIWEC Clinic Travel Medicine Center in Kathmandu, Nepal

Alan Siegel, Ph.D., president-elect of the Association for the Study of Dreams, an international organization based in Vienna, Virginia; a clinical psychologist in Berkeley and San Francisco; and co-author of *Dream Catching*

Harvey B. Simon, M.D., professor of preventive cardiology at Harvard Medical School

Joel Simon, M.D., assistant professor of medicine at the University of California, San Francisco, School of Medicine

Richard Simon, M.D., an orthopedic surgeon and sports medicine specialist at the Orthopaedic Center of South Florida in Plantation

R. J. Simonds, M.D., a medical epidemiologist in the division of HIV/AIDS prevention at the Centers for Disease Control and Prevention in Atlanta

Blake Simpson, M.D., assistant professor of otolaryngology/ head and neck surgery at the University of Texas Health Science Center at San Antonio

Laura E. Skellchock, M.D., associate clinical professor of dermatology at the University of California, San Francisco, School of Medicine; senior physician at Kaiser Permanente Medical Center in South San Francisco; and editor in chief of *Skin Care Today*

Barbara Smith, M.D., Ph.D., assistant professor of surgery at Harvard Medical School and co-director of the Women's Cancers Program at Massachusetts General Hospital, both in Boston

David V. Smith, Ph.D., professor and the vice chairman of the department of anatomy and neurobiology at the University of Maryland School of Medicine in Baltimore

DAVID SNOWDON, M.D., director of the Nun Study at the Sanders-Brown Center on Aging at the University of Kentucky in Lexington

ARTHUR J. SOBER, M.D., professor of dermatology at Harvard Medical School and associate chief of dermatology at Massachusetts General Hospital, both in Boston

ROSE ANN SOLOWAY, R.N., administrator of the American Association of Poison Control Centers in Washington, D.C.

STEPHEN SONIS, D.M.D., professor of oral medicine at the Harvard School of Dental Medicine

ROBERT SPERDUTO, M.D., chief of epidemiology in the division of biometry and epidemiology of the National Eye Institute at the National Institutes of Health

DAVID A. SPIEGEL, M.D., medical director of the Center for Anxiety and Related Disorders at Boston University

GENE SPILLER, D.Sc., PH.D., director of the Health Research and Studies Center in Los Altos, California, and author of *Eat Your Way to Better Health*

MARTIN B. SPRAY, PH.D., executive director of the Victoria Life Enrichment Society in British Columbia, Canada

DONNA STACH, a registered dental hygienist and associate professor of dental hygiene at the University of Colorado School of Dentistry in Denver

CHERI STANLEY, a former public education specialist in Arvada, Colorado, who created a "Babysitting Checklist" for concerned parents

HARRY STEINBERG, M.D., chief of pulmonary medicine at Long Island Jewish Medical Center in New Hyde Park, New York

RANDOLPH STEINHAGEN, M.D., associate professor of surgery at Mount Sinai Medical Center and a colon and rectal surgeon in New York City

CHRISTINA STEMMLER, M.D., director of the Center for Integrated Medicine in Houston

STUART STOLOFF, M.D., clinical associate professor of family and community medicine at the University of Nevada School of Medicine and a physician in Reno

JENNY STONE, a certified athletic trainer and the manager of clinical programs in the division of sports medicine for the U.S. Olympic Committee in Colorado Springs

CHRISTINA M. SURAWICZ, M.D., professor of medicine and chief of gastroenterology at the Harborview Medical Center at the University of Washington in Seattle, and president-elect of the American College of Gastroenterology

KIM SUTTON-TYRRELL, DR.P.H., an epidemiologist at the University of Pittsburgh

RANDY SWART, director of the Bicycle Helmet Safety Institute in Arlington, Virginia

LINDA TATE, R.N., a health education specialist location in Denver and author of the booklet *Gun Safety in the Home*

BARRY TAYLOR, a naturopathic doctor with the New England Family Health Center in Weston, Massachusetts

W. SCOTT TERRY, PH.D., professor of psychology at the University of North Carolina at Charlotte

ROBERT THAYER, PH.D., professor of psychology at California State University in Long Beach and author of *The Origin of Everyday Moods*

LILIAN U. THOMPSON, PH.D., professor of nutritional sciences at the University of Toronto in Ontario

YVONNE THORNTON, M.D., director of perinatal diagnostic testing at Morristown Memorial Hospital in New Jersey

MICHAEL THORPY, M.D., associate professor of neurology at Albert Einstein College of Medicine of Yeshiva University and director of the Sleep/Wake Disorders Center at Montefiore Medical Center, both in Bronx, New York

SHARON THORSON, injury prevention specialist and coordinator of the Brain Injury Prevention Program for the Colorado Department of Public Health and Environment in Denver

CHARLES TIFFT, M.D., associate professor of medicine at Boston University School of Medicine

BESSIE JO TILLMAN, M.D., a doctor specializing in wellness and preventive medicine with a private practice in Redding, California, and author of *The Natural Healing Cookbook*

THEODORE TSANGARIS, M.D., chief of breast surgery at Georgetown University Medical Center in Washington, D.C.

NADU TUAKLI, M.D., a preventive medicine specialist and a family practitioner in private practice in Columbia, Maryland

FRANCES TYSUS, a registered dietitian and consultant to the Cleveland Clinic Foundation

KARLIS ULLIS, M.D., assistant clinical professor of sports medicine at the University of California, Los Angeles, School of Medicine

ALAN UTTER, PH.D., assistant professor of health and exercise science at Appalachian State University in Boone, North Carolina

ARIANE VAN DER STRATEN, PH.D., a research scientist at the Center for AIDS Prevention Studies at the University of California, San Francisco

SHAMBU D. VARMA, PH.D., professor and director of ophthalmology research in the department of ophthalmology at the University of Maryland School of Medicine in Baltimore

MARK VEENSTRA, M.D., an orthopedic surgeon at K-Valley Orthopedics in Kalamazoo, Michigan

G. NICHOLAS VERNE, M.D., assistant professor of medicine in the division of gastroenterology, hematology, and nutrition at the University of Florida College of Medicine in Gainesville

JOHN VIOLANTI, PH.D., professor of preventive medicine at the University of Buffalo and professor of criminal justice at the Rochester Institute of Technology in Rochester, both in New York

MAY M. WAKAMATSU, M.D., an instructor at Harvard Medical

School and a urogynecologist at Massachusetts General Hospital, both in Boston

Brian Wallace, Ph.D., director of research, applied physiology, and nutrition at L. G. E. Sports Science International in Orlando, Florida

Kathe Wallace, a urogynecologic physical therapist in private practice in Seattle

Jack Walsh, executive director of the Danny Foundation, an organization located in Alamo, California, that was founded to educate the public about crib dangers

Kathleen Walsh, chief executive officer of PK Walsh, a women's hair replacement salon in Wellesley, Massachusetts

Stephen Warshafsky, M.D., assistant professor of medicine at New York Medical College in Valhalla

Guy F. Webster, M.D., Ph.D., professor of dermatology at the Jefferson Medical College of Thomas Jefferson University in Philadelphia

Martin E. Weisse, M.D., associate professor of pediatrics at West Virginia University in Morgantown

Robert Westermeyer, Ph.D., a psychologist in private practice in San Diego, California

Steven D. Wexner, M.D., chief of staff at the Cleveland Clinic Florida in Fort Lauderdale and professor of surgery at the Cleveland Clinic Foundation Health Sciences Center at Ohio State University in Cleveland

Emily White, Ph.D., associate professor in the division of public health sciences at the Fred Hutchinson Cancer Research Center and in the department of epidemiology at the University of Washington, both in Seattle

James White, Ph.D., exercise physiologist and professor emeritus in the department of physical education at the University of California, San Diego, and author of *Jump for Joy*

William B. White, M.D., professor of medicine and chief of the section of hypertension and clinical pharmacology at the University of Connecticut Health Center in Farmington

Robert E. C. Wildman, R.D., Ph.D., professor of human nutrition at the University of Delaware in Newark

Walter Willett, M.D., head of nutrition at Harvard School of Public Health

Redford Williams, M.D., professor of psychiatry and director of the Behavioral Medicine Research Center at Duke University Medical Center in Durham, North Carolina, and author of *Life Skills*

David Williamson, Ph.D., senior biomedical research scientist in the diabetes division at the Centers for Disease Control and Prevention in Atlanta

David Winston, founding member of the American Herbalist Guild and a clinical herbalist in Washington, New Jersey

Alan A. Winter, D.D.S., of Park Avenue Periodontal Associates in New York City

M. Michael Wolfe, M.D., chief of the section of gastroenterology at Boston University and Boston Medical Center

Michael Yapko, Ph.D., a clinical psychologist in Solana Beach, California, and author of *Breaking the Patterns of Depression*

Stephen B. Young, M.D., associate professor and director of urogynecology at the University of Masschusetts Medical Center in Worcester

Janice Yuwiler, director of the California Center for Childhood Injury Prevention at San Diego State University

Gary Zammit, Ph.D., director of the Sleep Disorders Institute at St. Luke's–Roosevelt Hospital in New York City

Irina Zhdanova, M.D., Ph.D., a research scientist in the department of brain and cognitive sciences at the Massachusetts Institute of Technology in Cambridge

Regina Ziegler, Ph.D., a nutritional epidemiologist at the National Cancer Institute in Bethesda, Maryland

Kendra Kaye Zuckerman, M.D., assistant professor of medicine at Allegheny University of the Health Sciences and director of the osteoporosis program at the Allegheny University Hospital in Philadelphia

Susan Zunt, D.D.S., associate professor of oral pathology at the Indiana University School of Dentistry in Indianapolis

INDEX

Underscored page references indicate boxed text. Prescription drug names are denoted with the symbol Rx.

HIV
infection, 38, 550
testing, 39, <u>40</u>, 41
Hives, 457–61, <u>460</u>, <u>641</u>
Hoarseness, 514–17, <u>515</u>
Homocysteine levels, 451, 487
Hormone replacement therapy
(HRT)
estrogen in, <u>588–89</u>
fibrocystic changes and, 151
menopause problems and,
538–41
in preventing
heart disease, <u>412</u>
loss of smell, <u>684</u>
loss of taste, <u>684</u>
memory loss, 534–35
osteoporosis, 92–93, 106,
539–40, <u>588</u>
stroke, 719
Hormones. *See also specific types*
carbohydrates and, 395–96
female, 395
oily hair and, 578
pregnancy and, 745
stress, 70, 151, 572
Hornet stings, 129
Hosiery, 520, 744, 751–52
Hot flashes, 538, 543
HPV, 191–92
HRT. *See* Hormone
replacement therapy
H₂-blockers (histamine-
blockers), 355, 406,
697–98
Human papillomavirus (HPV),
191–92
Humidifiers in preventing

chapped lips, 194
colds, <u>211</u>
dry mouth, 298
dry skin and winter itch,
303–4
insomnia, 480
postnasal drip, 621
sinusitis, 669
sore throat, 694
warts, 746
Hydrocortisone hemorrhoid
agent, <u>435</u>
Hydrocortisone
ointment/cream, 254,
647
Hydrogen peroxide, 727–28
Hydrogen sulfide, 108
Hydroxazine, 461
Hygiene
dental, 183–85, 186, 358–61
loofah and, 303
in preventing
acne, 24–27, 28, <u>29</u>
anal itching, 79
athlete's foot, 100
bedsores, 113–14
body odor, 137
colds, 210
conjunctivitis, 226
dry skin and winter itch,
304
eczema, 254
flu, 324
foot odor, 345–46
hepatitis, 439
jock itch, 502
oily skin, 579–82
pneumonia, 617